Marine Anti-inflammatory Agents

Marine Anti-inflammatory Agents

Special Issue Editors

Elena Talero
Javier Ávila-Román

MDPI • Basel • Beijing • Wuhan • Barcelona • Belgrade

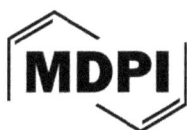

MDPI

Special Issue Editors

Elena Talero
Universidad de Sevilla
Spain

Javier Ávila-Román
Universitat Rovira i Virgili
Spain

Editorial Office
MDPI
St. Alban-Anlage 66
4052 Basel, Switzerland

This is a reprint of articles from the Special Issue published online in the open access journal *Marine Drugs* (ISSN 1660-3397) from 2018 to 2019 (available at: https://www.mdpi.com/journal/marinedrugs/special_issues/marine_anti-inflammatory_agents)

For citation purposes, cite each article independently as indicated on the article page online and as indicated below:

LastName, A.A.; LastName, B.B.; LastName, C.C. Article Title. *Journal Name* **Year**, *Article Number*, Page Range.

ISBN 978-3-03921-572-0 (Pbk)
ISBN 978-3-03921-573-7 (PDF)

Contents

About the Special Issue Editors vii

Preface to "Marine Anti-inflammatory Agents" ix

Azahara Rodríguez-Luna, Elena Talero, María del Carmen Terencio,
María Luisa González-Rodríguez, Antonio M. Rabasco, Carolina de los Reyes,
Virginia Motilva and Javier Ávila-Román
Topical Application of Glycolipids from *Isochrysis galbana* Prevents Epidermal Hyperplasia
in Mice
Reprinted from: *Mar. Drugs* **2018**, *16*, 2, doi:10.3390/md16010002 1

Azahara Rodríguez-Luna, JavierÁvila-Román, María Luisa González-Rodríguez,
María José Cózar, Antonio M Rabasco, Virginia Motilva and Elena Talero
Fucoxanthin-Containing Cream Prevents Epidermal Hyperplasia and UVB-Induced Skin
Erythema in Mice
Reprinted from: *Mar. Drugs* **2018**, *16*, 378, doi:10.3390/md16100378 20

Shiu-Jau Chen, Ching-Ju Lee, Tzer-Bin Lin, Hsien-Yu Peng, Hsiang-Jui Liu, Yu-Shan Chen
and Kuang-Wen Tseng
Protective Effects of Fucoxanthin on Ultraviolet B-Induced Corneal Denervation and
Inflammatory Pain in a Rat Model
Reprinted from: *Mar. Drugs* **2019**, *17*, 152, doi:10.3390/md17030152 42

Azahara Rodríguez-Luna, JavierÁvila-Román, Helena Oliveira, Virginia Motilva and
Elena Talero
Fucoxanthin and Rosmarinic Acid Combination Has Anti-Inflammatory Effects through
Regulation of NLRP3 Inflammasome in UVB-Exposed HaCaT Keratinocytes
Reprinted from: *Mar. Drugs* **2019**, *17*, 451, doi:10.3390/md17080451 56

Sandeep B. Subramanya, Sanjana Chandran, Saeeda Almarzooqi, Vishnu Raj,
Aisha Salem Al Zahmi, Radeya Ahmed Al Katheeri, Samira Ali Al Zadjali, Peter D. Collin
and Thomas E. Adrian
Frondanol, a Nutraceutical Extract from *Cucumaria frondosa*, Attenuates Colonic Inflammation
in a DSS-Induced Colitis Model in Mice
Reprinted from: *Mar. Drugs* **2018**, *16*, 148, doi:10.3390/md16050148 70

Tarek B. Ahmad, David Rudd, Michael Kotiw, Lei Liu and Kirsten Benkendorff
Correlation between Fatty Acid Profile and Anti-Inflammatory Activity in Common Australian
Seafood by-Products
Reprinted from: *Mar. Drugs* **2019**, *17*, 155, doi:10.3390/md17030155 84

Jing-Shiun Jan, Chih-Hao Yang, Mong-Heng Wang, Fan-Li Lin, Jing-Lun Yen, Irene Hsieh,
Maksim Khotimchenko, Tzong-Huei Lee and George Hsiao
Hirsutanol A Attenuates Lipopolysaccharide-Mediated Matrix Metalloproteinase 9 Expression
and Cytokines Production and Improves Endotoxemia-Induced Acute Sickness Behavior and
Acute Lung Injury
Reprinted from: *Mar. Drugs* **2019**, *17*, 360, doi:10.3390/md17060360 104

Paul O. Guillen, Sandra Gegunde, Karla B. Jaramillo, Amparo Alfonso, Kevin Calabro,
Eva Alonso, Jenny Rodriguez, Luis M. Botana and Olivier P. Thomas
Zoanthamine Alkaloids from the Zoantharian *Zoanthus* cf. *pulchellus* and Their Effects
in Neuroinflammation
Reprinted from: *Mar. Drugs* **2018**, *16*, 242, doi:10.3390/md16070242 . . . . **125**

Fuyan Liu, Xiaofeng Zhang, Yuqiu Li, Qixin Chen, Fei Liu, Xiqiang Zhu, Li Mei, Xinlei Song,
Xia Liu, Zhigang Song, Jinhua Zhang, Wen Zhang, Peixue Ling and Fengshan Wang
Anti-Inflammatory Effects of a *Mytilus coruscus* α-D-Glucan (MP-A) in Activated Macrophage
Cells via TLR4/NF-κB/MAPK Pathway Inhibition
Reprinted from: *Mar. Drugs* **2017**, *15*, 294, doi:10.3390/md15090294 . . . . **135**

Seyeon Oh, Myeongjoo Son, Hye Sun Lee, Hyun-Soo Kim, You-Jin Jeon and
Kyunghee Byun
Protective Effect of Pyrogallol-Phloroglucinol-6,6- Bieckol from *Ecklonia cava* on
Monocyte-Associated Vascular Dysfunction
Reprinted from: *Mar. Drugs* **2018**, *16*, 441, doi:10.3390/md16110441 . . . . **151**

Xiaxia Di, Caroline Rouger, Ingibjorg Hardardottir, Jona Freysdottir, Tadeusz F. Molinski,
Deniz Tasdemir and Sesselja Omarsdottir
6-Bromoindole Derivatives from the Icelandic Marine Sponge *Geodia barretti*: Isolation and
Anti-Inflammatory Activity
Reprinted from: *Mar. Drugs* **2018**, *16*, 437, doi:10.3390/md16110437 . . . . **162**

Federica Di Costanzo, Valeria Di Dato, Adrianna Ianora and Giovanna Romano
Prostaglandins in Marine Organisms: A Review
Reprinted from: *Mar. Drugs* **2019**, *17*, 428, doi:10.3390/md17070428 . . . . **179**

Philip C. Calder
Intravenous Lipid Emulsions to Deliver Bioactive Omega-3 Fatty Acids for Improved
Patient Outcomes
Reprinted from: *Mar. Drugs* **2019**, *17*, 274, doi:10.3390/md17050274 . . . . **202**

Zaida Montero-Lobato, María Vázquez, Francisco Navarro, Juan Luis Fuentes,
Elisabeth Bermejo, Inés Garbayo, Carlos Vílchez and María Cuaresma
Chemically-Induced Production of Anti-Inflammatory Molecules in Microalgae
Reprinted from: *Mar. Drugs* **2018**, *16*, 478, doi:10.3390/md16120478 . . . . **216**

About the Special Issue Editors

Elena Talero, (Full Professor in Pharmacology, received her PhD degree with European Mention from the University of Seville (Spain) in 2009 under the supervision of Prof. V. Motilva and Dr. S. Sánchez-Fidalgo. During her predoctoral period, Elena joined the laboratory of Prof. Alfredo Martinez (Cellular, Molecular, and Developmental Neurobiology Department, Instituto Cajal, Madrid), for 5 months, as well as the Division of Pre-Clinical Oncology (School of Medical and Surgical Sciences, University of Nottingham, U.K.), for 3 months under the supervision of Prof. S. Watson. In 2011, she worked as a postdoc on several projects with Prof. Chris Paraskeva at Bristol University (U.K.) for 6 months. Her current research interests focus on the understanding of inflammation as an essential component in the multifactorial origin of different diseases, with a special emphasis on intestinal bowel disease and skin inflammation and associated tumor processes. Her challenge is to find new bioactive compounds of marine or terrestrial origin for the treatment and/or prevention of these pathologies.

Javier Ávila-Román, Researcher, graduated in Biology in 2008 and received his PhD in Pharmacy in 2014 from Universidad de Sevilla, Spain. He worked as Assistant Professor in the Faculty of Biology and as Researcher in Faculty of Pharmacy from 2010 to 2017. During this period, he studied the role of natural products isolated from microalgae, mainly oxylipins (OXL), in Inflammatory Bowel Diseases (IBD) and associated colon cancer. He moved in 2018 to the Universitat Rovira i Virgili in Tarragona, Spain and works since then in the Nutrigenomic Group in the Department of Biochemistry and Biotechnology in the Faculty of Chemistry. His current research interests focus on natural and nutritional products, and more specifically on the bioactivity of these bioactive products in Metabolic Syndrome (arterial pressure, insulin resistance, obesity, inflammation) and the deciphering of their role in circadian and circannual rhythms and their molecular mechanisms.

Preface to "Marine Anti-inflammatory Agents"

Acute inflammation is a highly regulated process, and its dysregulation can lead to the development of a chronic inflammatory state which is believed to play a main role in the pathogenesis of many diseases, including cancer. In recent years, the need to find new anti-inflammatory molecules has raised the scientific community's interest for marine natural products. In this regard, the marine environment represents a source for isolating a wealth of bioactive compounds. In this Special Issue, the reported products have been obtained from microalgae, sea cucumber, octopus, squid, red alga-derived fungus, cnidarians, hard-shelled mussel, and sponges.

This Special Issue of Marine Drugs covers both the in vitro and in vivo studies of marine agents with anti-inflammatory activities, as well as clinical trials conducted in humans. Among the bioactive molecules reported in the papers are lipid compounds, such as glycolipids, which, for the first time, demonstrated their preventive effects in an inflammatory model of skin hyperplasia. In addition, beneficial effects of the carotenoid fucoxanthin were shown in the same model of skin hyperplasia, in UVB-induced damage and in a model of inflammatory pain. Moreover, frondanol, a lipid extract from *Cucumaria frondosa*, attenuated inflammation in an acute colitis model. Another paper evaluated the fatty acid compositions of lipid extracts from some common seafood organisms, reporting the highest level of omega 3 polyunsaturated fatty acids and the highest anti-inflammatory activity in the extracts from octopus and squid byproducts.

Additionally, the anti-inflammatory effects of other marine compounds have been reported, including hirsutanol A, a sesquiterpene from the red alga-derived marine fungus *Chondrostereum* sp. NTOU4196, two zoanthamine alkaloids from the zoantharian *Zoanthus* cf. *pulchellus*, an α-D-glucan from the hard-shelled mussel of *Mytilus coruscus*, and the polyphenol pyrogallol-phloroglucinol-6,6-bieckol from an edible marine brown alga.

Finally, this Special Issue is supplemented by three reviews focused on the occurrence of prostaglandins in the marine environment and their anti-inflammatory role; fish lipid emulsions used to improve patient outcomes in an inflammatory environment, such as postoperative; and the chemically induced production of compounds with anti-inflammatory activity from microalgae.

Elena Talero, Javier Ávila-Román
Special Issue Editors

marine drugs

MDPI

Article

Topical Application of Glycolipids from *Isochrysis galbana* Prevents Epidermal Hyperplasia in Mice

Azahara Rodríguez-Luna [1], Elena Talero [1], María del Carmen Terencio [2,3],
María Luisa González-Rodríguez [4], Antonio M. Rabasco [4], Carolina de los Reyes [5],
Virginia Motilva [1] and Javier Ávila-Román [1,*]

[1]   Department of Pharmacology, Faculty of Pharmacy, Universidad de Sevilla, 41012 Sevilla, Spain;
      arodriguez53@us.es (A.R.-L.); etalero@us.es (E.T.); motilva@us.es (V.M.)
[2]   Department of Pharmacology, Faculty of Pharmacy, University of Valencia, 46010 Valencia, Spain;
      carmen.terencio@uv.es
[3]   Institute of Molecular Recognition and Technological Development (IDM), 46100 Valencia, Spain
[4]   Department of Pharmaceutical Technology, Faculty of Pharmacy, Universidad de Sevilla, 41012 Sevilla,
      Spain; malugoro@us.es (M.L.G.-R.); amra@us.es (A.M.R.)
[5]   Department of Organic Chemistry, Faculty of Marine and Environmental Sciences, University of Cadiz,
      11510 Puerto Real, Cádiz, Spain; carolina.dereyes@uca.es
*   Correspondence: javierravila@us.es; Fax: +34-954-556-074

Received: 25 November 2017; Accepted: 7 December 2017; Published: 25 December 2017

Abstract: Chronic inflammatory skin diseases such as psoriasis have a significant impact on society. Currently, the major topical treatments have many side effects, making their continued use in patients difficult. Microalgae have emerged as a source of bio-active molecules such as glycolipids with potent anti-inflammatory properties. We aimed to investigate the effects of a glycolipid (**MGMG-A**) and a glycolipid fraction (**MGDG**) obtained from the microalga *Isochrysis galbana* on a TPA-induced epidermal hyperplasia murine model. In a first set of experiments, we examined the preventive effects of **MGMG-A** and **MGDG** dissolved in acetone on TPA-induced hyperplasia model in mice. In a second step, we performed an in vivo permeability study by using rhodamine-containing cream, ointment, or gel to determinate the formulation that preserves the skin architecture and reaches deeper. The selected formulation was assayed to ensure the stability and enhanced permeation properties of the samples in an ex vivo experiment. Finally, **MGDG**-containing cream was assessed in the hyperplasia murine model. The results showed that pre-treatment with acetone-dissolved glycolipids reduced skin edema, epidermal thickness, and pro-inflammatory cytokine production (TNF-α, IL-1β, IL-6, IL-17) in epidermal tissue. The in vivo and ex vivo permeation studies showed that the cream formulation had the best permeability profile. In the same way, **MGDG**-cream formulation showed better permeation than acetone-dissolved preparation. **MGDG**-cream application attenuated TPA-induced skin edema, improved histopathological features, and showed a reduction of the inflammatory cell infiltrate. In addition, this formulation inhibited epidermal expression of COX-2 in a similar way to dexamethasone. Our results suggest that an **MGDG**-containing cream could be an emerging therapeutic strategy for the treatment of inflammatory skin pathologies such as psoriasis.

Keywords: glycolipids; **MGDG**; skin; inflammation; epidermal hyperplasia; microalgae; *Isochrysis galbana*

1. Introduction

Inflammatory skin diseases have a significant impact on the quality of life of patients; one of them is psoriasis, considered a common immune-mediated inflammatory skin disorder. It is estimated that 2–4% of the population suffers from psoriasis [1]. Although the exact mechanism of this pathology is not completely understood, it is known that both genetic predisposition and environmental factors such as stress, infection, trauma, and use of some drugs play an important role in its etiology [2]. This disease is associated with several comorbidities as cardiovascular diseases, metabolic syndrome, and psychiatric disorders.

Accumulating evidence has demonstrated that exposure of skin to the protein kinase C activator 12-O-tetradecanoylphorbol-13-acetate (TPA) induces a pleiotropic tissue response and promotes macroscopic lesions, peeling, and erythema, mimicking an apparent psoriasis phenotype. Furthermore, an increase in epidermal thickness has been observed due to the hyperproliferation and aberrant differentiation of keratinocytes as well as the infiltration of inflammatory leukocytes into the epidermis and dermis [3]. Activated leukocytes cause uncontrolled production of reactive oxygen species (ROS), leading to peroxidative damage to skin membranes and contributing to the exacerbation of lesions. Moreover, these immune cells release growth factors, chemokines, and pro-inflammatory cytokines such as tumor necrosis factor (TNF)-α, interleukin (IL)-6, IL-1β and IL-17, which interact as a network in the pathogenesis of psoriasis [4]. The inducible enzyme cyclooxygenase-2 (COX-2) has also been demonstrated to play a pivotal role in skin proliferative disorders through overproduction of pro-inflammatory prostaglandins such as PGE$_2$ [5]. Currently, the treatment of psoriasis includes topical agents (corticoids, vitamin D derivatives, retinoids, and calcineurin inhibitors), photo-chemo-therapy, and systemic treatments (immunosuppressants and biological drugs) [6]. However, many patients, especially those with moderate to severe generalized psoriasis, are not adequately treated with effective or long-term therapies and most of them have various degrees of side effects. Thus, the development of well-tolerated immune-modulatory topical agents can offer an alternative option for the treatment of psoriatic patients.

Microalgae have emerged as a source of bioactive compounds, including lipids, proteins, polysaccharides, and carotenoids, which have attracted the interest of the pharmaceutical industry based on their anti-oxidant, anti-inflammatory, or anti-carcinogenic activity in different skin inflammatory models [7]. Recently, the anti-inflammatory activity of galactosylglycerides isolated from the marine microalga *Isochrysis galbana* (*I. galbana*), including a monogalactosyldiacylglycerol (**MGDG**) fraction [8] and the pure compound monogalactosylmonoacylglyceride (2S)-1-O-[(6Z,9Z,12Z,15Z)-octadeca-6,9,12,15-tetraenoyl]-3-O-β-D-galactopyranosylglycerol (**MGMG-A**) (*data not shown*), has been reported through the inhibition of TNF-α production in LPS-stimulated THP-1 human macrophages. However, data on these compounds' effects on skin inflammatory pathologies have not yet been collected.

Given the interesting anti-inflammatory properties and their high yield of these products in this microalga, we evaluated the preventive effects of the galactosylglycerides **MGMG-A** and **MGDG** from *I. galbana* in a murine model of TPA-induced epidermal hyperplasia by using a topical application of acetone-dissolved glycolipids. However, acetone application onto the skin has been reported to exhibit several drawbacks such as the amount of this organic solvent remaining in contact with the skin, spreading of the formulation and loss of sample, heterogeneity of the dose contacting with the skin, and difficulty of applying the sample [9]. It is well known that the topical application of bio-compounds requires their incorporation into a carrier that offers stability, good permeation, and sufficient time in contact with the skin. Currently, microalgae products are being used as cosmeceuticals through their incorporation in face and skin care products [10]. Therefore, our next objective was to use a pharmaceutical carrier to solve the above limitations of glycolipid solutions. The formulation of these substances involves the selection of appropriate combinations of formula ingredients with the aim of exerting a desirable local or systemic effect. Among them, topical formulations of different natures are used, including ointments, creams, and hydrophilic gels, in which the active compound is suspended or dissolved. In the present study, once a topical formulation was selected, we finally aimed to study its effect on a TPA-induced hyperplasia model and determinate its benefit to epidermal skin.

2. Results

2.1. Effects of Glycolipids on IL-6 and IL-8 Production in TNF-A-Stimulated HaCaT Human Keratinocytes

Non-cytotoxic concentrations of the monogalactosylmonoacylglyceride (2*S*)-1-*O*-[(6*Z*,9*Z*,12*Z*,15*Z*) -octadeca-6,9,12,15-tetraenoyl]-3-*O*-β-D-galactopyranosylglycerol (**MGMG-A**) and the monogalactosyldiacylglycerol fraction (**MGDG**) were selected to evaluate their effects on pro-inflammatory cytokines IL-6 and IL-8 production in HaCaT cells. The cytotoxic effect of **MGMG-A** and **MGDG** fraction was studied using the SRB method, resulting in 100% viability at the tested concentrations (Table S1).

TNF-α-stimulated HaCaT cells manifested high IL-6 and IL-8 levels in comparison with unstimulated control cells ($p < 0.001$) (Figure 1). Pre-treatment with the reference compound dexamethasone (Dex) as well as **MGMG-A** (10, 30, and 50 μM) and **MGDG** fraction (10, 30, and 50 μg/mL) significantly inhibited IL-6 and IL-8 production, with no significant differences between the different tested concentrations.

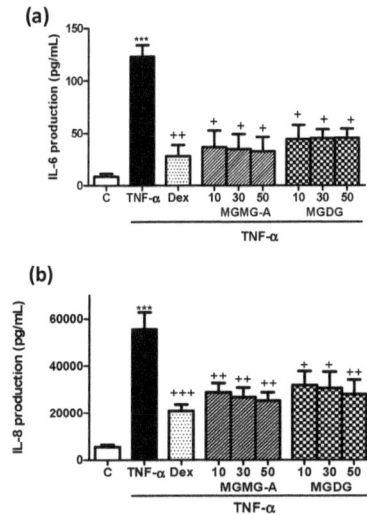

Figure 1. Effects of glycolipids from *I. galbana* on IL-6 and IL-8 production in TNF-α-stimulated HaCaT human keratinocytes. (**a**) IL-6 levels and (**b**) IL-8 levels in TNF-α-stimulated HaCaT human keratinocytes. Cells were pre-incubated with the glycolipid **MGMG-A** (10, 30, 50 μM) and the fraction **MGDG** (10, 30, 50 μg/mL) for 1 h, and then stimulated with TNF-α (10 ng/mL) for 24 h. Dexamethasone (Dex) was used as a positive reference compound at 1 μM. After 24 h, the production of cytokines in the supernatants was measured by ELISA assay. Results are representative of six independent experiments ($n = 6$). Values are means with standard errors represented by vertical bars. Mean value was significantly different compared with the control group (*** $p < 0.001$; Student *t* test). Mean value was significantly different compared with the TNF-α group (+ $p < 0.05$, ++ $p < 0.01$, +++ $p < 0.001$; one-way ANOVA followed by Bonferroni's Multiple Comparison test).

2.2. Topical Application of Acetone-Dissolved Glycolipids Inhibits Skin Inflammation and Hyperplasia in the Murine TPA-Induced Model

We studied the effect of **MGMG-A** and **MGDG** on the murine TPA-induced epidermal hyperplasia model, which reproduces certain biochemical and histopathological parameters typical of human psoriasis [11]. TPA administration to mouse skin resulted in the development of macroscopic lesions (Figure 2a) and skin edema, confirmed by a higher weight of the 1 cm² punch biopsies compared with the sham group ($p < 0.001$) (Figure 2b). Topical treatment with Dex (200 μM), **MGMG-A** and **MGDG** (200 μM or 200 μg/mL, respectively) 30 min prior to TPA application inhibited macroscopic damage and the skin punch weight ($p < 0.001$ and $p < 0.05$, respectively), suggesting an inhibition of skin edema (Figure 2b). We next examined hematoxylin- and eosin-stained sections of mouse skin (Figure 2c). Consistent with macroscopic changes, TPA-treated animals exhibited a clear evidence of edema, epidermal hyperplasia, and massive neutrophilic infiltration compared with the sham (Figure 2c). Moreover, a marked increase in epidermal thickness was evident in the TPA group ($p < 0.001$) (Figure 2d). These results correlated with increased MPO activity, an established marker for inflammatory cell infiltration into the skin (Figure 2e). Treatment with the pure compound and glycolipid fraction markedly prevented epidermal hyperplasia ($p < 0.01$ and $p < 0.001$, respectively) (Figure 2c,d), which was associated with a reduction in MPO activity, being significant for **MGMG-A** ($p < 0.01$) (Figure 2e).

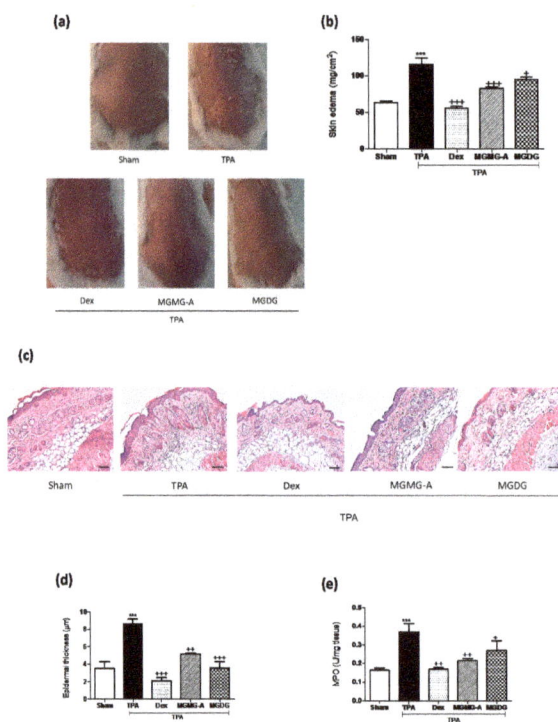

Figure 2. Topical application of acetone-dissolved glycolipids from *I. galbana* inhibits skin inflammation and hyperplasia on the murine 12-*O*-tetradecanoylphorbol-13-acetate (TPA)-induced model. The glycolipid **MGMG-A** (200 μM per site) or the fraction **MGDG** (200 μg/mL per site) were topically administered 30 min before TPA application (2 nmol per zone) during three consecutive days. Dex was used as a positive reference compound (200 μg per site). (**a**) Representative images of macroscopic appearance of the dorsal skin; (**b**) skin edema as punch biopsy; weight of edema (mg/cm^2) was employed as marker of inflammatory skin process; (**c**) histological appearance of mouse dorsal skin after H&E-staining ($n = 4$); Bar = 100 μm. Original magnification 100×. (**d**) Epidermal thickness assessment in H&E-stained skin slides; (**e**) yeloperoxidase (MPO) activity in dorsal skin. Values are means with standard errors represented by vertical bars. Data are means ± SEM ($n = 10$ mice/group). Mean value was significantly different compared with the sham group (*** $p < 0.001$; Student t test). Mean value was significantly different compared with TPA group (+ $p < 0.05$, ++ $p < 0.01$, +++ $p < 0.001$; one-way ANOVA followed by Bonferroni's Multiple Comparison test).

To support the beneficial effects of glycolipids on skin inflammation, we analyzed the production of several pro-inflammatory cytokines that are highly involved in psoriasis as well as the anti-inflammatory cytokine IL-10. Immune cell infiltration detected in the histological examination of the skin from TPA-treated mice correlated with increased levels of the pro-inflammatory cytokines TNF-α, IL-1β, IL-6 and IL-17, in comparison with the sham group ($p < 0.05$, $p < 0.01$, $p < 0.01$, and $p < 0.001$, respectively) (Figure 3). In accordance with the reduction of the skin edema, the production of TNF-α, IL-6, and IL-17 was significantly reduced in animals treated with the glycolipid **MGMG-A** ($p < 0.05$, $p < 0.001$, $p < 0.05$, respectively) (Figure 3a–d). Regarding the fraction **MGDG**, its application resulted in a strong significant suppression of TNF-α and IL-6 levels ($p < 0.01$, and $p < 0.001$) comparable to Dex (Figure 3a,c). IL-10 production analysis revealed increased levels in the TPA group when compared with the sham ($p < 0.05$). Nevertheless, pre-treatments showed lower IL-10 levels when compared to the TPA group, reflecting similar values to the sham (Figure 3e).

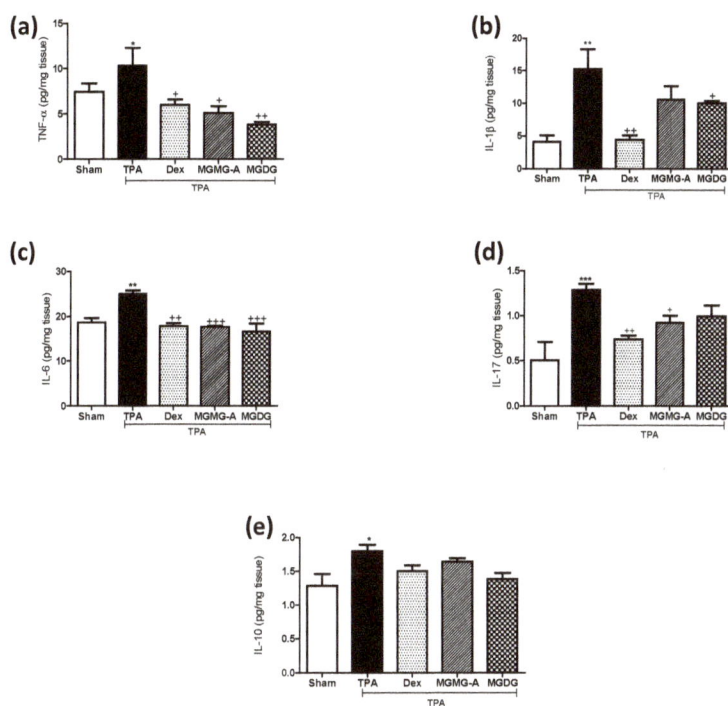

Figure 3. Effect of the glycolipid **MGMG-A** and the fraction **MGDG** from *I. galbana* on the production of cytokines in skin homogenates in the murine 12-*O*-tetradecanoylphorbol-13-acetate (TPA)-induced hyperplasia model. (**a**) TNF-α (pg/mg tissue); (**b**) IL-1β (pg/mg tissue); (**c**) IL-6 (pg/mg tissue); (**d**) IL-17 (pg/mg tissue); and (**e**) IL-10 (pg/mg tissue). Values are means with standard errors represented by vertical bars. Data are means $\pm$ SEM ($n = 10$). Mean value was significantly different compared with the sham group (* $p < 0.05$, ** $p < 0.01$, *** $p < 0.001$; Student t test). Mean value was significantly different compared with TPA group (+ $p < 0.05$, ++ $p < 0.01$, +++ $p < 0.001$; one-way ANOVA followed by Bonferroni's Multiple Comparison test).

2.3. Effect of the Formulation

The development of topical formulations implies the selection of excipients leading to improvement in the drug skin delivery. In order to evaluate the skin accumulation and penetration properties of the examined formulations, sections of the mice skin were analyzed by confocal laser scanning microscopy (CLSM) at the end of permeation experiments. For these studies, rhodamine 6G, a fluorescent hydrophobic probe, was added as a model drug [12]. The penetration depth of the fluorescent probe and the relative intensity of fluorescence in the skin layers were compared in three types of semisolid formulations (gel, cream, and ointment described in Section 4.10). Confocal images revealed that all the examined formulations penetrated deeply into the *stratum corneum* (*SC*) and diffused into the whole skin thickness, except for the ointment (Figure 4a). Cream showed the higher probe permeation in 24 h, following the control formulation containing only ethanol and incorporated into Carbopol® gels. However, the rhodamine 6G incorporated into the lipid ointment was observed to show a low penetration capacity. In addition to the effect of the carrier nature, deeper skin layers were more easily visualized when ethanol was present in the composition, as occurred in all the formulations except for the ointment, where the labeling probe was dissolved in propylene glycol.

The quantitative parameters of histogram distribution revealed a higher fluorescent intensity and accumulation of rhodamine 6G in the presence of ethanol (Figure 4b). Among all the samples, the cream system offered the higher fluorescence intensity and adequate symmetry of the normal distribution of histogram.

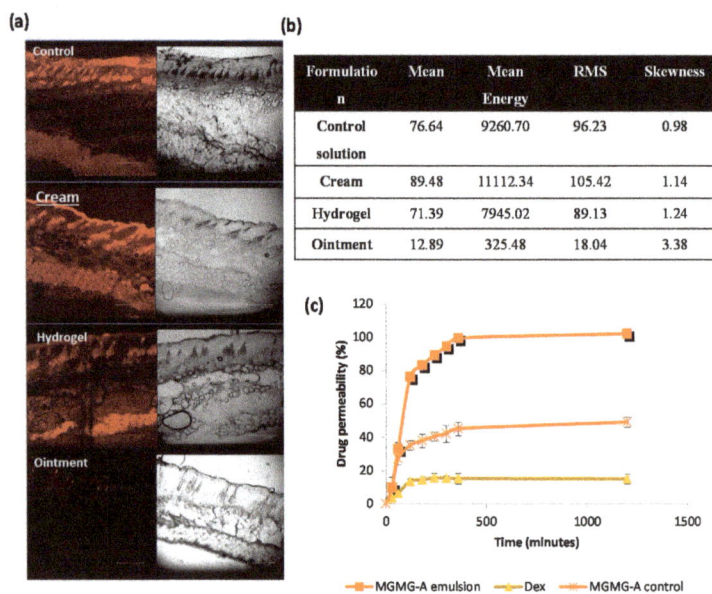

Formulation	Mean	Mean Energy	RMS	Skewness
Control solution	76.64	9260.70	96.23	0.98
Cream	89.48	11112.34	105.42	1.14
Hydrogel	71.39	7945.02	89.13	1.24
Ointment	12.89	325.48	18.04	3.38

Figure 4. Effect of the vehicle composition and physicochemical properties of the drug on the permeation characteristics. (**a**) Confocal micrographs of mice skin cross sections corresponding to rhodamine-loaded ethanolic control solution, cream, hydrogel, and ointment. Bar = 200 μm. Original magnification 100×; (**b**) Numerical data corresponding to the intensity histogram for each sample. Mean: arithmetical mean value; mean energy: average image energy; RMS: root mean square value; skewness: skewness of the distribution; (**c**) Ex vivo permeability percentages of **MGDG** formulations in 24 h (ethanolic control solution, cream, and ointment).

2.4. *Ex Vivo Permeation Studies*

Permeation profiles of **MGDG** from the ethanol solution and cream through mice skin membranes were obtained from the equation described in Section 4.11. Dex-loaded cream was used as the control formulation. Results showed that permeation of **MGDG** from the cream (100 ± 1.9% of the applied dose) was twice that observed from the ethanolic control solution (49.3 ± 3.5%). On the other hand, the permeated amount of Dex from cream was lower (15 ± 3.1%) in comparison with the other preparations (Figure 4c). This value can be attributed to the lower partition coefficient of this molecule (logP 1.83) compared to **MGDG**, whose lipophilicity resembled a reference diacylglycerol in terms of lipophilic acyl groups (logP 3.85) [13]. It is well known that the partition coefficient has been widely used as a measurement for defining the lipophilicity of a drug and the diffusion efficiency across the membranes [14].

2.5. Topical Pre-Treatment with MGDG-Cream Decreases Skin Inflammation and Hyperplasia in the Murine TPA-Induced Model

We evaluated the effect of the **MGDG**-cream formulation on the murine TPA-induced epidermal hyperplasia model. This cream formulation enabled lipid preservation and high permeation in comparison with the acetone vehicle. After treatment with TPA for three consecutive days, mice exhibited the expected psoriasis phenotype, including peeling, erythema, and thickening of the back skin, accompanied by a marked increase in dorsal skin thickness, weight, and substantial inflammatory cell infiltration in the dermis ($p < 0.001$) (Figure 5). Pre-treatment with **MGDG**-cream (100 mg per site containing 200 µg of **MGDG**) attenuated the macroscopic lesions formation (Figure 5a) and significantly reduced skin edema ($p < 0.001$) when compared with the cream-TPA group (Figure 5b). These results were accompanied by a clear inhibition of MPO activity following **MGDG**-cream administration ($p < 0.001$); interestingly, the glycolipid formulation was as effective as the reference topical treatment with Dex-cream, reaching similar levels to those in the healthy group (Figure 4e). Histological analysis of H&E-stained skin lesions confirmed an improvement in the microscopic features of hyperplasia in mice treated with **MGDG**-cream, evidenced by a reduction of epidermal thickness ($p < 0.05$) in relation to the cream-TPA group (Figure 5c,d). It is known that COX-2 plays an important role in skin pathologies. Immunohistochemical analysis of this enzyme showed that stimulation with TPA significantly increased COX-2-positive cell numbers ($p < 0.001$), predominantly localized in the epidermal layer (Figure 6a), when compared with the sham group. As shown in Figure 6b, skin from **MGDG**-cream-treated mice revealed a significant downregulation in the number of epidermal COX-2-positive stained cells in comparison with the cream-TPA group ($p < 0.001$).

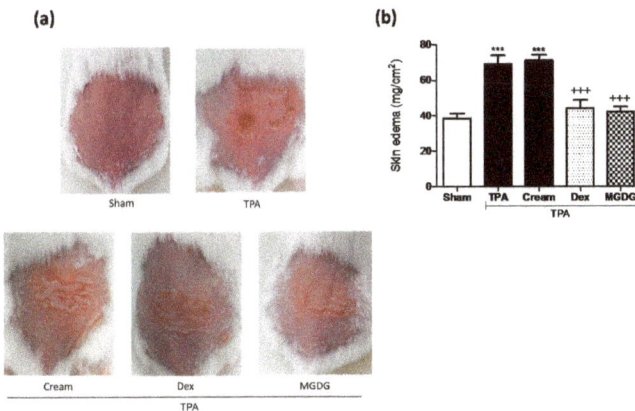

Figure 5. *Cont.*

(c)

(d) **(e)**

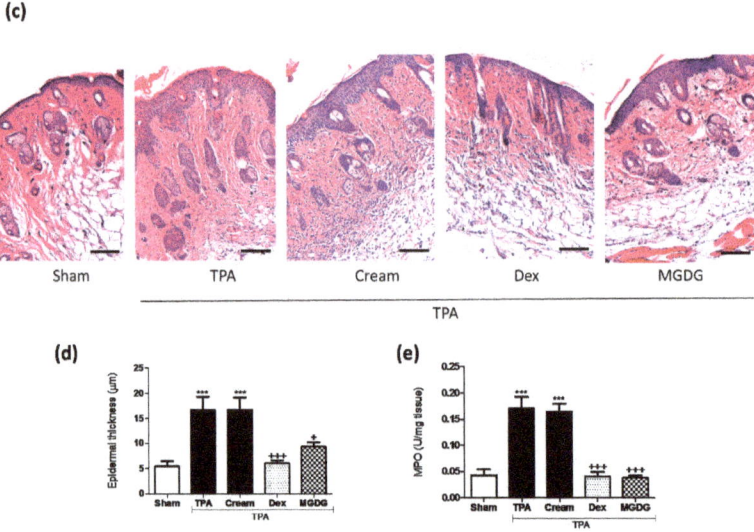

Figure 5. Topical pre-treatment with cream containing the glycolipid fraction **MGDG** from *I. galbana* decreases skin inflammation and hyperplasia on the murine 12-*O*-tetradecanoylphorbol-13-acetate (TPA)-induced model. Glycolipid cream formulation (100 mg per site containing 200 µg of **MGDG**), dexamethasone (Dex) (100 mg per site, equivalent at 200 µg of compound), or vehicle (cream with a comparable volume of ethanol) was topically administered from two days before hyperplasia induction and 30 min after each TPA application (2 nmol per zone for three consecutive days). Dex was used as the positive reference compound. (**a**) Representative images of macroscopic appearance of the dorsal skin; (**b**) determination of skin edema as punch biopsy weight; (**c**) histological appearance of mouse dorsal skin after H&E-staining ($n = 4$); Bar = 100 µm. Original magnification 100×. (**d**) Epidermal thickness assessment in H&E-stained skin slides; (**e**) myeloperoxidase (MPO) activity. Values are means with standard errors represented by vertical bars. Data are means ± SEM ($n = 10$ mice/group). Mean value was significantly different compared with the sham group (*** $p < 0.001$; Student *t* test). Mean value was significantly different compared with cream-TPA group (+ $p < 0.05$, +++ $p < 0.001$; one-way ANOVA followed by Bonferroni's Multiple Comparison test).

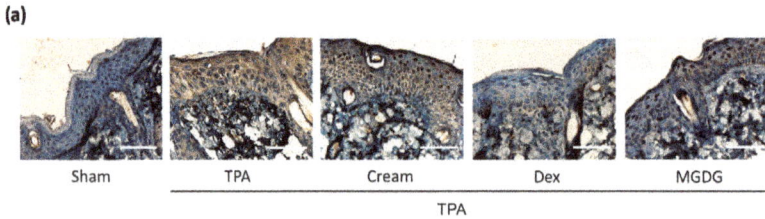

(a)

Figure 6. *Cont.*

(b)

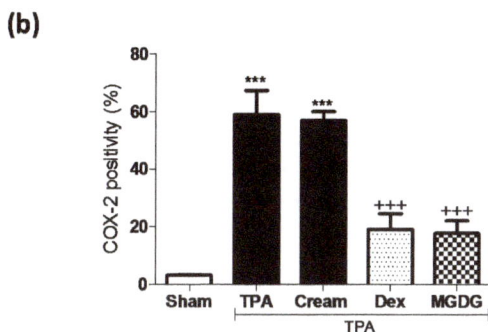

Figure 6. Topical pre-treatment with cream containing the glycolipid fraction **MGDG** from *I. galbana* attenuates 12-*O*-tetradecanoylphorbol-13-acetate (TPA)-induced COX-2 expression in mouse skin. (a) Representative photographs of epidermal COX-2 distribution by immunohistochemical detection; Bar = 200 μm. Original magnification 200×. (b) Positive COX-2 epidermal layer was assessed by counting the COX-2 positive cells versus total cells in different immunostained dorsal skin sections per animal. Representative photomicrographs showing positive epidermal COX-2 staining yielded a brown product. Values are means with standard errors represented by vertical bars. Data are means ± SEM (*n* = 4). Mean value was significantly different compared with the sham group (*** $p < 0.001$; Student's *t* test). Mean value was significantly different to the cream-TPA group (+++ $p < 0.001$; one-way ANOVA followed by Bonferroni's Multiple Comparison test).

3. Discussion

Inflammatory skin diseases have a significant impact on society, with atopic dermatitis, acne, sunburn, and psoriasis being the most common manifestations. Psoriasis is a chronic, autoimmune, and multisystem inflammatory disease that affects 2–4% of the population [15]. Currently, conventional treatments for this disease are based on the degree of severity and range from topical therapy and systemic agents through to phototherapy or combinations of those. However, many of these therapies are not recommended for the vast majority of patients afflicted with mild forms of psoriasis due to their potential risk [16]. Therefore, other treatment approaches for mild psoriasis that require topical therapy only are still needed. In this regard, natural products provide some options for increasing the safety and efficacy in the management of this pathology [17]. Microalgae species are a promising source of a variety of bioactive molecules, including polar lipids such as glycolipids. Lipid-enriched extracts or pure glycolipids have previously demonstrated their in vitro anti-inflammatory [18,19] and antitumor properties [20], which make them suitable candidates for further investigation. However, the use of galactosylglycerides to prevent skin pathologies such as psoriasis has not been previously evidenced. In this sense, we have recently observed that this kind of metabolite protects human HaCaT keratinocytes against UVB radiation through inhibition of ROS generation and a decrease in the production of the pro-inflammatory cytokine IL-6 (*data not shown*). These findings suggest that this type of molecule could play a main role not only in protecting the skin from UVB exposure but also in preventing the skin inflammatory process. In this context, we aimed to evaluate the anti-inflammatory effects of the glycolipid **MGMG-A** and **MGDG** fraction in an experimental TPA-induced hyperplasia model in mice. Moreover, we used different semisolid formulations in which the glycolipid was loaded in order to facilitate its topical application and to enhance the permeation mechanism compared to conventional liquid preparations.

Firstly, we tried to demonstrate the anti-inflammatory potential of the compounds under study in the in vitro model of TNF-α-stimulated HaCaT keratinocytes. This cytokine plays a crucial role in the pathogenesis of skin inflammatory diseases such as psoriasis [21]. We observed that pre-treatment with the compound **MGMG-A** or the fraction **MGDG** significantly reduced the production of the pro-inflammatory cytokines IL-6 and IL-8 in stimulated HaCaT keratinocytes. These results encouraged us to evaluate the preventive effects of these products on TPA-induced hyperplasia in murine skin using two experimental approaches. In the first model, glycolipids dissolved in acetone were topically administered to dorsal skin 30 min before TPA administration. Our data showed that TPA clearly caused peeling, erythema, and a strong inflammatory reaction produced by a marked influx of mononuclear and polymorphonuclear leukocytes in epidermis and dermis. Treatment of mice with the compound **MGMG-A** or the fraction **MGDG** from *I. galbana* reduced the hyperplasia manifestations and the inflammation grade, presumably due to an inhibition of inflammatory cells infiltration, as revealed by an MPO study. These findings are interesting since the cellular infiltrate has a pathogenic role in psoriasis and its control is extremely important for the attenuation of this disease [22]. Microscopic analysis of the dorsal skin was in accordance with a macroscopic study reflecting the attenuation of keratinocytes hyperproliferation in the epidermis after treatment with acetone-dissolved glycolipids. Our results are in line with a previous report that showed that topical pre-treatment with the glycoglycerolipids **MGDG**, **DGDG**, or **SQDG**, obtained from a blue-green alga, reduced inflammation in croton-oil-induced ear edema and in carrageenan-induced paw edema models [23].

The role of TNF-α, IL-17 and IL-1β in psoriasis pathogenesis has been well documented [24], being a particularly effective strategy to block their production [25]. In the present study, dorsal skin samples from TPA group showed increased levels of the pro-inflammatory cytokines TNF-α, IL-1β, IL-6, and IL-17, which were decreased in mice treated with **MGMG-A** or **MGDG** fraction. On the other hand, IL-10 is considered an anti-inflammatory cytokine since it inhibits T cells and macrophages' pro-inflammatory cytokine production [26]. In this sense, IL-10 is a rapid-response cytokine that ameliorates the acute immune response that occurs in recurrent diseases such as psoriasis or IBD [27,28]. In this acute experimental epidermal hyperplasia model, dorsal skin reacted to TPA by increasing IL-10 production versus a sham, but treatments interestingly prevented this production. These results are in line with a previous study of murine recurrent colitis in which it is proposed that pre-treatment with an oxylipin-containing lyophilized biomass from microalgae kept levels of pro-inflammatory cytokines low, thus the production of IL-10 was not required, supporting a less hyperactive immune response in the recurrent colitis model [29].

After examining the preventive effects of the compound **MGMG-A** and fraction **MGDG** obtained from *I. galbana*, we aimed to optimize the permeation behavior of these substances with respect to previously acetone-dissolved preparations. In skin diseases such as psoriasis, local topical delivery can be improved by following two main approaches. Firstly, the suitable choice of formulation can optimize the local targeting. Secondly, the physicochemical parameters of the drug itself, such as lipophilicity, can also affect the degree of delivery.

Concerning the choice of carrier composition, different formulations, including hydrophilic gel, cream, and ointment, were prepared and analyzed. For these studies, a fluorescent hydrophobic marker such as rhodamine 6G, with an oil/water partition coefficient of 2.62, was added as a model drug [30]. The in vivo CLSM study defined the cream as the best vehicle to dig deeper into the skin, preserving the entity of different tissue layers. This may be due to the fact that the surfactant-like properties of this heterogeneous disperse system could enhance the amount of permeated rhodamine 6G. On the other hand, a control solution using ethanol as solvent and hydroalcoholic Carbopol® gels also exhibited high drug permeation. This could also be attributed to the presence of ethanol in the formulation, which was used as a solubilizer and permeation enhancer. On the contrary, the deposition of the fluorophore from lipid ointment onto the skin was very low. This would be ascribed to the hydrophobic nature of the vehicle, which, being insoluble, did not penetrate through the skin but remained on the surface, as visualized in Figure 4. Usually, the permeation pathway across the SC resides in the intercellular lipid domains. Conversely, at the viable epidermis level, the fluorophore is not only restricted to the cell membranes but also accumulates in the cytosol. In this study, a relationship between the lipophilicity of the applied formulation on the accumulation of the fluorophore in SC and viable epidermis was observed. Although the fluorescent label was applied to the SC of mice, only low relative accumulation in the deeper layers of the skin was observed for the most lipophilic vehicle, the ointment. This can be explained since the lipid lamellae constitute only a small region of the *SC* compared to the corneocytes. However, the adjacent viable epidermis is much more brightly stained than *SC* in samples from the rhodamine-loaded cream and hydrogel formulations, because in this layer the label can distribute throughout the entire epidermis, which results in a brighter appearance [31].

Once we selected the cream for further studies, an ex vivo permeation process was planned for comparison of **MGDG**-loaded cream with **MGDG** reference solution and Dex-cream. In this assay, the permeation through mice excised skin was determined using a Franz diffusion apparatus and degassed absolute ethanol. Since the goal of this study was to find the experimental conditions that allowed a fast and accurate method to evaluate the permeability properties of different formulations across the skin, we decided to use ethanol as the solvent forming the receiving compartment because the assayed molecules (**MGDG** and Dex) are freely soluble in this medium. This solvent has been used for analyzing the skin diffusion kinetic of other molecules, such as α-tocopherol acetate [32]. However, the use of this solvent has the potential to extract lipids from the *SC* and to artificially increase skin permeability. Since all the formulations tested in these experiments had ethanol as the penetration enhancer interacting with skin constituents to increase drug flux, this would not affect the relative results.

The formulations were detected in the receiver medium in a time-dependent manner and cumulative amount permeated curves were plotted. Concerning **MGDG** cream with respect to the **MGDG** ethanolic solution, the difference in the permeability percentage may be attributed to the surfactant-like properties of emulsion components and their affinity for the phospholipids of the skin membrane [33]. A common mechanism of action of surfactants as penetration enhancers involves firstly a "push" effect to increase the drug solubility and hence to create a high concentration gradient. Secondly, a "pull" effect is related to the flux of the permeation enhancer through the skin, which can induce skin structural transformations [34]. In addition, findings from our study indicate that the cream exerted the best effect in increasing the skin permeation of **MGDG** compared to Dex, in which the permeated amount was lower ($15 \pm 3.1\%$). In accordance with other studies [35], this behavior can be attributed to the lower partition coefficient of this molecule (logP 1.83) with respect to **MGDG** [13]. The interaction of the drug between the water and oil phase can determine the extent of lowering of the thermodynamic activity in external phase, which is in contact with the skin. Partitioning of the drug into internal oily phase (higher logP) is due to the hydrophobic characteristic of the drug. As both molecules are highly lipophilic substances, the extremely slow permeation of Dex from the emulsion through the mice skin can be explained by the fact that the diffusion of drug through the oily phase is the limiting step for drug permeation [36].

An important consideration in psoriasis is the skin's condition. Topical formulations may be applied either to opened lesions that have lost *SC* barrier properties or to thickened lesions that represent an additional barrier to absorption [37]. Thus, our findings suggest that a hydrophilic vehicle (cream) could be an interesting alternative to improved topical delivery of **MGDG** in both conditions.

Based on the results above, we carried out a second TPA-induced hyperplasia model in mice using **MGDG**-cream. In this experimental model, TPA was applied 1 h before the administration of **MGDG**-containing cream to ensure the correct absorption of the product as well as increase its permeation and protect the lipid integrity. Our data showed that dorsal application of TPA caused similar manifestations to those detected in the previous model. Consistent with the anti-inflammatory activity of glycolipids, pre-treatment with **MGDG**-cream ameliorated macroscopic cutaneous lesions, skin edema, and MPO activity induced by repetitive application of TPA, which was correlated with the histological study. Interestingly, the reduction of skin edema and MPO activity was higher with **MGDG**-cream than that detected in the **MGDG** dissolved in acetone, reaching similar levels to those of the reference corticosteroid Dex-cream.

It has been shown that topical application of TPA activates intracellular transduction signals, enhancing aberrant expression of COX-2 in mouse skin [38,39]. To further elucidate the mechanisms for the anti-inflammatory role of **MGDG**-cream in damaged skin, we detected this protein expression by immunohistochemistry. The results evidenced that pre-treatment with **MGDG**-cream markedly attenuated COX-2 expression in TPA-stimulated mouse skin, reaching similar levels to Dex-cream. Furthermore, this effect was confirmed in TNF-α-stimulated HaCaT human keratinocytes pre-treated with different concentrations of **MGDG**, showing that this glycolipid fraction reduced COX-2 levels at 50 μg/mL (*data not shown*). These findings at least partly suggest that suppression of COX-2 expression may be involved in the preventive effect of this glycolipid fraction on TPA-induced epidermal hyperplasia.

4. Materials and Methods

4.1. Glycolipids

The extraction of dried biomass of *I. galbana* with acetone/methanol and the separation of the extract to obtain the fraction glycolipids has been previously described [8]. The pure compound **MGMG-A** was isolated during the microalgae products separation by C18 SPE cartridges (Supelco, Bellefonte, PA, USA), the elution with MeOH/H_2O (90:10, *v/v*) and the separation by reverse-phase HPLC (Merck, Darmstadt, Germany) using MeOH/H_2O (98:2, *v/v*). The spectroscopic data obtained for this compound, which matched those described in the literature, led to its identification as monogalactosylmonoacylglyceride (2*S*)-1-*O*-[(6*Z*,9*Z*,12*Z*,15*Z*)-octadeca-6,9,12,15-tetraenoyl]-3-*O*-β-D-galactopyranosylglycerol (**MGMG-A**) [40]. On the other hand, the separation of the extract of *I. galbana* previously described led to obtaining a fraction of monogalactosyldiacylglycerides (**MGDG**). In the **MGDG** fraction 10 compounds have been identified and the major **MGDG**s are (2*S*)-1-[(3*Z*,6*Z*,9*Z*,12*Z*,15*Z*)-octadeca-3,6,9,12,15-pentaenoyl]-2-*O*-[(6*Z*,9*Z*,12*Z*,15*Z*)-octadeca-6,9,12,15-tetraenoyl]-*O*-3-*O*-β-D-galactopyranosylglycerol, and (2*S*)-1-*O*-tetradecanoyl-2-*O*-[(6*Z*,9*Z*,12*Z*,15*Z*)-octadeca-6,9,12,15-tetraenoyl]-3-*O*-β-D-galactopyranosylglycerol [9].

4.2. Cell Culture

HaCaT human keratinocytes were obtained from the American Type Culture Collection and maintained in high glucose Dulbecco's modified Eagle's medium (DMEM, GIBCO, Grand Island, NY, USA) supplemented with 10% fetal bovine serum, 2 mM L-glutamine, 100 U/mL penicillin, and 100 mg/mL streptomycin in an atmosphere of 5% CO_2 at 37 °C.

4.3. Cell Viability Assay

Viability of HaCaT cells upon exposure to glycolipid compounds was determined by the sulforhodamine B (SRB) assay [41]. Briefly, the cells were seeded into 96-well plates at 1×10^4 cells/well. After 24 h, cells were incubated with compounds at the final concentrations range of 10–100 μM or 10–100 μg/mL (100 μL/well) that were prepared by dilution of stock solutions (10 mM) in DMSO in fresh medium. After 24, 48, and 72 h, cells were fixed with 50 μL of trichloroacetic acid (TCA 50% *v/v*) at 4 °C for 1 h and processed as described in the literature.

4.4. Determination of IL-6 and IL-8 Production

HaCaT cells were seeded in six-well plates (2 mL/well) at 5×10^5 cells/well. After 24 h, the cells were treated with different concentrations of **MGMG-A** (10, 30 and 50 μM) and **MGDG** (10, 30 and 50 μg/mL) and dexamethasone (Dex) (1 μM) for 1 h, and then stimulated with TNF-α (10 ng/mL) for 24 h. Then, supernatant fluids were collected and stored at −80 °C until IL-6 and IL-8 measurements. Controls contained a medium with equivalent amounts of solvent compared to treatments, and were incubated with and without TNF-α. Commercial enzyme-linked immunosorbent assay (ELISA) kits (Diaclone GEN-PROBE, Besançon, France) were used to quantify cytokines according to the manufacturer's protocol. The absorbance at 450 nm was read by a microplate reader.

4.5. Animals

For the present study, eight-week-old female Swiss CD-1 mice (25–30 g) were supplied by Janvier-Labs (Le Genest St. Isle, France). Mice were maintained in our animal laboratory under standard conditions (temperature of 24–25 °C, humidity of 70–75% and 12 h light–12 h dark cycle). Mice were allowed free access to a standard diet (Panlab, Barcelona, Spain) and water ad libitum. Dorsal hair of the mice was removed using electric clippers and depilatory skin cream (Deliplus, Barcelona, Spain) in order to maintain a hair-free skin area to carry out the topical treatments. All studies were performed in accordance with the recommendations of the European Union regarding animal experimentation (Directive of the European Council 2010/63/EU). The experiments followed a protocol approved by the Animal Ethics Committee of the University of Seville.

4.6. TPA-Induced Epidermal Hyperplasia Model and Glycolipid Treatments

We evaluated the effect of glycolipids from *I. galbana* on TPA-induced hyperplasia in murine skin. Briefly, dorsal skin of female Swiss mice was shaved and 24 h later, animals that displayed no evidence of hair regrowth or injury were assigned to the different groups.

In a first set of experiments (n = 10 per group), **MGMG-A** and **MGDG** dissolved in acetone (10 µg/µL, 200 µg per site) or the reference agent Dex dissolved in acetone (10 µg/µL, 200 µg per site) were topically administered to the shaved dorsal skin of animals in an area of 1 cm^2 by using a micropipette (total volume, 20 µL). Vehicle (acetone) was administered in a comparable volume to sham and TPA group. After 30 min, TPA (2 nmol per site, dissolved in acetone) was topically applied to the same areas, except the sham, which received a comparable volume of acetone (day 0). This procedure was repeated for two consecutive days [2]. Mice were sacrificed on day 3 by cervical dislocation and punch biopsies from the treated dorsal skin were weighed to evaluate edema before further processing for histology and biochemical parameters.

4.7. MPO Activity

Myeloperoxidase (MPO) activity was assayed as a marker of neutrophil infiltration according to the method of Grisham et al. [42]. The tissue was thawed, weighed, and homogenized in 10 volumes of 50 mM-PBS (pH 7.4). The homogenate was centrifuged at $20,000 \times g$ for 20 min at 4 °C. The pellet was again homogenized in 10 volumes of 50 mM-PBS (pH 6) containing hexadecyl trimethylammonium bromide (0.5%) and 10 mM-EDTA. This homogenate was subjected to one cycle of freezing/thawing and a brief period of sonication. A sample of the homogenate (50 µL) was added to a 96-well microplate and incubated at 37 °C for 3 min with a mixture containing *o*-dianisidine dihydrochloride (0.067%), hexadecyl trimethyl-ammonium bromide (0.5%) and 0.3 mM-H_2O_2. Changes in absorbance at 450 nm were measured with a microplate reader (Labysystem Multiskan EX, Thermo Scientific, New York, NY, USA). One unit of MPO activity was defined as the amount of enzyme present that produced a change in absorbance of 1.0 unit/min at 37 °C in the final reaction volume containing the acetate. Results are expressed as units/mg tissue.

4.8. Histological Study

Tissue samples from the dorsal skin of four animals were fixed in 4% buffered paraformaldehyde, dehydrated by increasing concentrations of ethanol and embedded in paraffin. Tissue sections cut to 7 µm on a rotary microtome (Leica Microsystems, Wetzlar, Germany) were mounted on slides, deparaffinized with xylene, rehydrated through graded alcohols, and stained with hematoxylin and eosin (H&E) according to standard protocols. The tissues were analyzed by a blinded observer under an Olympus BH-2 microscope (GMI Inc., Ramsey, MN, USA) for determination of histopathological changes. Epidermal thickness was measured using Scientific Imaging Systems (Biophotonics ImageJ Analysis Software; National Institutes of Health, Rockville, MD, USA).

4.9. Measurement of Cytokines in Skin Homogenates

Frozen skin biopsies were homogenized in three volumes of ice-cold tissue lysis buffer containing PBS (pH 7.2) with 0.1 M of EDTA, 1 mg/mL of leupeptin, 1 mg/mL of pepstatin, 1 mg/mL of aprotinin, and 1 mM phenylmethylsulfonyl fluoride. Homogenates were centrifuged at $12,000\times g$ for 10 min at 4 °C. Supernatant fluids were stored at -80 °C until measurements. Levels of TNF-α, IL-1β, IL-6, IL-17 and IL-10 were measured by quantitative Enzyme-Linked ImmunoSorbent Assay kits (ELISA) (Peprotech, Hamburg, Germany), according to the manufacturer's instructions. Data are reported as pg/mg tissue.

4.10. Skin Topical Formulations

Hydrophilic gel. Carbopol® 934P (Lubrizol, Cleveland, OH, USA) was selected as a gelling agent at 1% (w/v) due to its widespread use in pharmaceutical formulations and fast dispersion in water. Rhodamine 6G solution in ethanol absolute (10 µg/µL) was gradually added to the polymer dispersion under magnetic stirring. The dispersion was neutralized with triethanolamine to obtain an adequate consistency suitable for topical application.

Cream. This O/W emulsion was prepared by gradually adding rhodamine (10 µg/µL), **MGDG** (10 µg/µL) or Dex (10 µg/µL) solution in ethanol absolute to a cold mix excipient composed of Caprylic/Capric Triglycerides, Glycol Stearate, PEG-3 Glyceryl Cocoate and Steareth-7 previously heated to improve the drug interposition. The final formulations contained 0.2% (w/w) **MGDG**.

Lipophilic ointment. This formulation was obtained using melt emulsification combined with stirring. Briefly, Brij® 72 (5% w/w) and white soft paraffin (77.3% w/w) were blended under gentle stirring in a water bath at 70 °C to form the lipid phase. Successively, liquid paraffin (5% w/w) and α-tocopherol (0.002% w/w) were added into the lipid phase until complete interposition at 60 °C. Then, rhodamine dissolved in propylene glycol (10 µg/µL) was added to the mixture. Meanwhile, two solutions of EDTA (0.0065% w/w) and disodium phosphate dihydrate (0.026% w/w) were prepared with distilled water at 60 °C and added dropwise to the lipid phase, with moderate magnetic stirring at 150 rpm for 20 min. Finally, the rhodamine-loaded ointment was maintained at room temperature for further use.

4.11. Permeation Studies

In vivo skin depth permeation by confocal laser scanning microscopy (CLSM). Confocal studies were performed in order to investigate the penetration ability of several formulations through the different skin layers [43]. Towards this aim, Carbopol® hydrogel, cream, and ointment were prepared by adding a hydrophobic fluorescent probe, i.e., rhodamine 6G (100 mg per site, equivalent at 200 µg of compound dissolved in ethanol), in the lipid or in the water-ethanol phase, according to the composition of formulations. Rhodamine 6G was selected as an equivalent marker for **MGDG** or Dex due to their comparable lipophilic properties. Appropriate samples of these formulations were taken and placed on SC of mice and maintained in contact with the skin for 24 h. At the end of the experiment, the remaining preparation was carefully washed with purified water from the skin surface. Then, dorsal skin was excised and rinsed with pH 7.4 phosphate buffer solution, rapidly frozen in liquid nitrogen and then stored at -80 °C. Sections of skin (50 µm thickness) were then perpendicularly cut with a cryomicrotome and examined to investigate the fluorescent marker distribution in the different skin layers. Analysis was carried out using a Leica TCS SP II CLSM (Leica, Heidelberg, Germany) equipped with a Kr-Ar-He-Ne ion laser and a Leica DM IRE 2 microscope endowed with HCPL Fluotar Leica 10× and 20× dry objectives and HCXPLAN APO Leica X40 multi-immersion objective (numeric aperture 0.85). For excitation of the fluorescent label the 488 nm wavelength was used and the fluorescence emission was detected at 520 nm.

From the confocal images, a mathematical treatment was carried out in order to evaluate the intensity of fluorescence in the samples, as appeared in the histogram curve provided from Leica software. Statistical calculations were as follows:

$$\text{Arithmetical mean value}: \ \mu(I) = \frac{1}{N_{\text{pixel}}} \times \sum I_i, \tag{1}$$

$$\text{Average image energy}: \ I_{\text{mean}}^2 = \frac{1}{N_{\text{pixel}}} \times \sum_{\text{pixel}} I_i^2, \tag{2}$$

$$\text{Root mean square value}: \ I_{\text{mean}}^2 = \sqrt{\frac{1}{N_{\text{pixel}}} \sum_{\text{pixel}} I_i^2}, \tag{3}$$

$$\text{Skewness of the distribution}: \ \frac{1}{N} \sum_i \left[\frac{I_i - \mu(I)}{\sqrt{VAR(I)}} \right]^3, \tag{4}$$

where I is the energy intensity, I_i is the energy intensity of each pixel, I_{mean} is the mean value of energy intensity, N_{pixel} is the number of pixels of the image, $\mu(I)$ is the arithmetical mean of the energy intensity and VAR is the variance.

Ex vivo permeation studies. Diffusion studies were carried out using a Franz diffusion cell apparatus (SES-Gmgh Analyses system, Bechenheim, Germany) with an effective diffusional area of $3.14 \ cm^2$. Excised mice skin was used as a membrane. Animals were sacrificed and full thickness dorsal skin was excised. A specific portion of the skin was cut and used for the permeation study after washing it with distilled water. The study was carried out following the methodology previously reported [44]. Animal skin was inserted between the donor and receiving compartments and adjusted by means of a pinch clamp. The receiving chamber was filled with 14.5 mL of degassed ethanol absolute and thermostated by means of a water bath circulator and a jacket surrounding the cell, maintaining 32 °C in the skin surface. The receiving medium was continuously stirred to avoid the diffusion layer effect.

Once we selected the cream carrier from the previous study, **MGDG**-cream (0.2% *w/w*), **MGDG** control solution (0.2% *w/w*), and Dex-cream (0.2% *w/w*) were accurately measured and placed on *SC* in the donor compartment and sealed with parafilm. Aliquots of 0.5 mL were withdrawn from the receiving medium at predetermined time intervals (0, 0.5, 1, 2, 3, 4, 5, 6 and 24 h) according to international guidelines and the same volume was replaced with fresh ethanol absolute at the same temperature. These samples were quantified by HPLC (Hitachi Elite LaChrom, Barcelona, Spain) for **MGDG** quantification and spectrophotometry UV-visible (Agilent 8453, Barcelona, Spain) was used for Dex quantification. HPLC system is equipped with an L-2130 isocratic pump, a diode array detector L-2455 and L-2200 autosampler. The chromatographic separation was performed on a reverse-phase LichroCART® C18 column (5 µm, 4.6 mm ID × 150 mm, Agilent, Santa Clara, CA, USA) using as mobile phase acetonitrile (ACN, solution A): formic acid solution ((0.1% *v/v*), solution B) adjusted to pH 2.67 in the following gradient (*v/v*): 0–6 min, 90% A, 10% B, flux 1 mL/min; 6–15 min, 100% A. The injection volume was 30 µL. The cumulative amount of drug in receptor chamber for the three formulations (**MGDG**-cream, **MGDG** control solution and Dex control solution) was plotted as a function of time (*t*, h). The cumulative amount (%) of drug permeated through the skin (*P*%) was determined as per the following equation [45]:

$$P\% = \frac{C_n \times V + \sum_{i=1}^{n-1} C_i \times V_i}{M} \times 100, \tag{5}$$

where C_n is the drug concentration of the nth sampling point (mg/mL), C_i is the drug concentration of the ith sample point (mg/mL), V is the total volume (14.5 mL) of liquid in receiving pool, V_i is the volume (0.5 mL) of the ith sampling points and M is the mass of drug (**MGDG** or Dex).

*4.12. TPA-Induced Epidermal Hyperplasia Model and **MGDG**-Cream Treatment*

Given acetone is considered moderately toxic and irritant and we aim to elaborate an optimal glycolipid-containing pharmacological formulation, we evaluated the effect of **MGDG**-cream on TPA-induced hyperplasia in murine skin. The dorsal skin of female Swiss mice was shaved as described above.

In this second experimental model (n = 10 per group), a pre-treatment was carried out two days (day −2 and day −1) before the first TPA challenge (day 0). **MGDG**-cream formulation (100 mg per site, containing 200 µg of **MGDG** dissolved in ethanol at 10 µg/µL), Dex-cream (100 mg per site, equivalent at 200 µg of compound dissolved in ethanol at 10 µg/µL) or vehicle (cream with a comparable volume of ethanol) were applied to the shaved dorsal skin of the animals in an area of 1 cm^2 using a syringe. On day 0, TPA (2 nmol per site, dissolved in ethanol) was topically applied to the same areas using a micropipette (total volume of 20 µL). After 1 h, **MGDG**-cream, Dex-cream, or vehicle was topically administered. Mice were anesthetized with ketamine (100 mg/kg of animal) and diazepam (5 mg/kg of animal) during treatments and TPA challenge. This protocol was repeated for two consecutive days. Mice were sacrificed on day 3 by cervical dislocation and punch biopsies from the treated dorsal skin were weighed to evaluate edema, before further processing for MPO activity and histology.

4.13. Immunohistochemical Analysis

Staining of COX-2 was performed using a streptavidin-biotin-peroxidase method [46]. Paraffin-embedded dorsal skin sections (7 µm) were mounted on slides, deparaffinized with xylene, and rehydrated through graded alcohols. These sections were boiled (10 mM citrate buffer, pH 6.0 for 3 min) for antigen retrieval, followed by cooling at room temperature for 20 min. Endogenous peroxidase was quenched with 0.3% (v/v) hydrogen peroxide for 20 min. Sections were rinsed with PBS for 10 min. Nonspecific adsorption was minimized by incubating sections in normal horse serum (Vectastain Kit; Vector Laboratories, Burlingame, CA, USA) for 20 min. Subsequently, slides were incubated with rabbit polyclonal anti-COX-2 antibody (Cayman Chemical, Ann Arbor, MI, USA) (1:300) overnight at 4 °C. Then, slides were treated with anti-mouse IgG antibody for 30 min and incubated with the streptavidin–peroxidase complex for 30 min at room temperature (Vectastain Kit; Vector Laboratories, CA, USA). The enzymatic activities were developed with 3,3′-diaminobenzidine (DAB), and the sections were counterstained with hematoxylin. Negative control sections were treated in the same way, omitting the primary antibody [47]. COX-2 immunoreactivity was examined on all sections using a microscope Olympus BX61 (Olympus Optical Co. Ltd., Tokyo, Japan). The quantification of immunohistochemical data was done by counting the number of immunostained brown cells as the percent of total epidermal cells from 10 microscopic fields of immunostained tissues per animal.

4.14. Statistical Analysis

All values in the figures and text are expressed as arithmetic means ± SEM. Data were evaluated with GraphPad Prism version 5.00 software (GraphPad Software, Inc., San Diego, CA, USA). In all cases, the Shapiro–Wilk test was used to verify the normality of the data. The Mann–Whitney U-test was chosen for non-parametric values. The parametric values groups were analyzed by one-way analysis of variance (ANOVA) followed by Bonferroni's Multiple Comparison Test. p values < 0.05 were considered statistically significant. In the histological experiment, results shown are representative of at least four independent experiments performed on different days.

5. Conclusions

In conclusion, our study demonstrates for the first time the preventive effects of topical administration of the glycolipid **MGMG-A** or a fraction **MGDG** from *I. galbana*, in the inflammatory model of TPA-induced skin hyperplasia. These actions may be associated with a reduction of edema, leukocyte infiltration, pro-inflammatory cytokines production and COX-2 expression in skin mouse. Topical application of **MGDG**-cream enhanced the sample permeability and consequently, increased the preventive effects of this product. Future studies are needed to expand the vision of the mechanisms by which these lipid products improve skin inflammation and will support their potential use in the development of effective therapeutic strategies for skin pathologies as psoriasis.

Supplementary Materials: The following are available online at www.mdpi.com/1660-3397/16/1/2/s1, Table S1: Viability of HaCaT human keratinocytes treated with different concentrations of **MGMG-A** and **MGDG** fraction isolated from the microalgae *Isochrysis galbana*.

Acknowledgments: This study was supported by grants from Ministerio de Economía y Competitividad MICIIN INNPACTO-IPT-2012-1370-060000 and Consejería de Innovación, Ciencia y Empresa-Junta de Andalucía POLFANAT-P12-AGR-430. The authors thank "Centro de Investigación, Tecnología e Innovación" of the University of Seville for providing technical assistance.

Author Contributions: María del Carmen Terencio, Elena Talero, Virginia Motilva, and Javier Ávila-Román designed the study protocol; Carolina de los Reyes performed chemical characterization of glycolipids from *I. galbana*; Azahara Rodríguez-Luna, Elena Talero, and Javier Ávila-Román conducted in vivo and histological experiments and analyzed the data; Azahara Rodríguez-Luna, María Luisa González-Rodríguez, and Antonio M. Rabasco executed technologic experiments; Azahara Rodríguez-Luna, Elena Talero, María Luisa González-Rodríguez, Virginia Motilva, and Javier Ávila-Román wrote the draft of the manuscript. All the authors critically reviewed and approved the final version of the manuscript.

Conflicts of Interest: The authors declare no conflict of interest.

Abbreviations

CLSM	confocal laser scanning microscopy
Dex	dexamethasone
IL	Interleukin
I. galbana	*Isochrysis galbana*
MGDG	Monogalactosyldiacylglycerol fraction
MGMG-A	Monogalactosylmonoacylglyceride (2*S*)-1-*O*-[(6*Z*,9*Z*,12*Z*,15*Z*)-octadeca-6,9,12,15-tetraenoyl]-3-*O*-β-D-galactopyranosylglycerol
MPO	myeloperoxidase
RMS	root mean square
SC	*stratum corneum*
TNF-α	Tumor Necrosis Factor alpha
TPA	12-*O*-tetradecanoylphorbol-13-acetate

References

1. An, J.; Li, Z.; Dong, Y.; Ren, J.; Huo, J. Amentoflavone protects against psoriasis-like skin lesion through suppression of NF-κB-mediated inflammation and keratinocyte proliferation. *Mol. Cell. Biochem.* **2016**, *413*, 87–95. [CrossRef] [PubMed]

2. Arasa, J.; Martos, P.; Terencio, M.C.; Valcuende-Cavero, F.; Montesinos, M.C. Topical application of the adenosine A2A receptor agonist CGS-21680 prevents phorbol-induced epidermal hyperplasia and inflammation in mice. *Exp. Dermatol.* **2014**, *23*, 555–560. [CrossRef] [PubMed]

3. Liu, R.F.; Wang, F.; Wang, Q.; Zhao, X.C.; Zhang, K.M. Mesenchymal stem cells from skin lesions of psoriasis patients promote proliferation and inhibit apoptosis of HaCaT cells. *Genet. Mol. Res.* **2015**, *14*, 17758–17767. [CrossRef] [PubMed]

4. Lowes, M.A.; Bowcock, A.M.; Krueger, J.G. Pathogenesis and therapy of psoriasis. *Nature* **2007**, *445*, 866–873. [CrossRef] [PubMed]

5. Zulfakar, M.H.; Porter, R.M.; Heard, C.M. In vivo response of GsdmA3(Dfl)/+ mice to topically applied fish oil—Effects on cellular markers and macrophages. *FEBS. Open Bio* **2016**, *6*, 827–834. [CrossRef] [PubMed]

6. Guerra, I.; Pérez-Jeldres, T.; Iborra, M.; Algaba, A.; Monfort, D.; Calvet, X.; Chaparro, M.; Mañosa, M.; Hinojosa, E.; Minguez, M.; et al. Incidence, clinical characteristics, and management of psoriasis induced by anti-tnf therapy in patients with inflammatory bowel disease. *Inflamm. Bowel Dis.* **2016**, *22*, 894–901. [CrossRef] [PubMed]

7. Talero, E.; García-mauriño, S.; Ávila-román, J.; Rodríguez-luna, A.; Alcaide, A.; Motilva, V. Bioactive compounds isolated from microalgae in chronic inflammation and cancer. *Mar. Drugs* **2015**, *13*, 6152–6209. [CrossRef] [PubMed]

8. De los Reyes, C.; Ortega, M.J.; Rodríguez-Luna, A.; Talero, E.; Motilva, V.; Zubía, E. Molecular characterization and anti-inflammatory activity of galactosylglycerides and galactosylceramides from the microalga *Isochrysis galbana*. *J. Agric. Food Chem.* **2016**, *64*, 8783–8794. [CrossRef] [PubMed]

9. Rowe, R.C.; Sheskey, P.J.; Owen, S.C.; American Pharmacists Association. *Handbook of Pharmaceutical Excipients*; APhA/Pharmaceutical Press: London, UK, 2009; pp. 7–8.

10. Martins, A.; Vieira, H.; Gaspar, H.; Santos, S. Marketed marine natural products in the pharmaceutical and cosmeceutical industries: Tips for success. *Mar. Drugs* **2014**, *12*, 1066–1101. [CrossRef] [PubMed]

11. Andrés, R.M.; Montesinos, M.C.; Navalón, P.; Payá, M.; Terencio, M.C. NF-κB and STAT3 inhibition as a therapeutic strategy in psoriasis: In vitro and in vivo effects of BTH. *J. Investig. Dermatol.* **2013**, *133*, 2362–2371. [CrossRef] [PubMed]

12. Mura, P.; Maestrelli, F.; González-Rodríguez, M.L.; Michelacci, I.; Ghelardini, C.; Rabasco, A.M. Development, characterization and in vivo evaluation of benzocaine-loaded liposomes. *Eur. J. Pharm. Biopharm.* **2007**, *67*, 86–95. [CrossRef] [PubMed]

13. Maréchal, E.; Block, M.A.; Joyard, J.; Douce, R. Comparison of the kinetic properties of MGDG synthase in mixed micelles and in envelope membranes from spinach chloroplast. *FEBS Lett.* **1994**, *352*, 307–310. [CrossRef]

14. Qiu, Y.; Chen, Y.; Zhang, G. *Developing Solid Oral Dosage Forms: Pharmaceutical Theory and Practice*; Academic Press: London, UK, 2009; pp. 282–283.

15. Anand, S.; Gupta, P.; Bhardwaj, R.; Narang, T.; Dogra, S.; Minz, R.W.; Saikia, B.; Chhabra, S. Is psoriasis an autoimmune disease: Interpretations from an immunofluorescence-based study. *J. Cutan. Pathol.* **2017**, *44*, 1–6. [CrossRef] [PubMed]

16. Malatestinic, W.; Nordstrom, B.; Wu, J.J.; Goldblum, O.; Solotkin, K.; Lin, C.Y.; Kistler K.; Fraeman, K.; Johnston, J.; Hawley, L.L.; et. al. Characteristics and medication use of psoriasis patients who may or may not qualify for randomized controlled trials. *J. Manag. Care Spec. Pharm.* **2017**, *23*, 370–381. [CrossRef] [PubMed]

17. Herman, A.; Herman, A.P.; Herman, A. Topically used herbal products for the treatment of psoriasis—Mechanism of action, drug delivery, clinical studies. *Planta Med.* **2016**, *82*, 1447–1455. [CrossRef] [PubMed]

18. Robertson, R.C.; Guihéneuf, F.; Bahar, B.; Schmid, M.; Stengel, D.B.; Fitzgerald, G.F.; Ross, R.P.; Stanton, C. The anti-inflammatory effect of algae-derived lipid extracts on lipopolysaccharide (LPS)-stimulated human THP-1 macrophages. *Mar. Drugs* **2015**, *13*, 5402–5424. [CrossRef] [PubMed]

19. Banskota, A.H.; Stefanova, R.; Sperker, S.; Lall, S.P.; Craigie, J.S.; Hafting, J.T.; Critchley, A.T. Polar lipids from the marine macroalga Palmaria palmata inhibit lipopolysaccharide-induced nitric oxide production in RAW264.7 macrophage cells. *Phytochemistry* **2014**, *101*, 101–108. [CrossRef] [PubMed]

20. Hossain, Z.; Kurihara, H.; Hosokawa, M.; Takahashi, K. Growth inhibition and induction of differentiation and apoptosis mediated by sodium butyrate in caco-2 cells with algal glycolipids. *In Vitro Cell. Dev. Biol.-Anim.* **2005**, *41*, 154–159. [CrossRef] [PubMed]

21. Amigó, M.; Payá, M.; De Rosa, S.; Terencio, M.C. Antipsoriatic effects of avarol-3′-thiosalicylate are mediated by inhibition of TNF-alpha generation and NF-kappaB activation in mouse skin. *Br. J. Pharmacol.* **2007**, *152*, 353–365. [CrossRef] [PubMed]

22. Yazici, C.; Köse, K.; Utaş, S.; Tanrikulu, E.; Taşlidere, N. A novel approach in psoriasis: First usage of known protein oxidation markers to prove oxidative stress. *Arch. Dermatol. Res.* **2016**, *308*, 207–212. [CrossRef] [PubMed]

23. Bruno, A.; Rossi, C.; Marcolongo, G.; Di Lena, A.; Venzo, A.; Berrie, C.P.; Corda, D. Selective in vivo anti-inflammatory action of the galactolipid monogalactosyldiacylglycerol. *Eur. J. Pharmacol.* **2005**, *524*, 159–168. [CrossRef] [PubMed]

24. Mahil, S.K.; Capon, F.; Barker, J.N. Update on psoriasis immunopathogenesis and targeted immunotherapy. *Semin. Immunopathol.* **2016**, *38*, 11–27. [CrossRef] [PubMed]

25. Campa, M.; Mansouri, B.; Warren, R.; Menter, A. A review of biologic therapies targeting IL-23 and IL-17 for use in moderate-to-severe plaque psoriasis. *Dermatol. Ther.* **2016**, *6*, 1–12. [CrossRef] [PubMed]

26. Geginat, J.; Larghi, P.; Paroni, M.; Nizzoli, G.; Penatti, A.; Pagani, M.; Gagliani, N.; Meroni, P.; Abrignani, S.; Flavell, R.A. The light and the dark sides of Interleukin-10 in immune-mediated diseases and cancer. *Cytokine Growth Factor Rev.* **2016**, *30*, 87–93. [CrossRef] [PubMed]

27. Traupe, H. Psoriasis and the interleukin-10 family: Evidence for a protective genetic effect, but not an easy target as a drug. *Br. J. Dermatol.* **2017**, *176*, 1438–1439. [CrossRef] [PubMed]

28. Fonseca-Camarillo, G.; Furuzawa-Carballeda, J.; Llorente, L.; Yamamoto-Furusho, J.K. IL-10- and IL-20-Expressing Epithelial and Inflammatory Cells are Increased in Patients with Ulcerative Colitis. *J. Clin. Immunol.* **2013**, *33*, 640–648. [CrossRef] [PubMed]

29. Ávila-Roman, J.; Talero, E.; Rodríguez-Luna, A.; García-Mauriño, S.; Motilva, V. Anti-inflammatory effects of an oxylipin-containing lyophilised biomass from a microalga in a murine recurrent colitis model. *Br. J. Nutr.* **2016**, *116*, 1–9. [CrossRef] [PubMed]

30. Wang, J.D.; Douville, N.J.; Takayama, S.; Elsayed, M. Quantitative analysis of molecular absorption into PDMS microfluidic channels. *Ann. Biomed. Eng.* **2012**, *40*, 1862–1873. [CrossRef] [PubMed]

31. Aggarwal, N.; Goindi, S.; Mehta, S.D. Preparation and evaluation of dermal delivery system of griseofulvin containing vitamin E-TPGS as penetration enhancer. *AAPS PharmSciTech* **2012**, *13*, 67–74. [CrossRef] [PubMed]

32. Mahamongkol, H.; Bellantone, R.A.; Stagni, G.; Plakogiannis, F.M. Permeation study of five formulations of alpha-tocopherol acetate through human cadaver skin. *J. Cosmet. Sci.* **2005**, *56*, 91–103. [PubMed]

33. Williams, A.C.; Barry, B.W. Penetration enhancers. *Adv. Drug Deliv. Rev.* **2012**, *64*, 128–137. [CrossRef]

34. Puglia, C.; Bonina, F. Effect of polyunsaturated fatty acids and some conventional penetration enhancers on transdermal delivery of atenolol. *Drug Deliv.* **2008**, *15*, 107–112. [CrossRef] [PubMed]

35. Wang, M.Y.; Yang, Y.Y.; Heng, P.W.S. Role of solvent in interactions between fatty acids-based formulations and lipids in porcine stratum corneum. *J. Control. Release* **2004**, *94*, 207–216. [CrossRef] [PubMed]

36. Grams, Y.Y.; Alaruikka, S.; Lashley, L.; Caussin, J.; Whitehead, L.; Bouwstra, J.A. Permeant lipophilicity and vehicle composition influence accumulation of dyes in hair follicles of human skin. *Eur. J. Pharm. Sci.* **2003**, *18*, 329–336. [CrossRef]

37. Garnier, T.C.S. Topical treatment for cutaneous leishmaniasis. *Curr. Opin. Investig. Drugs* **2002**, *3*, 538–544. [PubMed]

38. Kundu, J.K.; Hwang, D.M.; Lee, J.C.; Chang, E.J.; Shin, Y.K.; Fujii, H.; Sun, B.; Surh, Y.J. Inhibitory effects of oligonol on phorbol ester-induced tumor promotion and COX-2 expression in mouse skin: NF-κB and C/EBP as potential targets. *Cancer Lett.* **2009**, *273*, 86–97. [CrossRef] [PubMed]

39. Passos, G.F.; Medeiros, R.; Marcon, R.; Nascimento, A.F.Z.; Calixto, J.B.; Pianowski, L.F. The role of PKC/ERK1/2 signaling in the anti-inflammatory effect of tetracyclic triterpene euphol on TPA-induced skin inflammation in mice. *Eur. J. Pharmacol.* **2013**, *698*, 413–420. [CrossRef] [PubMed]

40. Hiraga, Y.; Shikano, T.; Widianti, T.; Ohkata, K. Three new glycolipids with cytolytic activity from cultured marine dinoflagellate Heterocapsa circularisquama. *Nat. Prod. Res.* **2008**, *22*, 649–657. [CrossRef] [PubMed]

41. Skehan, P.; Storeng, R.; Scudiero, D.; Monks, A.; McMahon, J.; Vistica, D.; Warren, J.T.; Bokesch, H.; Kenney, S.; Boyd, M.R. New colorimetric cytotoxicity assay for anticancer-drug screening. *J. Natl. Cancer Inst.* **1990**, *82*, 1107–1112. [CrossRef] [PubMed]

42. Grisham, M.B.; Benoit, J.N.; Granger, D.N. Assessment of leukocyte involvement during ischemia and reperfusion of intestine. *Methods Enzymol.* **1990**, *186*, 729–742. [PubMed]

43. Álvarez-Roman, R.; Naik, A.; Kalia, Y.N.; Fessi, H.; Guy, R.H. Visualization of skin penetration using confocal laser scanning microscopy. *Eur. J. Pharm. Biopharm.* **2004**, *58*, 301–316. [CrossRef] [PubMed]

44. López-Pinto, J.M.; González-Rodríguez, M.L.; Rabasco, A.M. Effect of cholesterol and ethanol on dermal delivery from DPPC liposomes. *Int. J. Pharm.* **2005**, *298*, 1–12. [CrossRef] [PubMed]

45. Li, Z.; Liu, M.; Wang, H.; Du, S. Increased cutaneous wound healing effect of biodegradable liposomes containing madecassoside: Preparation optimization, in vitro dermal permeation, and in vivo bioevaluation. *Int. J. Nanomed.* **2016**, *11*, 2995–3007. [CrossRef] [PubMed]

46. Talero, E.; Sánchez-Fidalgo, S.; Villegas, I.; de la Lastra, C.A.; Illanes, M.; Motilva, V. Role of different inflammatory and tumor biomarkers in the development of ulcerative colitis-associated carcinogenesis. *Inflamm. Bowel Dis.* **2011**, *17*, 696–710. [CrossRef] [PubMed]

47. Talero, E.; Di Paola, R.; Mazzon, E.; Esposito, E.; Motilva, V.; Cuzzocrea, S. Anti-inflammatory effects of adrenomedullin on acute lung injury induced by Carrageenan in mice. *Mediat. Inflamm.* **2012**, *2012*. [CrossRef]

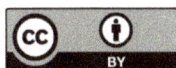

marine drugs

MDPI

Article

Fucoxanthin-Containing Cream Prevents Epidermal Hyperplasia and UVB-Induced Skin Erythema in Mice

Azahara Rodríguez-Luna [1], Javier Ávila-Román [1], María Luisa González-Rodríguez [2], María José Cózar [2], Antonio M Rabasco [2], Virginia Motilva [1] and Elena Talero [1,*]

[1] Department of Pharmacology, Faculty of Pharmacy, Universidad de Sevilla, 41012 Seville, Spain; arodriguez53@us.es (A.R.-L.); javieravila@us.es (J.Á.-R.); motilva@us.es (V.M.)

[2] Department of Pharmaceutical Technology, Faculty of Pharmacy, Universidad de Sevilla, 41012 Seville, Spain; malugoro@us.es (M.L.G.-R.); cozar@us.es (M.J.C.); amra@us.es (A.M.R.)

* Correspondence: etalero@us.es; Tel.: +34-954-559879

Received: 20 September 2018; Accepted: 8 October 2018; Published: 10 October 2018

Abstract: Microalgae represent a source of bio-active compounds such as carotenoids with potent anti-inflammatory and antioxidant properties. We aimed to investigate the effects of fucoxanthin (FX) in both in vitro and in vivo skin models. Firstly, its anti-inflammatory activity was evaluated in LPS-stimulated THP-1 macrophages and TNF-α-stimulated HaCaT keratinocytes, and its antioxidant activity in UVB-irradiated HaCaT cells. Next, in vitro and ex vivo permeation studies were developed to determine the most suitable formulation for in vivo FX topical application. Then, we evaluated the effects of a FX-containing cream on TPA-induced epidermal hyperplasia in mice, as well as on UVB-induced acute erythema in hairless mice. Our results confirmed the in vitro reduction of TNF-α, IL-6, ROS and LDH production. Since the permeation results showed that cream was the most favourable vehicle, FX-cream was elaborated. This formulation effectively ameliorated TPA-induced hyperplasia, by reducing skin edema, epidermal thickness, MPO activity and COX-2 expression. Moreover, FX-cream reduced UVB-induced erythema through down-regulation of COX-2 and iNOS as well as up-regulation of HO-1 protein via Nrf-2 pathway. In conclusion, FX, administered in a topical formulation, could be a novel natural adjuvant for preventing exacerbations associated with skin inflammatory pathologies as well as protecting skin against UV radiation.

Keywords: fucoxanthin; inflammation; epidermal hyperplasia; UVB; photoprotection

1. Introduction

Skin is the organ that acts as main defence against external environment factors, protecting the organism from harmful substances, mechanical damage, pathological invasion and radiations. Nonetheless, the normal structure and functionality could be altered by external factors such as toxic compounds or ultraviolet (UV) radiation, or by internal factors including genetic predisposition, immune and hormone disorders, or stress. The result of these skin perturbations could trigger an inflammatory process, an oxidative stress status, an unbalanced epidermal homeostasis, or a limited immune response, among others [1].

In this respect, inflammatory skin diseases such as psoriasis, atopic dermatitis or rosacea have harsh clinical implications because of their chronic curse and lead to develop comorbidities that make difficult their treatment and have a remarkable impact on the quality-of-life of patients [2]. Nowadays, UV skin exposure to treat these inflammatory conditions is recommended due to its beneficial effects. In this line, UV radiation achieves long remission periods in psoriasis through activation of immunosuppressive pathways and keratinocyte apoptosis [3]. On the other hand, detrimental effects of UVB radiation exposure (280–315 nm) have been extensively reported: it promotes a strong acute inflammatory response characterized by activation and recruitment of innate immune cells such as neutrophils and macrophages to the epidermis and dermis. In addition, UVB radiation is the main source of reactive oxygen species (ROS) production, which increases the inflammatory response, causing DNA oxidative damage in keratinocytes [4]. For this reason, new approaches to modulate the skin inflammation and protect against UV radiation are necessary to supplement the existing skin anti-inflammatory therapies.

Currently, marine resources are recognized for their variety of biologically active substances [5], which are becoming important ingredients in skin care products due to their potent anti-inflammatory and antioxidant actions as well as the safety and low risk in their administration [6]. In this sense, carotenoids have shown antioxidant, anti-inflammatory or anti-carcinogenic properties in different skin inflammatory models [7]. Fucoxanthin (FX) is an orange carotenoid present in brown seaweeds, diatoms and microalgae [8], whose antioxidant activity has been well demonstrated in previous studies [9,10]. Particularly, FX has shown to enhance AKT/ nuclear factor (erythroid-derived 2)-like 2 (Nrf2)/glutathione (GSH)-dependent antioxidant response in keratinocytes [11]. Moreover, this carotenoid reduces wrinkle formation and epidermal hypertrophy in mice [12] and suppresses melanogenesis and prostaglandin synthesis [13]. In addition, FX has been proposed as a photoprotective compound by stimulating restoration of the skin barrier in UVA-induced sunburn [14]. However, the protective effect of a FX-containing topical formulation has not been described yet on a skin inflammatory model. The possibility to administer FX topically has been subjected to several drawbacks because of its molecular weight and lipophilicity. As it is known, the compound must diffuse across *stratum corneum* and tight junctions to achieve effective permeation. In this sense, topical dosage forms such as creams, ointments, lotions and gels are commonly used for enhancing the cutaneous penetration. Thus, their composition will affect the drug permeation [15]. Concerning FX, several preparations have been studied with this aim [16,17]; in all of them, the evaluation of cutaneous penetration is a useful approach to predict the safety and efficacy of formulations [18]. To date, previous papers have developed topical experiments in mice applying acetone-dissolved compounds on skin [12,19]. With the aim of solving the irritant effect of acetone for its use in humans, a previous study from our group recently evaluated a glycolipid fraction-containing cream formulation on the murine 12-O-tetradecanoylphorbol 13-acetate (TPA)-induced epidermal hyperplasia model. Our findings reported an anti-inflammatory effect of this formulation with no signs of toxicity [20].

In the present study, we evaluated the anti-inflammatory and antioxidant properties of FX-containing cream in both in vitro and in vivo models in order to justify its use as adjuvant in inflammatory skin pathologies in which sun exposition is recommended. Firstly, we carried out two in vitro models to elucidate its anti-inflammatory and antioxidant activity. Then, FX was dissolved in absolute ethanol to further be incorporated into several common topical formulations (ointment, cream or hydrophilic gel). Once a topical formulation was selected, we finally aimed to study its effect on the TPA-induced hyperplasia model in mice, which mimics psoriatic parameters in dorsal murine skin, and on the UVB-induced erythema model in hairless mice, which reproduces the consequences expected in humans receiving acute UVB radiation.

2. Results

2.1. Effect of FX on Cell Viability

The effect of FX on THP-1 macrophages and HaCaT cells viability was measured by using the sulforhodamine B (SRB) assay. Results from cytotoxicity study showed that none of the tested concentrations affected cell viability. The inhibitory concentration 50 (IC_{50}) (half maximal inhibitory concentration) was above 100 μM at 24 h after treatment (Table S1).

2.2. Effects of FX on TNF-α Production in LPS-Stimulated THP-1 Macrophages and IL-6 and IL-8 Production in TNF-α-Stimulated HaCaT Human Keratinocytes

Non-cytotoxic concentrations of FX were used to determinate its effect on pro-inflammatory cytokines in both THP-1 macrophages and human keratinocytes. As shown in Figure 1, all concentrations tested significantly reduced the production of inflammatory cytokines in both cell models. Interestingly, the pre-treatment with the carotenoid at 50 μM showed a significant reduction of tumor necrosis factor alpha (TNF-α) production in lipopolysaccharide (LPS)-stimulated THP-1 macrophages, reaching similar values to dexamethasone (Dex) ($p < 0.001$) (Figure 1A). In relation to interleukin (IL)-6 and IL-8 production in HaCaT keratinocytes, similar results were exhibited in cells pretreated with the highest dose of FX ($p < 0.001$) (Figure 1B,C).

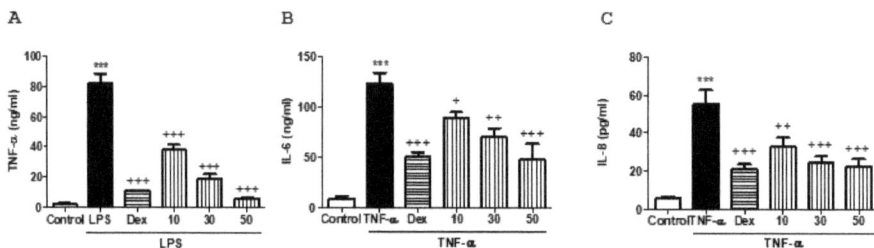

Figure 1. Effects of fucoxanthin (FX) on pro-inflammatory cytokines production in THP-1 macrophages and HaCaT keratinocytes. (**A**) Tumor necrosis factor alpha (TNF-α) in lipopolysaccharide (LPS)-stimulated THP-1 macrophages. (**B**) Interleukin (IL)-6 and (**C**) IL-8 in TNF-α-stimulated HaCaT keratinocytes. Cells were treated with FX (10, 30 and 50 μM) for 1 h, and then stimulated with LPS (1 μg/mL) in THP-1 macrophages or TNF-α (10 ng/mL) in HaCaT cells for 24 h. Dexamethasone (Dex) was used as positive reference compound at 1 μM. Production of cytokines in supernatant was measured by ELISA assay. Results are representative of six independent experiments. Values are means with standard errors represented by vertical bars. The mean value was significantly different compared with the control group (*** $p < 0.001$; Student t test). Mean value was significantly different compared with the LPS or TNF-α group (+ $p < 0.05$, ++ $p < 0.01$, +++ $p < 0.001$; one-way ANOVA followed by Bonferroni's Multiple Comparison test).

2.3. In Vitro Permeation Studies of BC from Different Topical Formulations

The objective of this study was to evaluate the in vitro permeation through artificial membranes of β-carotene (BC) from different topical formulations. BC was selected because of its structural similarity with FX. The formulations tested were: ethanolic solution as control, hydrogel, cream and ointment. BC was detected in the receiver medium in a time-dependent manner and profiles of cumulative amount of drug permeated have been obtained (Figure 2).

The permeation profiles showed the cream as the most favourable vehicle as penetration enhancer. When compared with the ethanolic control solution, a high percentage of BC permeated was obtained at a flux very similar to the control solution, as reported in Table 1. However, the ointment and hydrogel preparations made it difficult the pass through the membrane, probably due to their lipophilic and hydrophilic nature, respectively. This was visualized in terms of lower permeation percentages and flux rates. Hydrophilic cream provided the highest release of BC in comparison with lipophilic ointment or hydrogels, as previously reported for flavonoids [21]. Therefore, the hydrophilic cream (oil-in-water (OW) emulsion base) was chosen for incorporating FX and Dex for further studies. As these emulsions have hydrophilic external phase, they are miscible with water and skin secretions, thus they are not occlusive and are easily removed from skin.

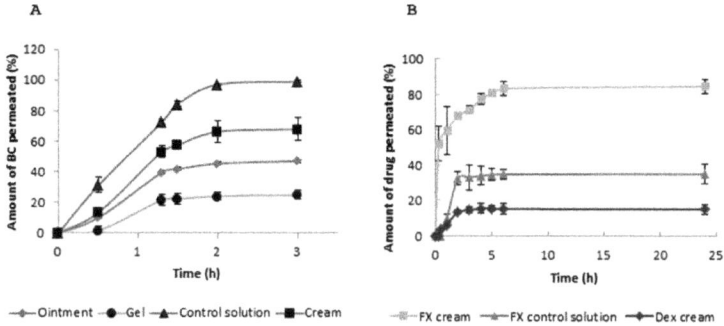

Figure 2. Permeation profiles. (**A**) In vitro permeation profile of β-Carotene (BC) from different topical formulations: cream, ointment and gel. BC dissolved in absolute ethanol was used as control solution. Artificial membranes impregnated with N-dodecanol mimicked the skin barrier. Absolute ethanol was used as release medium. (**B**) In vitro permeation profiles of fucoxanthin (FX) and dexamethasone (Dex) from cream formulation. FX dissolved in absolute ethanol was used as control solution. Dex-loaded cream was used as positive control. The experimental procedure was similar to that for BC. The percentages of drug release were obtained from the amount of drug that reached the receiver medium with time. These values are expressed in percentage, where 100% corresponds to the theoretical amount of drug added to the formulation. Data are represented as the mean ± standard error (*n* = 3).

Table 1. Total percentage permeated across artificial lipophilic membrane of β-carotene (BC) from different topical formulations, and flux rate (Jss) ($\mu g/cm^2 \cdot min$) calculated from the slope of amount permeated per area versus time.

Formulation	% Permeation (180 min)	Flux (Jss) ($\mu g/cm^2 \cdot min$)	r^2
Cream	68.38	0.1159	0.9795
Ointment	47.31	0.0548	0.9704
Hydrogel	25	0.0383	0.9403
Control	100	0.1350	0.9862

2.4. Ex Vivo Permeation Studies of FX-Containing Cream

Once the cream was selected as the vehicle for drug formulation, FX-loaded cream was prepared following the same methodology that for BC. In addition, Dex-loaded cream was formulated as positive control for the in vivo assay. The permeation profiles of FX contained in the hydrophilic cream were evaluated with the aim of analyzing the permeation behavior in the mice skin compared to an ethanolic control solution and Dex-cream.

Results showed a clear improvement of FX permeation with time (Figure 2). As evidenced from the area under the drug permeation curve (AUC) calculated (48,610, 19,914 and 8671%/h for FX-cream, FX control and Dex-cream, respectively), the cream vehicle offered a higher amount of FX permeated with time, whereas the control solution of this molecule showed a lower percentage. Although the ethanol acts as permeation enhancer, the cream composition, rich in surfactants, made the formulation improve the amount of FX to cross the membrane. Surprisingly, the permeation profile of Dex-cream showed 15%, approximately, of drug permeation. This lack of diffusion across the membrane could be attributed to a lower partition coefficient than FX (1.83 vs. 14.76). Dex has a lower molecular weight than FX, but the lipophilic nature of the carotenoid makes it a better candidate to interact with the surfactant components of the cream, which aids the solubilized molecule to reach the receiver medium.

2.5. Topical Application of FX-Containing Cream Decreases Skin Inflammation and Hyperplasia on the Murine TPA-Induced Model

To analyze whether topical pre-treatment with FX could reduce the in vivo inflammation, we studied this carotenoid on the murine TPA-induced epidermal hyperplasia model. Topical pre-treatment with FX-cream (100 mg per site containing 200 µg of FX) and Dex (100 mg per site containing 200 µg of Dex) was administered from 2 days before TPA-induced hyperplasia and 1 h after each TPA application (2 nmol per zone for three consecutive days). Then, 24 h after the last application of TPA, mice were sacrificed and skin biopsies were removed and weighted. Mice treated with TPA or TPA-cream resulted in the development of macroscopic lesions as peeling (Figure 3A), confirmed by an increase of weight of the 1 cm^2 punch biopsies of dorsal skin, in comparison with sham group ($p < 0.001$), with no significant differences between both groups (Figure 3B). This comparison led us to confirm that cream did not interfere in TPA action in our experiment. As expected, pre-treatment with the reference compound Dex significantly reduced the skin punch weight ($p < 0.001$). Similarly, mice treated with FX-cream showed a significant attenuation of skin edema when compared with TPA-cream group ($p < 0.001$) (Figure 3B). We next analyzed the skin homogenates to evaluate myeloperoxidase (MPO) activity as a neutrophil infiltration parameter with important relevance in hyperplasia model (Figure 3E). Our results confirm that this marker significantly increased after TPA application in comparison with sham group ($p < 0.01$). Dex application markedly diminished MPO activity in relation to TPA-cream group ($p < 0.01$). In a similar way, this parameter was reduced by FX-cream ($p < 0.05$) (Figure 3E). These results were confirmed with histological analysis of hematoxylin and eosin (H&E)-stained skin lesions in mice (Figure 3C), which showed that TPA administration produced a massive neutrophilic infiltration and an epidermal hyperplasia, because of uncontrolled and abnormal keratinocyte production. This effect was evidenced by a marked increase of epidermal thickness in this group ($p < 0.001$). Animals pre-treated with Dex and FX-cream evidenced a significant improvement in epidermal hyperplasia in relation to TPA-cream group ($p < 0.001$, and $p < 0.01$, respectively) (Figure 3C,D).

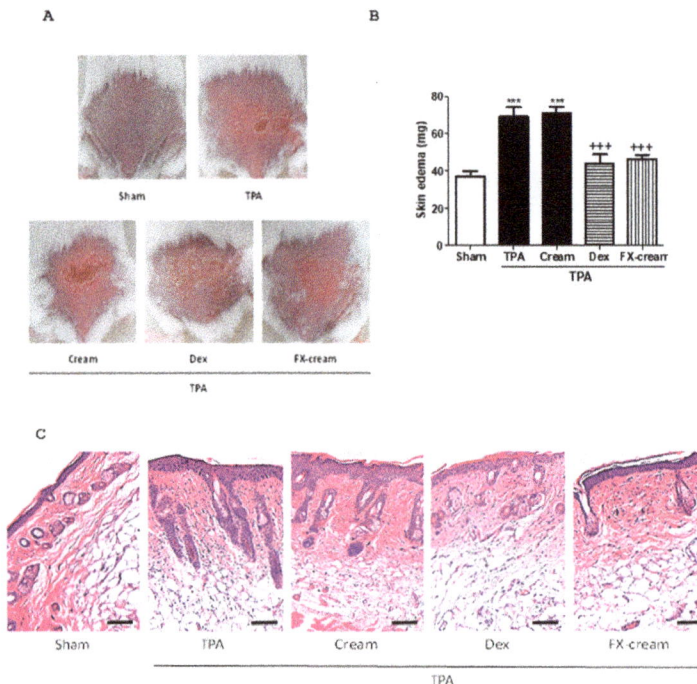

Figure 3. *Cont.*

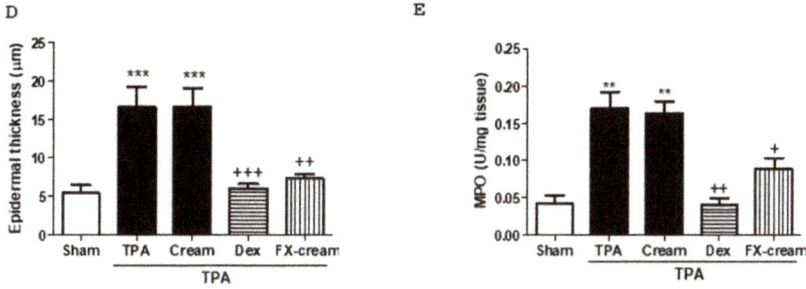

Figure 3. Fucoxanthin (FX) ameliorates skin hyperplasia and inflammation induced by 12-O-tetradecanoylphorbol-13-acetate (TPA) in mice (n = 10 mice/group). FX-cream formulation (100 mg per site at 200 μg), dexamethasone (Dex, 100 mg per site at 200 μg) or vehicle (cream with 0.2% ethanol) were topically administered as described in Material and methods. (**A**) Macroscopic mice back appearance at the end of experiment. (**B**) Skin edema as punch biopsy. (**C**) Histological appearance of mouse dorsal skin after hematoxylin/eosin (H&E)-staining; Bar = 10 mm. Original magnification 100× (**D**) Epidermal thickness assessment in H&E-stained skin slides. (**E**) Myeloperoxidase (MPO) activity. Values are means with standard errors represented by vertical bars. The mean value was significantly different compared with the sham group (** $p < 0.01$, *** $p < 0.001$; Student t test). The mean value was significantly different compared with TPA-cream group (+ $p < 0.05$, ++ $p < 0.01$, +++ $p < 0.001$; one-way ANOVA followed by Bonferroni's Multiple Comparison test).

To support the beneficial effects of FX on skin inflammation and explore its possible mechanism of action, we measured cyclooxygenase-2 (COX-2) expression in skin samples (Figure 4). This enzyme has been shown to have an important role in pathogenesis of skin diseases. Immunohistochemical analysis of this enzyme exhibited that TPA-induced hyperplasia significantly enhanced COX-2-positive cell numbers ($p < 0.001$), principally located in epidermal layer, in comparison with sham (Figure 4B). Figure 4 shows that the results of mice pre-treated with Dex confirmed the anti-inflammatory effect of this corticoid ($p < 0.001$). Interestingly, pre-treatment with FX-cream resulted in a marked decrease in the number of epidermal COX-2-positive stained cells related with TPA-cream group, reaching expression levels lower than those in Dex group ($p < 0.001$).

A

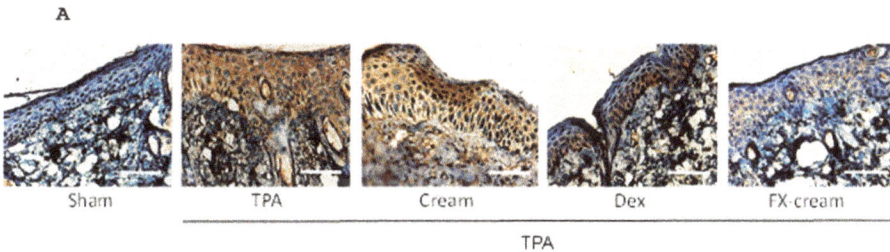

Figure 4. *Cont.*

B

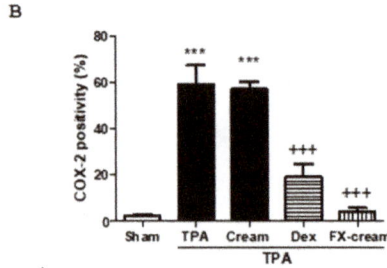

Figure 4. Topical application of fucoxanthin (FX) reduced 12-O-tetradecanoylphorbol-13-acetate (TPA)-induced epidermal cyclooxygenase-2 (COX-2) expression in mice. (**A**) Representative photographs of epidermal COX-2 distribution by immunohistochemical detection; Bar = 12.7 mm. Original magnification 200×. (**B**) Percentage of COX-2 positivity in epidermal layer was assessed by counting the number of COX-2 positive cells vs. total cells from 10 equal sections of immunostained dorsal skin per animal ($n = 3$). Values are means with standard errors represented by vertical bars. The mean value was significantly different compared with the sham group (*** $p < 0.001$; Student *t* test). The mean value was significantly different compared with TPA-cream group (+++ $p < 0.001$; one-way ANOVA followed by Bonferroni's Multiple Comparison test).

2.6. FX Protects Human HaCaT Keratinocytes against UVB-Caused Damage

To examine the protective effect of FX in irradiated HaCaT cells, we evaluated cell viability by lactate dehydrogenase (LDH) enzyme activity, ROS levels and IL-6 production after UVB exposure. As expected, UVB irradiation significantly increased LDH activity, ROS content and IL-6 production in HaCaT keratinocytes compared to unirradiated control ($p < 0.001$) (Figure 5A–C). Pre-treatment of cells with FX 1 h prior to UVB exposure significantly decreased UVB-induced mortality, preserving cell membrane integrity in a dose-dependent manner at all concentrations used (10, 30 and 50 μM, $p < 0.05$, $p < 0.01$, $p < 0.001$, respectively) (Figure 5A). We next evaluated intracellular ROS levels in UVB-irradiated cells based on the dichlorofluorescein diacetate (DCF-DA) assay (Figure 5B). FX markedly reduced ROS levels by 23, 31 and 32% at the concentration of 10, 30 and 50 μM, respectively ($p < 0.01$, $p < 0.001$, $p < 0.001$) (Figure 5B).

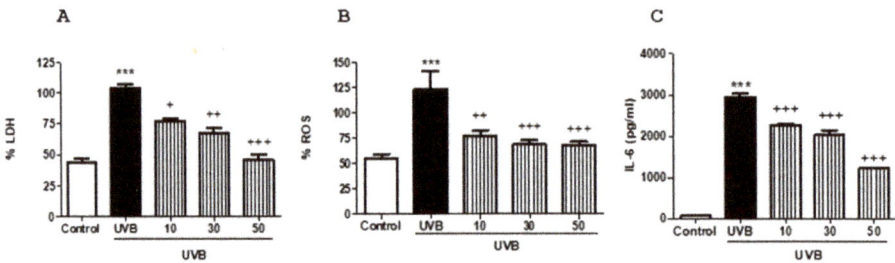

Figure 5. Protective effect of fucoxanthin (FX) on UVB-induced damage in HaCaT cells. Keratinocytes were preincubated with FX (10, 30 and 50 μM) for 1 h prior to UVB (50 mJ/cm^2) exposure. (**A**) After 24 h, cell viability was assessed by using lactate dehydrogenase (LDH) assay. (**B**) Intracellular reactive oxygen species (ROS) generation was measured 30 min after UVB irradiation by relative fluorescence intensity using dichlorofluorescin-diacetate (DCF-DA) assay. (**C**) Interleukin (IL)-6 production was evaluated by ELISA assay, 24 after UVB exposure. Cell viability and ROS production are expressed as percentage respect to UVB-irradiated cells and IL-6 levels as pg/mL. Results are representative of four independent experiments. Values are means with standard errors represented by vertical bars. The mean value was significantly different compared with the control group (*** $p < 0.001$; Student *t* test). The mean value was significantly different compared with UVB group (+ $p < 0.05$, ++ $p < 0.01$, +++ $p < 0.001$; one-way ANOVA followed by Bonferroni's Multiple Comparison test).

It is known that UVB exposure induces abnormally augmented cytokine production from keratinocytes, leading to inflammatory skin disorders. To evaluate the effect of FX on IL-6 production, HaCaT cells were pre-treated for 1 h with this carotenoid, and then were exposed to UVB. Pre-treatment with FX at the concentrations tested of 10, 30 and 50 µM substantially inhibited this cytokine levels by 23, 31 and 59%, respectively ($p < 0.001$) (Figure 5C).

2.7. Topical Application of FX-Containing Cream Protects against UVB-Induced Skin Erythema in SKH-1 Hairless Mice

The possible photoprotective effect of the topical pre-treatment with FX-cream in hairless mice was assayed using an acute proinflammatory UVB dose (360 mJ/cm^2) [22]. BC-cream was employed as reference compound due to its antioxidant and photoprotective activity [23]. Animals were examined with a dermatoscope for five days, evaluating UVB-induced skin alterations. As shown in Figure 6A, a single acute UVB exposure accelerated skin damage, showing typical symptoms such as peeling, loss of moisture, reduction of elasticity and increase of melanin production in comparison with sham controls (Figure 6A–D). The progressive evaluation of mice showed that pre-treatment with FX-cream increased the skin moisture (Figure 6B) and elasticity (Figure 6C) and decreased the production of melanin (Figure 6D), with similar values to BC-cream. In order to confirm the protective profile of FX, 48 h after UVB irradiation, the mice were sacrificed and dorsal skin was examined. Our data reflected significant increases of skin edema and MPO activity in UVB-irradiated group when compared with sham ($p < 0.001$). The reference group, BC-cream, showed pronounced lower levels of these parameters when compared to UVB-irradiated group ($p < 0.001$, $p < 0.05$, respectively) (Figure 6E,F). Similar results were found after pre-treatment with FX-cream (Figure 6E,F). These findings were confirmed by histological study by using H&E staining. Histologically, a significant increase in superficial skin layer thickness due to unregulated keratinocytes proliferation was detected in UVB-irradiated animals in comparison to sham ($p < 0.001$) (Figure 6G,H). FX-cream treatment was as effective as topical application of BC-cream; our data revealed a decrease in keratinocytes proliferation when compared to UVB-irradiated group, evidenced by a significant reduction of epidermal thickness ($p < 0.001$) (Figure 6G,H).

To further explore the possible mechanisms of action of FX, we examined the expression levels of different inflammatory and antioxidant proteins in dorsal skin samples. Exposure of skin to UVB induced a significant increase in the pro-inflammatory enzymes iNOS ($p < 0.001$) and COX-2 ($p < 0.001$) expression (Figure 7B,C). Neither of these proteins changed significantly in animals treated with the reference compound BC-cream. However, pre-treatment with FX-cream resulted in a significant downregulation of COX-2 expression levels in irradiated mice ($p < 0.05$) in comparison with UVB-irradiated animals. As regards the iNOS protein, although its expression tended to decrease in FX-cream-treated animals, no significant differences were observed in relation to UVB-treated mice. UVB exposure significantly down-regulated the expression of Nrf-2 protein ($p < 0.05$). BC-cream application induced a marked increase in Nrf2 levels ($p < 0.001$) accompanied with a rise of its target gene heme oxygenase-1 (HO-1) ($p < 0.05$). In a similar way, FX-cream significantly increased the expression of these antioxidant proteins in UVB-exposed skin ($p < 0.01$ and $p < 0.05$, respectively) (Figure 7D,E).

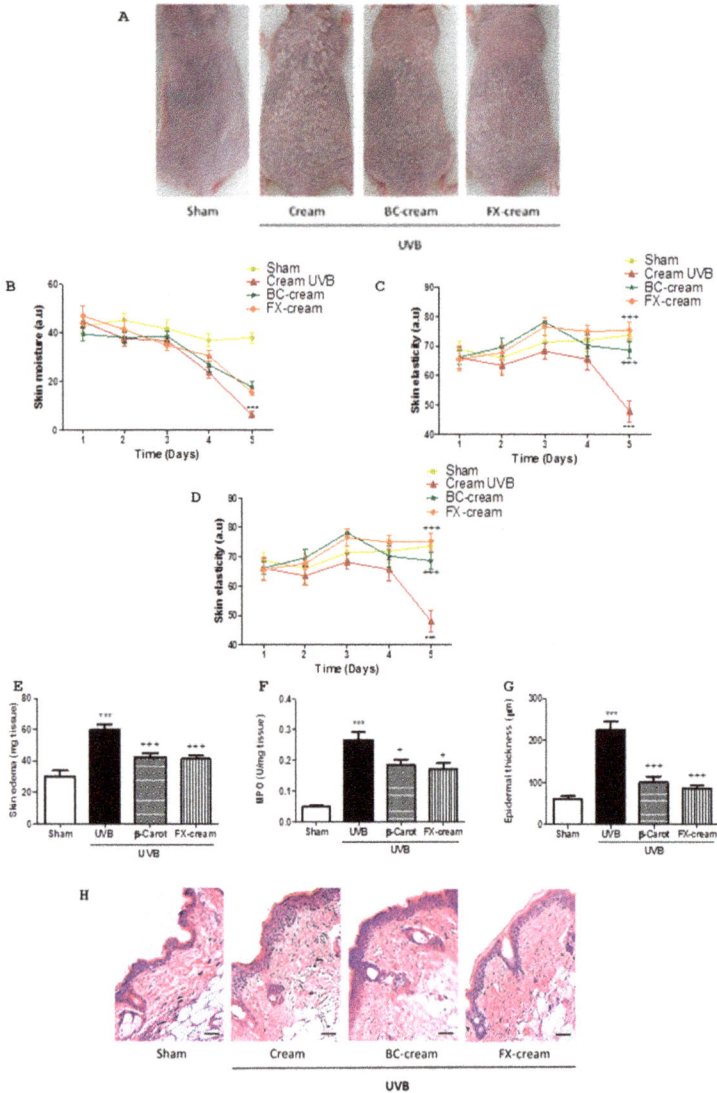

Figure 6. Fucoxanthin (FX) has photoprotective effects in UVB-induced erythema model in hairless mice (*n* = 8 mice/group). Mice received a single UVB radiation dose of 360 mJ/cm^2. FX-cream formulation (FX-cream, 100 mg per site at 200 µg), β-carotene-cream (BC-cream, 100 mg per site at 200 µg) or vehicle (cream with 0.2% ethanol) were topically administered as described in Material and methods. (**A**) Macroscopic mice back appearance at the end of experiment. (**B**) Skin moisture, (**C**) skin elasticity and (**D**) melanin index were evaluated during all experiment. (a.u), arbitrary units. (**E**) Determination of skin edema as punch biopsy weight. (**F**) Myeloperoxidase (MPO) activity. (**G**) Measurement of the epidermal thickness in hematoxylin/eosin (H&E)-stained skin slides. (**H**) Photomicrographs of mouse dorsal skin after H&E-staining; Bar = 10 mm. Original magnification 100×. Values are means with standard errors represented by vertical bars. The mean value was significantly different compared with the sham group (*** $p < 0.001$; Student *t* test). The mean value was significantly different compared with UVB-exposed group (+ $p < 0.05$, +++ $p < 0.001$; one-way ANOVA followed by Bonferroni's Multiple Comparison test).

A

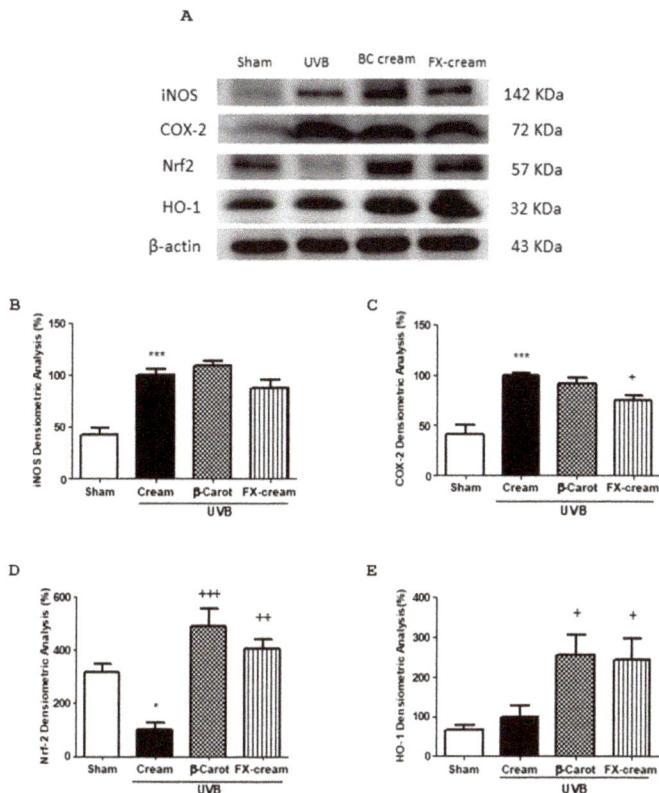

Figure 7. Anti-inflammatory and antioxidant effects of fucoxanthin (FX) in UVB-induced erythema model in hairless mice (n = 8 mice/group). Mice received a single UVB radiation dose of 360 mJ/cm^2. FX-cream formulation (100 mg per site at 200 μg), β-carotene-cream (BC-cream, 100 mg per site at 200 μg) or vehicle (cream with 0.2% ethanol) were topically administered as described in Material and methods. (**A**) Representative Western blot images of different skin proteins. Densitometric analysis of (**B**) inducible nitric oxide synthase (iNOS), (**C**) cyclooxygenase-2 (COX-2), (**D**) nuclear factor (erythroid-derived 2)-like 2 (Nrf2) and (**E**) heme oxygenase-1 (HO-1) proteins. Data were studied following normalization to the control (housekeeping gene, β-actin). Values are means with standard errors represented by vertical bars. The mean value was significantly different compared with the sham group (* $p < 0.05$, *** $p < 0.001$; Student t test). The mean value was significantly different compared with UVB-exposed group (+ $p < 0.05$, ++ $p < 0.01$, +++ $p < 0.001$ one-way ANOVA followed by Bonferroni's Multiple Comparison test).

3. Discussion

FX has formerly demonstrated in vitro and in vivo anti-inflammatory and antioxidant activities [11,14,24]. Nevertheless, the use of topical formulations such as cream/emulsion containing this carotenoid to prevent exacerbations related with skin inflammatory pathologies and provide a photoprotective effect has not been previously evidenced. Treatment of the skin with these topical formulations is a rational approach since avoids gastrointestinal degradation and preserves bioavailability [25].

Firstly, in the present study, we confirmed the in vitro anti-inflammatory activity of FX through decrease in TNF-α production in LPS-stimulated macrophages and reduction of IL-6 and IL-8 levels in TNF-α-stimulated HaCaT keratinocytes. These results led us to evaluate the possible preventive effects of this carotenoid on two in vivo acute skin inflammatory models: a hyperplasia model induced by multiple applications of TPA and an erythema model induced by a single UVB challenge.

Drug delivery across the skin remains as an important challenge in the development of drug delivery systems. This is mainly attributed to the highly organized intercellular lipids and poor permeability of *stratum corneum* [26]. It is also well-known that lipophilic molecules move across the barrier by a transcellular mechanism whereas hydrophilic agents are likely to follow a paracellular pathway to cross the skin. FX is lipophilic with a high partition coefficient (log P 6.83–7.54). To date, some studies with FX have been carried out by dissolving FX in ethanol for applying the drug dissolved onto the skin [12]. However, this solvent is known to produce dryness effect in the skin. To improve FX topical application, various hydrophilic and lipid-based formulations have been developed, firstly using BC as model drug because of its structural similarity to FX [27]. In this sense, new approaches are desirable in order to avoid the use of uncomfortable formulations such as paraffin [13]. In order to have a prediction of the in vivo permeation behaviour of the drug and to avoid the expensive cost of the use of animals or human skin, alternative artificial skin diffusion apparatus was used for conducting in vitro permeation studies. As regards the formulations tested (cream, ointment and hydrogel), it was found that lipid-based formulations improved most efficiently the diffusion of BC through the permeation membrane in a Franz diffusion cell. In contrast, water-based formulations, such as Carbopol gel, exhibited poor penetration. The composition of cream, which was highly charged in surfactants, makes it to act as a permeation enhancer that changes the atmosphere of the lipids to encourage the diffusion of lipid molecules (BC or FX) and/or influence their solubility [28]. The blend of agents with polar and non-polar properties, which probably mimic the complex lipid/polar nature of the *stratum corneum*, makes the cream thermodynamically similar to the *stratum corneum*, enabling the permeation of BC through the skin. Other authors incorporated surfactant-like molecules (D-α-tocopheryl polyethylene glycol 1000 succinate) into the formulations for synergistically acting with ethanol as solubilizing agents of griseofulvin [29]. This is the reason why formulations too occlusive and lipophilic (ointment) make difficult the permeation process of poorly water-soluble compounds. On the contrary, concerning the highly hydrophilic formulations (gel), it is known that water can generate a resistant boundary at the donor-skin interface (impregnated in our artificial membranes with dodecanol) and may prolong or delay the permeation of poorly water-soluble molecules such as BC.

Once we selected the cream as a vehicle for our studies, we proceeded to elucidate the FX behaviour in terms of permeation kinetics through a comparative study with control solution and Dex-cream. This carotenoid has been previously formulated in O/W formulations by other authors [16]. Our results showed that, under the experimental conditions used, FX-cream has a higher permeability though artificial membrane than the other formulations (control solution FX and Dex-cream). Other authors reported that the differences in penetration might be associated with the variation in the lipophilicity of the tested compounds [30], as obtained in this case. Although Dex has a lower molecular weight than FX, which might favour the diffusion across the membrane, its low lipophilicity (log P 1.83) compared to FX, makes more difficult this passage, showing permeation profiles more reduced [26]. The efficacy of FX-loaded O/W emulsions has been demonstrated as anti-obesity formulations being prepared by using medium chain triglyceride as an oil phase and l-α-phosphatidylcholine as an emulsifier [17,31]. This heterogeneous disperse system has been also used for incorporating other antioxidant molecules such as green tea polyphenols with the aim of preventing UVB-induced oxidation of lipids in mouse skin [21]. Thus, hydrophilic cream may serve as an optimal delivery system for FX use in animal models.

TPA is an activator of protein kinase C isoenzymes and a well-known inducer of inflammatory response in murine skin rising expression of the inflammation mediators [32]. TPA-induced hyperplasia model in dorsal murine skin reproduces typical manifestations of inflammatory skin pathologies as psoriasis. In this regards, TPA administration causes macroscopic lesions such as erythema or peeling, as well as increment of epidermis thickness by hyperproliferation and aberrant differentiation of keratinocytes or leukocytes infiltration into the dermis and consequent cytokines and chemokines production [33]. The pre-treatment with FX-cream ameliorated skin hyperplasia reducing MPO activity, as indicatory of leucocyte infiltration, and skin edema. These results were related with the improvement of histological damage by reducing epidermal thickness and neutrophil infiltration, getting similar levels to those of the reference corticosteroid Dex. The relation between epidermal differentiation and COX-2 expression has been strongly reported, as well as their connection with the pathogenesis of psoriasis [34]. In this sense, repeated applications of TPA in dorsal murine skin induce inflammation symptoms that are accompanied by COX-2 epidermal overexpression in relation with healthy group [35]. Our data evidenced a reduced COX-2 expression in mice treated with FX, presenting lower levels than those in Dex group. These findings, at least partly, suggest that suppression of COX-2 expression may be involved in the preventive effect of this carotenoid on TPA-induced epidermal hyperplasia. Our results are in agreement with previous in vitro studies that showed the capacity of FX to modulate inflammatory response through inhibition of COX-2 and iNOS expression and the consequent decrease of NO and prostaglandin E2 levels [24,36]. The molecular mechanisms underlying the anti-inflammatory properties of FX may be associated with the suppression of nuclear factor-kappaB and mitogen-activated protein kinase pathways, similar to those previously reported for Dex in skin inflammatory pathologies [37]. More recently, FX has shown to downregulate COX-2 levels in a murine model of high-fat-diet-induced obesity [38]. It is well known that inflammatory pathologies as psoriasis require long-term topical corticosteroids therapy, which is associated with both topical and systemic adverse effects. Moreover, the chronic use of these compounds may increase tendency to "steroid addiction syndrome", which forces to change the corticoid and select one more potent [39]. For these reasons, the use of a well-tolerated immune-modulatory topical formulation containing FX could offer a safer alternative to continued use of corticoids for the treatment of skin inflammatory disorders.

Additionally, it is worth highlighting that since these pathologies benefit from therapeutic sun exposure, it is very important to assure the photoprotection of exposed skin. Sunscreens are used to prevent the deleterious effects of UVB due to this radiation remains as an important risk factor to develop skin lesions [40]. In this sense, further therapeutic strategies targeting UVB-induced inflammation and oxidative stress are necessary. Thus, our next objective was to examine the photoprotective effects of FX in an UVB-induced cell damage model in HaCaT keratinocytes, as well as on an UVB-induced erythema model in hairless mice in order to complete the functional activity study of this compound as adjuvant treatment in skin inflammatory disorders. It is well known that UVB irradiation induces cell cytotoxicity through loss of cellular membrane integrity, which leads to liberation of LDH enzyme from cytosol to the culture medium [41]. Moreover, UVB radiation causes increased ROS production and DNA damage, as well as a strong inflammatory response, characterized by the production of inflammatory cytokines, such as IL-6, which leads to premature skin aging and carcinomas [42]. Recently, it has been demonstrated that the antioxidative role of FX in HaCaT keratinocytes is related to DNA protection against oxidative stress and the prevention of apoptosis [43,44]. According with these results, we have shown that pre-treatment of HaCaT keratinocytes with FX significantly attenuated UVB-induced damage by increasing cell viability and inhibiting ROS and IL-6 levels.

In relation to in vivo alterations, acute UVB radiation promotes erythema, edema and loss of skin moisture and elasticity, as well as increases melanin production, which is involved in melanogenesis. Recently, several studies have revealed the photoprotective effects of FX in UVB-irradiated mice by reducing melanogenesis parameters [13] and in UVA-induced sunburn by promotion of skin barrier formation [14]. In addition, this carotenoid prevented skin photoaging in hairless mice through its antiangiogenic and antioxidant effects [12]. Herein, we report that the topical pre-treatment with FX-cream formulation ameliorated erythema induced by UVB as well as edema and MPO activity, which are important inflammation and neutrophil recruitment parameters. Overexpression of COX-2 is highly related to some carcinomas including skin cancer [45]. In this regard, and in accordance to the above results from TPA model, we also reported the reduction of COX-2 expression by FX-cream pre-treatment on UVB-exposed skin, effect not observed upon BC administration.

It has been reported that excessive ROS generation results in oxidative stress in skin cells and plays a vital role in the initiation, promotion and progression of skin aging, carcinogenesis and many inflammatory disorders [46]. In this respect, Nrf2 is a transcription factor that perceives variation in cellular oxidative stress and promotes the transcription of antioxidant genes and detoxification enzymes such as HO-1 to protect against UVB-induced oxidative damage [47,48]. An in vitro study has elicited the antioxidant activity of FX by enhancing the Akt/Nrf2/GSH pathways in human keratinocytes [11]. Moreover, FX has been recently shown to be able to activate Nrf2 signalling pathway by inducing demethylation of CpG sites in Nrf2 [49]. In accordance with these results, our data reported that FX and BC offer a similar protection against oxidative stress caused by UVB exposure via increase of Nrf2 expression and its downstream target HO-1. However, in a previous paper FX was confirmed to have higher antioxidative effects than BC, due to its more polar nature and consequent placement in the cell membrane [50]. In the present study, although the two carotenoids have shown to have similar antioxidant properties, FX provides additional benefits, exhibiting an anti-inflammatory activity by downregulating COX-2 expression after UVB irradiation. These findings propose this carotenoid as a natural approach for protecting skin against UV radiation and modulating the inflammatory response associated.

4. Materials and Methods

4.1. Cell Culture

The THP-1 human monocytic leukemia cell line and HaCaT human keratinocytes were obtained from the American Type Culture Collection (ATCC, Manassas, VA, USA). THP-1 cells were cultured in RPMI 1640 medium (GIBCO, Grand Island, New York, NY, USA) containing 10% heat-inactivated fetal bovine serum (FBS), 100 U/mL penicillin and 100 µg/mL streptomycin. HaCaT human keratinocytes were maintained in high glucose Dulbecco's modified Eagle's medium (DMEM, GIBCO, Grand Island, New York, NY, USA). Both cell lines were grown in a humidified atmosphere containing 5% CO_2 at 37 °C [20].

4.2. Cell Viability Assay

SRB assay was used for determining the viability of THP-1 macrophages and HaCaT cells upon exposure to FX (Sigma-Aldrich, St. Louis, MO, USA) [51]. Firstly, for differentiation into macrophages, THP-1 cells were seeded into 96-well plates at 10^4 cells/well in presence of phorbol 12-myristate 13-acetate (PMA, Sigma-Aldrich, St. Louis, MO, USA) for a final concentration of 0.2 µM for 72 h in 96-well plates and HaCaT cells were seeded into 96-well plates in the growth medium at 10^4 cells/well for 24 h to ensure the adherence. Both cellular types were incubated in a humidified atmosphere of 5% CO_2 at 37 °C. After that, cells were treated with FX at final concentrations range of 10–100 µM in DMSO 0.1% (v/v) and the cytotoxicity was measured after 24, 48 and 72 h of incubation. The absorbance was determined at 492 nm in a microplate spectrophotometer (Sinergy HT, Biotek®, Bad Friedrichshall, Germany).

4.3. Determination of TNF-α Production

THP-1 monocytes were differentiated into macrophages in 96-well plates (10^4 cells/well). Then, cells were incubated for 1 h with FX (10, 30 and 50 µM). The positive reference compound used was Dex (1 µM) (Sigma-Aldrich, St. Louis, MO, USA). Inflammatory response was induced by addition of LPS (1 µg/mL) except for control group [52]. After 24 h, commercial enzyme-linked immunosorbent assay (ELISA) kit (Diaclone GEN-PROBE, Besançon, France) was used to quantify TNF-α according to the manufacturer's protocol.

4.4. Determination of IL-6 and IL-8 Production

HaCaT cells were seeded in 6-well plates (5×10^5 cells/well). After 24 h, cells were washed twice (PBS, 4 °C) and medium containing FX (10, 30 and 50 μM) or Dex (1 μM) was added for 1 h, and then cells were stimulated with TNF-α (10 ng/mL) except for control group. After 24 h, supernatant fluids were collected and stored −80 °C until measurements [20]. Commercial enzyme-linked immunosorbent assay (ELISA) kit (Diaclone GEN-PROBE, Besançon, France) was used to quantify IL-6 and IL-8 according to the manufacturer's protocol.

4.5. Preparation of Topical Formulations

Based on previous studies, topical formulations were performed following the methodology detailed in Rodríguez-Luna et al. [20]. Thus, three different preparations were developed: hydrogel, cream and ointment. Concerning the hydrogel, BC (Sigma-Aldrich, St. Louis, MO, USA) solution in ethanol absolute (10 mg/mL) was gradually added to the polymer dispersion (1% *w/v*) under magnetic stirring. The ointment was prepared using both the melt emulsification and stirring steps. BC dissolved in ethanol (10 mg/mL) was added to the lipid mixture. Regarding cream, three different preparations were made containing 2 mg/g of drug (BC, FX or Dex). In all of them, the drug was dissolved in absolute ethanol (10 mg/mL) and added to the excipient cold mixture.

4.6. In Vitro Permeation Studies from Topical Formulations

In vitro drug permeation studies from the topical formulations were performed using a Franz diffusion cell apparatus (SES-Gmgh Analyses system, Bechenheim, Germany), with 14.5 mL receptor volume and 3.14 cm^2 diffusion area. An appropriately conditioned cellulose nitrate membrane (Tuffryn®; Pall Corporation, Port Washington, New York, NY, USA), impregnated with lauryl alcohol (membrane weight increase 90–110%), was employed as artificial lipophilic membrane simulating the epidermal barrier [53,54]. The membrane was placed in the diffusion cell sandwiching the donor and receptor compartments. The receiver solution contained absolute ethanol and the donor chamber was filled with 1 g of formulation at 2 mg/g of BC (cream, ointment or hydrogel). In this study, BC was employed as reference compound because of its structural similarity with FX. The whole diffusion cell was thermostated maintaining the temperature at 32 °C. Aliquots of 0.5 mL were withdrawn from the receptor chamber after 0.5, 1, 1.5, 2 and 3 h and replaced with fresh ethanol. The concentrations of BC were spectrometrically assayed at 454 nm (UV/vis 1601 Shimadzu, Duisburg, Germany). The cumulative amounts of permeated drug per unit area in the receiver chamber (μg/cm^2) were plotted as a function of time (h). The slope of the linear portion of the plot was presented as steady state flux (Jss, μg/cm^2/h). From the permeation profiles, the AUC was calculated using the trapezoidal rule as a quantitative parameter for studying the permeation magnitude [55].

4.7. Animals

Female Swiss CD-1 mice (25–30 g) were purchased from Janvier-Labs (Le Genest St Isle, France) and female SKH-1 hairless mice (18–20 g) from Charles River Laboratories (Écully, France). Mice were maintained under standard conditions (temperature of 24–25 °C, humidity of 70–75% and 12 h light-12 h dark cycle) and were allowed free access to a standard diet (Panlab) and water *ad libitum*. All studies were performed in accordance with the recommendations of the European Union regarding animal experimentation (Directive of the European Council 2010/63/EU). The experiments followed protocols approved by the Animal Ethics Committee of the University of Seville (Protocol 06/04/2018/042).

4.8. Ex Vivo Permeation Studies from Creams

Once the cream carrier was chosen from the previous study, ex vivo diffusion studies were performed using excised mice skin as a membrane for evaluating the permeation behaviour of

FX-loaded cream. Moreover, Dex-cream was included because it was used as positive control in the in vivo hyperplasia study. Swiss CD-1 mice were sacrificed by cervical dislocation and full dorsal skin was excised. A specific portion of the skin was washed with distilled water and cut for the permeation assay. The study was carried out following the methodology previously reported [56]. Animal skin was inserted between the donor and receiving compartments and adjusted by means of a pinch clamp. The receiving chamber was filled with 14.5 mL of degassed ethanol absolute and was thermostated by means of a water bath circulator and a jacket surrounding the cell, maintaining 32 °C in the skin surface. The receiving medium was continuously stirred to avoid diffusion layer effect.

FX-cream (0.2% *w/w*), FX control solution in ethanol (0.2% *w/w*) and Dex-cream (0.2% *w/w*) were accurately measured and placed on stratum corneum in the donor compartment and sealed with parafilm. The same procedure as previously described was followed [56]. Absolute ethanol was used as solvent in the receiver compartment. The concentrations of Dex were spectrometrically assayed at 254 nm (UV/vis 1601 Shimadzu). The FX content in the ethanol solutions was analyzed by using HPLC method. The analysis was performed on a Hitachi Elite Lachron HPLC system equipped with a L-2130 isocratic pump, a diode array detector L-2455 and a L-2200 autosampler. Separation was carried out within a chromatographic C18 column (Merck, RP-18 LichroCART® 150 mm × 4 mm, 5 μm). For drug analysis, the injection volume was 10 μL, and the flow rate and column temperature were set at 1.0 mL/min and 25 °C, respectively. The mobile phase consisted of A (formic acid 0.1%) and B (acetonitrile). The elution program was: 6 min isocratic at 90% B, followed by a gradient to 100% B at 10 min. Afterwards, the column was re-equilibrated during 5 min at 90% B. The cumulative amount of drug in receptor chamber for the three formulations (FX-cream, FX control solution and Dex-cream) was measured as a function of time (t, h). The cumulative amount (%) of drug permeated through the skin (*P%*) was determined as per the following equation [57]:

$$P\% = \frac{C_n \cdot V + \sum_{i=1}^{n-1} C_i \cdot V_i}{M} \cdot 100 \tag{1}$$

where C_n is the drug concentration of the *n*th sampling point (mg/mL), C_i is the drug concentration of the *i*th sample point (mg/mL), V is the total volume (14.5 mL) of liquid in receiving pool, V_i is the volume (0.5 mL) of the *i*th sampling points and M is the mass of drug (FX or Dex) [20].

4.9. TPA-Induced Epidermal Hyperplasia Model and Treatments

Female Swiss CD-1 mice (*n* = 10 per group) were used to study the effect of FX on TPA-induced hyperplasia in mice dorsal skin. Briefly, the dorsal hair of animals was removed with an electric clipper and treated with depilatory cream (Deliplus, Barcelona, Spain) [35]. After 24 h, the animals were assigned to the different groups: Sham (vehicle: 100 mg of cream with 0.2% of ethanol); TPA control group; TPA-Cream (vehicle: 100 mg of cream with 0.2% of ethanol); Dex-cream (100 mg of cream per site, containing 200 μg of Dex dissolved in ethanol at 10 μg/mL); FX-cream formulation (100 mg of cream per site, containing 200 μg of FX dissolved in ethanol at 10 μg/mL). The creams were applied to the dorsal skin in an area of 1 cm² using a syringe, during 2 days before the hyperplasia induction. Mice were anesthetized with ketamine (100 mg/kg of animal) and diazepam (5 mg/kg of animal) during treatments and TPA challenge. On day 4, TPA (2 nmol of TPA, dissolved in 20 μL of ethanol) was topically applied to the same areas on all groups except in sham group. After 1 h, FX-cream, the Dex-cream or vehicle were administered following the mentioned protocol. This procedure was replicated during two consecutive days. After 24 h of the last TPA dorsal application (day 7), mice were sacrificed by cervical dislocation and punch biopsies from the treated dorsal skin were weighed to evaluate edema, before further processing for histology and biochemical parameters.

4.10. MPO Activity

The measurement of MPO activity was used as a marker of neutrophil infiltration [58]. The tissue was thawed, weighed and homogenized in 10 volumes of 50 mM-PBS (pH 7.4). Then, the homogenate was centrifuged at 20,000× g for 20 min at 4 °C and the pellet was again homogenized in 10 volumes of 50 mM-PBS (pH 6) containing hexadecyl trimethylammonium bromide (0.5%) and 10 mM-EDTA. This homogenate was subjected to one cycle of freezing/thawing and sonicated. The homogenate samples (50 μL) were added to 96-well microplate and incubated at 37 °C for 3 min with a measurement mix (*o*-dianisidine dihydrochloride (0.067%), hexadecyl trimethyl-ammonium bromide (0.5%) and 0.3 mM-H_2O_2). The changes in absorbance were monitorized at 450 nm with a microplate reader (Labysystem Multiskan EX, Thermo Scientific, New York, NY, USA). MPO activity unit was defined as the amount of enzyme present that produced a change in absorbance of 1.0 unit/min at 37 °C in the final reaction volume containing acetate. Results are expressed as units/mg tissue [20].

4.11. Histological Study

The samples were fixed in paraformaldehyde, dehydrated by increasing concentrations of ethanol and embedded in paraffin. For H&E stains, tissue sections were cut to 7 μm on a rotary microtome (Leica Microsystems, Wetzlar, Germany), mounted on slides, deparaffinized with xylene, rehydrated through graded alcohols and stained according to standard protocols. All tissue sections were examined under an Olympus BH-2 microscope (GMI Inc., Ramsey, MN, USA) for determination of histopathological changes. Epidermal thickness was measured by using Scientific Imaging Systems (Biophotonics ImageJ Analysis Software; National Institutes of Health, Rockville, MD, USA).

4.12. Immunohistochemical Analysis

COX-2 expression was measured by immunohistochemical analysis by using a streptavidin-biotin-peroxidase method [59]. Paraffin-embedded dorsal skin sections (7 μm) were mounted on slides, deparaffinized with xylene and rehydrated through graded alcohols. These sections were boiled (10 mM citrate buffer (pH 6.0) for 3 min) for antigen retrieval, followed by cooling at room temperature for 20 min. Endogenous peroxidase was quenched with 0.3% (v/v) hydrogen peroxide for 20 min and the sections were washed (PBS, 10 min). To minimize the non-specific adsorption the sections were incubated in normal horse serum (Vectastain Kit; Vector Laboratories, Burlingame, CA, USA) for 20 min. Afterwards, slides were incubated with rabbit polyclonal anti-COX-2 antibody (Cayman Chemical, Ann Arbor, MI, USA) (1:300) overnight at 4 °C. Then, the samples were treated with anti-mouse IgG antibody. After 30 min, the cells were incubated with the streptavidin–peroxidase complex for 30 min, at room temperature (Vectastain Kit; Vector Laboratories, Burlingame, CA, USA). The enzymatic activities were developed with 3,3′-diaminobenzidine (DAB), and the sections were counterstained with hematoxylin. Negative control sections were treated in the same way, omitting the primary antibody. To examine COX-2 immunoreactivity, the microscope Olympus BX61 was used (Olympus Optical Co. Ltd., Tokyo, Japan). The quantification of immunohistochemical data was done by counting the number of immunostained cells as percent of total epidermal cells from 10 microscopic fields of immunostained tissues per animal.

4.13. UVB Irradiation of HaCaT Keratinocytes

Human keratinocytes were exposed to UVB radiation as previously described [60]. Briefly, the cells were grown to confluence and were treated with different concentrations of FX (10, 30 and 50 μM) for 1 h. Then, the medium was removed and a thin layer of PBS was added. Cells were exposed to a single dose of UVB radiation (50 mJ/cm^2) for 1 min. The UVB source was a CL-1000M UV Crosslinker (UVP, Upland, CA, USA), which was used to deliver an energy spectrum of UVB light (280–315 nm; peak intensity, 302 nm). After UVB irradiation, the cells were supplied with fresh complete medium and incubated for 24 h.

4.14. Analysis of Intracellular LDH Activity

The measure of cytosolic enzyme LDH is one of the commonly used methods for assessing loss of cellular membrane integrity. The assay is based on the conversion of lactate to pyruvate in the presence of LDH with the consequence oxidation of NADH as previously described [61]. HaCaT cells were seeded in 6-well plates (5×10^5 cells/well). After 24 h, cells were treated with FX (10, 30 and 50 μM) for 1 h and then, were irradiated with UVB. After 24 h, cell-free supernatants and cell lysates were mixed in a 96-well plate and the absorbance was read by using a microplate reader system (Sinergy HT, Biotek®, Bad Friedrichshall, Germany). LDH leakage was estimated calculating the LDH activity in the cell-free medium and LDH activity in lysates ratio. Results were represented as the percentage (%) of change in activity compared with the control cells.

4.15. Intracellular ROS Scavenging Activity

For quantification of ROS in HaCaT cells, the DCF-DA assay was employed [62]. HaCaT cells were seeded in nin96-well plates (10^4 cells/well). Non-irradiated cells were used as negative control. After 24 h, cells were treated with FX (10, 30 and 50 μM) for 1 h and then, were exposed to UVB. Post irradiation, cells were incubated with 2′,7′-dichlorodihydrofluorescein diacetate (DCFH-DA) solution (5 mg/mL) in PBS for 30 min [63]. The fluorescence of the 2′,7′-dichlorofluorescein (DCF) product was determined using a fluorescence plate reader (Sinergy HT, Biotek®, Bad Friedrichshall, Germany) at 485 nm for excitation and 535 nm for emission.

4.16. Determination of IL-6 Production in UVB-Exposed HaCaT Keratinocytes

HaCaT cells (5×10^5 cells/well) were seeded in 6-well plates. After 24 h, cells were treated with FX (10, 20 and 50 μM) for 1 h and then, were exposed to UVB. After 24 h, supernatant fluids were collected and ELISA kit (Diaclone GEN-PROBE, Besançon, France) was employed to quantify IL-6 according to the manufacturer's protocol. The absorbance at 450 nm was read by a microplate reader (Labysystem Multiskan EX, Thermo Scientific, New York, NY, USA).

4.17. UVB-Induced Erythema in Hairless Mice

Female SKH-1 hairless mice ($n = 8$ per group) were used to study the effect of FX on UVB-induced erythema. Animals were distributed to the different groups: Sham (vehicle: 100 mg of cream with 0.2% of ethanol); UVB (100 mg of cream with 0.2% of ethanol); BC-cream (100 mg of cream per site, containing 200 μg of BC dissolved in ethanol at 10 μg/μL) as reference control; FX-cream (100 mg per site, containing 200 μg of FX dissolved in ethanol at 10 μg/μL). The formulations were applied on the dorsal skin (1 cm²/area) by using a syringe, and starting 2 days before irradiation. On day 3, 30 min after application of the substances, all groups except the sham control were exposed to an acute UVB dose (360 mJ/cm²) as previously described [22]. Then, 48 h after UVB exposure, mice were macroscopically evaluated and sacrificed. At this end-point time, a pronounced UVB-induced cutaneous inflammation was shown [4].

4.18. Dermatoscope Measurements

Dorsal skin was macroscopically examined every day by using a multi-dermatoscope (Dermatoscope MDS 800, Microcaya, Bilbao, Spain). Corneometer® was used to determinate the hydration in the *stratum corneum* through electrical capacitance of the skin surface [64]. A Cutometer® probe was used as suction method to analyse the real elasticity of skin [65]. In the last step, Mexameter® was employed to analyse the redness skin by melanin index [66]. Every day, dorsal skin of mice was assessed twice and finally the results were expressed in arbitrary units (a. u.) or by a melanin index scale (1-36).

4.19. Western Blot Assay

Frozen dorsal skin tissues from UVB-induced erythema model were randomly selected (6 per group), weighed and homogenized in ice-cold buffer (50 mM Tris-HCl, pH 7.5, 8 mM MgCl₂, 5 mM ethylene glycol bis (2-aminoethyl ether)-N,N,N′,N′-tetra acetic acid, 0.5 mM EDTA, 0.01 mg/mL leupeptin, 0.01 mg/mL pepstatin, 0.01 mg/mL aprotinin, 1 mM phenylmethylsulfonyl fluoride, and 250 mM NaCl). The homogenates were centrifuged ($12,000 \times g$, 15 min, 4 °C), and the supernatants were collected and stored at −80 °C. To determinate the protein concentration of the homogenates was used the Bradford colorimetric method [67]. Samples of the supernatants with equal amounts of protein (25 µg) were separated on 10% acrylamide gel by sodium dodecyl sulfate polyacrylamide gel electrophoresis. Then, the proteins were electrophoretically transferred onto a nitrocellulose membrane and incubated with specific primary antibodies: rabbit anti-inducible nitric oxide synthase (iNOS) (1:1000; Stressgen-Enzo Life Sciences, Farmingdale, NY, USA); rabbit anti-COX-2 (1:3000; Cayman Chemical®, Ann Arbor, MI, USA); rabbit anti-Nrf2, rabbit anti-HO-1 (1:1000; Cell Signaling, Danvers, MA, USA) overnight at 4 °C. After rinsing, the membranes were incubated with the horseradish peroxidase-linked (HRP) secondary antibody anti-rabbit (1:1000; Cayman Chemical®, Ann Arbor, MI, USA) or anti-mouse (1:1000; Dako®, Atlanta, GA, USA) containing blocking solution for 1 h at room temperature. To prove equal loading, the blots were analyzed for β-actin expression using an anti-β-actin antibody (1:1000; Sigma Aldrich®, St. Louis, MO, USA). Immunodetection was performed using an enhanced chemiluminescence light-detecting kit (SuperSignal West Pico Chemiluminescent Substrate, Pierce, IL, USA). Then, the immunosignals were monitorized by using LAS-3000 Imaging System (Fujifilm Image Reader, Valhalla, NY, USA) and densitometric data were studied after normalization to the control (housekeeping gene). The signals were analyzed and quantified with a Scientific Imaging Systems (Biophotonics ImageJ Analysis Software, National Institute of Mental Health, Bethesda, MD, USA) and expressed as percentage respect to sham control group [68].

4.20. Statistical Analysis

All values in the figures and text are expressed as arithmetic means ± SEM. Data were evaluated with GraphPad Prism version 5.00 software (GraphPad Software, Inc., San Diego, CA, USA). In all cases, the Shapiro-Wilk test was used to verify the normality of the data. The Mann-Whitney U-test was chosen for non-parametric values. The parametric values groups were analyzed by one-way analysis of variance (ANOVA) followed by Bonferroni's Multiple Comparison Test. p values < 0.05 were considered statistically significant.

5. Conclusions

In conclusion, the in vitro anti-inflammatory, antioxidant and protective activity of FX has been confirmed in human keratinocytes. Furthermore, we have demonstrated for the first time the anti-inflammatory activity of a topical formulation containing FX in hyperplasic skin, reducing cell infiltrate and epidermal COX-2 expression, which has a main role in the progression of hyperplasia and the consequent skin damage. In addition, this carotenoid protects mice against superficial skin damage induced by UVB through inhibition of inflammatory mediators and promotion of antioxidant responses through Nrf2 pathway. For these reasons, FX, administered in a well-tolerated topical formulation and that improves its permeation, could be a novel natural adjuvant for preventing exacerbations associated with skin inflammatory pathologies as well as protecting skin against UV radiation.

Supplementary Materials: The following is available online at http://www.mdpi.com/1660-3397/16/10/378/s1, Table S1: Viability of THP-1 human macrophages and HaCaT human keratinocytes cells treated with different concentrations of fucoxanthin (FX). Values are mean ± ES (%) of three independent experiments ($n = 3$).

Author Contributions: The authors' contributions are follows: E.T., V.M. and J.Á.-R. designed the study protocol; A.R.-L., J.Á.-R. and E.T., conducted the in vivo and histological experiments and analysed the data; A.R.-L., M.J.C., A.M.R. and M.L.G.-R. executed technologic experiments; A.R.-L., E.T., J.Á.-R., V.M. and M.L.G.-R. wrote the draft of the manuscript. All the authors critically reviewed and approved the final version of the manuscript. None of the authors has any conflicts of interest to declare.

Funding: This study was supported by grants from Consejería de Innovación, Ciencia y Empresa-Junta de Andalucía POLFANAT-P12-AGR-430. The authors thank "Centro de Investigación, Tecnología e Innovación" of the University of Seville for providing technical assistance.

Conflicts of Interest: The authors have no conflict of interest to declare.

Abbreviations

BC	β-carotene
COX-2	cyclooxygenase-2
DCF	2′,7′-dichlorofluorescein
DCF-DA	dichlorofluorescein diacetate
DCFH-DA	2′,7′-dichlorodihydrofluorescein diacetate
Dex	dexamethasone
FX	fucoxanthin
H&E	hematoxylin and eosin
HO-1	heme oxygenase-1
IL	interleukin
LDH	lactate dehydrogenase
LPS	lipopolysaccharide
MPO	myeloperoxidase
Nrf2	nuclear factor E2-related factor 2
ROS	reactive oxygen species
SRB	sulforhodamine B
TNF-α	tumor necrosis factor alpha
TPA	12-O-tetradecanoylphorbol-13-acetate
UV	ultraviolet

References

1. Fernández-García, E. Function Skin protection against UV light by dietary antioxidants. *Food Funct.* **2014**, *5*, 1994–2003. [CrossRef] [PubMed]
2. Nijsten, T. Atopic dermatitis and comorbidities: Added value of comprehensive dermatoepidemiology. *J. Investig. Dermatol.* **2017**, *137*, 1009–1011. [CrossRef] [PubMed]
3. Hart, P.H.; Norval, M.; Byrne, S.N.; Rhodes, L.E. Exposure to ultraviolet radiation in the modulation of human diseases. *Annu. Rev. Pathol. Mech. Dis.* **2018**, *14*, 421058260. [CrossRef] [PubMed]
4. Duncan, F.; Martin, J.; Wulff, B.; Stoner, G.; Tober, K.; Oberyszyn, T.; Kusewitt, D.; Van Buskirk, A. Topical treatment with black raspberry extract reduces cutaneous UVB-induced carcinogenesis and inflammation. *Cancer Prev. Res.* **2009**, *2*, 54–56. [CrossRef] [PubMed]
5. Berthon, J.-Y.; Nachat-Kappes, R.; Bey, M.; Cadoret, J.-P.; Renimel, I.; Filaire, E. Marine algae as attractive source to skin care. *Free Radic. Res.* **2017**, *51*, 555–567. [CrossRef] [PubMed]
6. Brunt, E.G.; Burgess, J.G. The promise of marine molecules as cosmetic active ingredients. *Int. J. Cosmet. Sci.* **2018**, *40*, 1–15. [CrossRef] [PubMed]
7. Milani, A.; Basirnejad, M.; Shahbazi, S.; Bolhassani, A. Carotenoids: Biochemistry, pharmacology and treatment. *Br. J. Pharmacol.* **2017**, *174*, 1290–1324. [CrossRef] [PubMed]
8. Zhang, H.; Tang, Y.; Zhang, Y.; Zhang, S.; Qu, J.; Wang, X.; Kong, R.; Han, C.; Liu, Z. Fucoxanthin: A promising medicinal and nutritional ingredient. *Evid. Based. Complement. Alternat. Med.* **2015**, *2015*, 723515. [CrossRef] [PubMed]
9. D'Orazio, N.; Gemello, E.; Gammone, M.A.; de Girolamo, M.; Ficoneri, C.; Riccioni, G. Fucoxantin: A treasure from the sea. *Mar. Drugs* **2012**, *10*, 604–616. [CrossRef] [PubMed]
10. Jang, E.J.; Kim, S.C.; Lee, J.-H.; Lee, J.R.; Kim, I.K.; Baek, S.Y.; Kim, Y.W. Fucoxanthin, the constituent of Laminaria japonica, triggers AMPK-mediated cytoprotection and autophagy in hepatocytes under oxidative stress. *BMC Complement. Altern. Med.* **2018**, *18*, 97. [CrossRef] [PubMed]
11. Zheng, J.; Piao, M.J.; Kim, K.C.; Yao, C.W.; Cha, J.W.; Hyun, J.W. Fucoxanthin enhances the level of reduced glutathione via the Nrf2-mediated pathway in human keratinocytes. *Mar. Drugs* **2014**, *12*, 4214–4230. [CrossRef] [PubMed]
12. Urikura, I.; Sugawara, T.; Hirata, T. Protective effect of fucoxanthin against UVB-induced skin photoaging in hairless mice. *Biosci. Biotechnol. Biochem.* **2011**, *75*, 757–760. [CrossRef] [PubMed]

13. Shimoda, H.; Tanaka, J.; Shan, S.-J.; Maoka, T. Anti-pigmentary activity of fucoxanthin and its influence on skin mRNA expression of melanogenic molecules. *J. Pharm. Pharmacol.* **2010**, *62*, 1137–1145. [CrossRef] [PubMed]

14. Matsui, M.; Tanaka, K.; Higashiguchi, N.; Okawa, H.; Yamada, Y.; Tanaka, K.; Taira, S.; Aoyama, T.; Takanishi, M. Protective and therapeutic effects of fucoxanthin against sunburn caused by UV irradiation. *J. Pharmacol. Sci.* **2016**, *132*, 55–64. [CrossRef] [PubMed]

15. Marwah, H.; Garg, T.; Goyal, A.K.; Rath, G. Permeation enhancer strategies in transdermal drug delivery. *Drug Deliv.* **2016**, *23*, 564–578. [CrossRef] [PubMed]

16. Dai, J.; Kim, J.-C. Chemical stability and skin permeation of fucoxanthin-loaded microemulsions. *J. Drug Deliv. Sci. Technol.* **2013**, *23*, 597–601. [CrossRef]

17. Dai, J.; Kim, J.-C. In vivo anti-obesity efficacy of fucoxanthin-loaded emulsions stabilized with phospholipid. *J. Pharm. Investig.* **2016**, *46*, 669–675. [CrossRef]

18. Freitas, J.V.; Praça, F.S.G.; Bentley, M.V.L.B.; Gaspar, L.R. Trans-resveratrol and beta-carotene from sunscreens penetrate viable skin layers and reduce cutaneous penetration of UV-filters. *Int. J. Pharm.* **2015**, *484*, 131–137. [CrossRef] [PubMed]

19. Arasa, J.; Martos, P.; Terencio, M.C.; Valcuende-Cavero, F.; Montesinos, M.C. Topical application of the adenosine A2A receptor agonist CGS-21680 prevents phorbol-induced epidermal hyperplasia and inflammation in mice. *Exp. Dermatol.* **2014**, *23*, 555–560. [CrossRef] [PubMed]

20. Rodríguez-Luna, A.; Talero, E.; Terencio, M.C.; González-Rodríguez, M.L.; Rabasco, A.M.; de los Reyes, C.; Motilva, V.; Ávila-Román, J. Topical Application of Glycolipids from isochrysis galbana prevents epidermal hyperplasia in mice. *Mar. Drugs* **2017**, *16*, 2. [CrossRef] [PubMed]

21. Bernatoniene, J.; Masteikova, R.; Davalgiene, J.; Peciura, R.; Gauryliene, R.; Bernatoniene, R.; Majiene, D.; Lazauskas, R.; Civinskiene, G.; Velziene, S.; et al. Topical application of calendula officinalis (L.): Formulation and evaluation of hydrophilic cream with antioxidant activity. *J. Med. Plants Res.* **2011**, *5*, 868–877.

22. Sirerol, J.A.; Feddi, F.; Mena, S.; Rodriguez, M.L.; Sirera, P.; Aupí, M.; Pérez, S.; Asensi, M.; Ortega, A.; Estrela, J.M. Topical treatment with pterostilbene, a natural phytoalexin, effectively protects hairless mice against UVB radiation-induced skin damage and carcinogenesis. *Free Radic. Biol. Med.* **2015**, *85*, 1–11. [CrossRef] [PubMed]

23. Stahl, W.; Sies, H. β-Carotene and other carotenoids in protection from sunlight 1–3. *Am. J. Clin. Nutr.* **2012**, *96*, 1179–1184. [CrossRef] [PubMed]

24. Kim, K.-N.; Heo, S.-J.; Yoon, W.-J.; Kang, S.-M.; Ahn, G.; Yi, T.-H.; Jeon, Y.-J. Fucoxanthin inhibits the inflammatory response by suppressing the activation of NF-κB and MAPKs in lipopolysaccharide-induced RAW 264.7 macrophages. *Eur. J. Pharmacol.* **2010**, *649*, 369–375. [CrossRef] [PubMed]

25. Martinez, R.M.; Pinho-Ribeiro, F.A.; Vale, D.L.; Steffen, V.S.; Vicentini, F.T.M.C.; Vignoli, J.A.; Baracat, M.M.; Georgetti, S.R.; Verri, W.A.; Casagrande, R. Trans-chalcone added in topical formulation inhibits skin inflammation and oxidative stress in a model of ultraviolet B radiation skin damage in hairless mice. *J. Photochem. Photobiol. B Biol.* **2017**, *171*, 139–146. [CrossRef] [PubMed]

26. Xie, F.; Chai, J.-K.; Hu, Q.; Yu, Y.-H.; Ma, L.; Liu, L.-Y.; Zhang, X.-L.; Li, B.-L.; Zhang, D.-H. Transdermal permeation of drugs with differing lipophilicity: Effect of penetration enhancer camphor. *Int. J. Pharm.* **2016**, *507*, 90–101. [CrossRef] [PubMed]

27. Mahamongkol, H.; Bellantone, R.A.; Stagni, G.; Plakogiannis, F.M. Permeation study of five formulations of alpha-tocopherol acetate through human cadaver skin. *J. Cosmet. Sci.* **2005**, *56*, 91–103. [PubMed]

28. Williams, A.C.; Barry, B.W. Penetration enhancers. *Adv. Drug Deliv. Rev.* **2012**, *64*, 128–137. [CrossRef]

29. Aggarwal, N.; Goindi, S.; Mehta, S.D. Preparation and evaluation of dermal delivery system of griseofulvin containing vitamin E-TPGS as penetration enhancer. *AAPS PharmSciTech* **2012**, *13*, 0–7. [CrossRef] [PubMed]

30. Taofiq, O.; González-Paramás, A.; Barreiro, M.; Ferreira, I. Hydroxycinnamic acids and their derivatives: cosmeceutical significance, challenges and future perspectives, a review. *Molecules* **2017**, *22*, 281. [CrossRef] [PubMed]

31. Maeda, H.; Hosokawa, M.; Sashima, T.; Funayama, K.; Miyashita, K. Effect of medium-chain triacylglycerols on anti-obesity effect of fucoxanthin. *J. Oleo Sci.* **2007**, *56*, 615–621. [CrossRef] [PubMed]

32. Laihia, J.K.; Taimen, P.; Kujari, H.; Leino, L. Topical cis-urocanic acid attenuates oedema and erythema in acute and subacute skin inflammation in the mouse. *Br. J. Dermatol.* **2012**, *167*, 506–513. [CrossRef] [PubMed]

33. Perera, G.K.; Di Meglio, P.; Nestle, F.O. Psoriasis. *Annu. Rev. Pathol. Mech. Dis.* **2012**, *7*, 385–422. [CrossRef] [PubMed]

34. Ikai, K. Psoriasis and the arachidonic acid cascade. *J. Dermatol. Sci.* **1999**, *21*, 135–146. [CrossRef]

35. Andrés, R.M.; Montesinos, M.C.; Navalón, P.; Payá, M.; Terencio, M.C. NF-κB and STAT3 inhibition as a therapeutic strategy in psoriasis: In vitro and in vivo effects of BTH. *J. Investig. Dermatol.* **2013**, *133*, 2362–2371. [CrossRef] [PubMed]

36. Zhao, D.; Kwon, S.H.; Chun, Y.S.; Gu, M.Y.; Yang, H.O. Anti-neuroinflammatory effects of fucoxanthin via inhibition of Akt/NF-κB and MAPKs/AP-1 pathways and activation of PKA/CREB pathway in lipopolysaccharide-activated BV-2 Microglial. *Cells Neurochem. Res.* **2017**, *42*, 667–677. [CrossRef] [PubMed]

37. Fan, H.J.; Xie, Z.P.; Lu, Z.W.; Tan, Z.B.; Bi, Y.M.; Xie, L.P.; Wu, Y.T.; Zhang, W.T.; Liu-Kot, K.; Liu, B.; et al. Anti-inflammatory and immune response regulation of Si-Ni-San in 2,4-dinitrochlorobenzene-induced atopic dermatitis-like skin dysfunction. *J. Ethnopharmacol.* **2018**, *222*, 1–10. [CrossRef] [PubMed]

38. Tan, C.P.; Hou, Y.H. First evidence for the anti-inflammatory activity of fucoxanthin in high-fat-diet-induced obesity in mice and the antioxidant functions in PC12 cells. *Inflammation* **2014**, *37*, 443–450. [CrossRef] [PubMed]

39. Hajar, T.; Leshem, Y.A.; Hanifin, J.M.; Nedorost, S.T.; Lio, P.A.; Paller, A.S.; Block, J.; Simpson, E.L. (the National Eczema Association Task Force) A systematic review of topical corticosteroid withdrawal ("steroid addiction") in patients with atopic dermatitis and other dermatoses. *J. Am. Acad. Dermatol.* **2015**, *72*, 541–549. [CrossRef] [PubMed]

40. Saewan, N.; Jimtaisong, A. Natural products as photoprotection. *J. Cosmet. Dermatol.* **2015**, *14*, 47–63. [CrossRef] [PubMed]

41. Lakatos, P.; Szabó, É.; Hegedus, C.; Haskó, G.; Gergely, P.; Bai, P.; Virág, L. 3-Aminobenzamide protects primary human keratinocytes from UV-induced cell death by a poly(ADP-ribosyl)ation independent mechanism. *Biochim. Biophys. Acta Mol. Cell Res.* **2013**, *1833*, 743–751. [CrossRef] [PubMed]

42. Leerach, N.; Yakaew, S.; Phimnuan, P.; Soimee, W.; Nakyai, W.; Luangbudnark, W.; Viyoch, J. Effect of Thai banana (Musa AA group) in reducing accumulation of oxidation end products in UVB-irradiated mouse skin. *J. Photochem. Photobiol. B Biol.* **2017**, *168*, 50–58. [CrossRef] [PubMed]

43. Heo, S.-J.; Jeon, Y.-J. Protective effect of fucoxanthin isolated from Sargassum siliquastrum on UV-B induced cell damage. *J. Photochem. Photobiol. B.* **2009**, *95*, 101–107. [CrossRef] [PubMed]

44. Zheng, J.; Piao, M.J.; Keum, Y.S.; Kim, H.S.; Hyun, J.W. Fucoxanthin protects cultured human keratinocytes against oxidative stress by blocking free radicals and inhibiting apoptosis. *Biomol. Ther.* **2013**, *21*, 270–276. [CrossRef] [PubMed]

45. Kanekura, T.; Higashi, Y.; Kanzaki, T. Inhibitory effects of 9-cis-retinoic acid and pyrrolidinedithiocarbamate on cyclooxygenase (COX)-2 expression and cell growth in human skin squamous carcinoma cells. *Cancer Lett.* **2000**, *161*, 177–183. [CrossRef]

46. Fehér, P.; Ujhelyi, Z.; Váradi, J.; Fenyvesi, F.; Róka, E.; Juhász, B.; Varga, B.; Bombicz, M.; Priksz, D.; Bácskay, I.; et al. Efficacy of pre- and post-treatment by topical formulations containing dissolved and suspended silybum marianum against UVB-induced oxidative stress in guinea pig and on HaCaT keratinocytes. *Molecules* **2016**, *21*, 1269. [CrossRef] [PubMed]

47. Zhong, J.; Li, L. Skin-derived precursors against UVB-induced apoptosis via Bcl-2 and Nrf2 upregulation. *Biomed. Res. Int.* **2016**, *2016*, 6894743. [CrossRef] [PubMed]

48. Furue, M.; Uchi, H.; Mitoma, C.; Hashimoto-Hachiya, A.; Chiba, T.; Ito, T.; Nakahara, T.; Tsuji, G. Antioxidants for healthy skin: The emerging role of aryl hydrocarbon receptors and nuclear factor-erythroid 2-related factor-2. *Nutrients* **2017**, *9*, 223. [CrossRef] [PubMed]

49. Yang, Y.; Yang, I.; Cao, M.; Su, Z.-Y.; Wu, R.; Guo, Y.; Fang, M.; Kong, A.-N. Fucoxanthin elicits epigenetic modifications, Nrf2 activation and blocking transformation in mouse skin JB6 P+ cells. *AAPS J.* **2018**, *20*, 32. [CrossRef] [PubMed]

50. Sangeetha, R.K.; Bhaskar, N.; Baskaran, V. Comparative effects of beta-carotene and fucoxanthin on retinol deficiency induced oxidative stress in rats. *Mol. Cell. Biochem.* **2009**, *331*, 59–67. [CrossRef] [PubMed]

51. Skehan, P.; Storeng, R.; Scudiero, D.; Monks, A.; McMahon, J.; Vistica, D.; Warren, J.T.; Bokesch, H.; Kenney, S.; Boyd, M.R. New colorimetric cytotoxicity assay for anticancer-drug screening. *J. Natl. Cancer Inst.* **1990**, *82*, 1107–1112. [CrossRef] [PubMed]

52. De los Reyes, C.; Ortega, M.J.; Rodríguez-Luna, A.; Talero, E.; Motilva, V.; Zubía, E. Molecular characterization and anti-inflammatory activity of galactosylglycerides and galactosylceramides from the microalga isochrysis galbana. *J. Agric. Food Chem.* **2016**, *64*, 8783–8794. [CrossRef] [PubMed]

53. Mura, P.; Celesti, L.; Murratzu, C.; Corsi, S.; Furlanetto, S.; Corti, P. In vitro studies of simulated percutaneous absorption: influence of artificial membrane impregnation agent. *Acta Technol. Leg. Med.* **1993**, *4*, 121–136.

54. Maestrelli, F.; González-Rodríguez, M.L.; Rabasco, A.M.; Mura, P. Preparation and characterisation of liposomes encapsulating ketoprofen-cyclodextrin complexes for transdermal drug delivery. *Int. J. Pharm.* **2005**, *298*, 55–67. [CrossRef] [PubMed]

55. Cirri, M.; Maestrelli, F.; Mennini, N.; Mura, P. Combined use of bile acids and aminoacids to improve permeation properties of acyclovir. *Int. J. Pharm.* **2015**, *490*, 351–359. [CrossRef] [PubMed]

56. López-Pinto, J.M.; González-Rodríguez, M.L.; Rabasco, A.M. Effect of cholesterol and ethanol on dermal delivery from DPPC liposomes. *Int. J. Pharm.* **2005**, *298*, 1–12. [CrossRef] [PubMed]

57. Li, Z.; Liu, M.; Wang, H.D.S. Increased cutaneous wound healing effect of biodegradable liposomes containing madecassoside: preparation optimization, in vitro dermal permeation, and in vivo bioevaluation. *Int. J. Nanomed.* **2016**, *11*, 2995–3007. [CrossRef] [PubMed]

58. Grisham, M.B.; Benoit, J.N.; Granger, D.N. Assessment of leukocyte involvement during ischemia and reperfusion of intestine. *Methods Enzymol.* **1990**, *186*, 729–742. [PubMed]

59. Talero, E.; Alvarez de Sotomayor, M.; Sánchez-Fidalgo, S.; Motilva, V. Vascular contribution of adrenomedullin to microcirculatory improvement in experimental colitis. *Eur. J. Pharmacol.* **2011**, *670*, 601–607. [CrossRef] [PubMed]

60. Huang, J.-H.; Huang, C.-C.; Fang, J.-Y.; Yang, C.; Chan, C.-M.; Wu, N.-L.; Kang, S.-W.; Hung, C.-F. Protective effects of myricetin against ultraviolet-B-induced damage in human keratinocytes. *Toxicol. In Vitro* **2010**, *24*, 21–28. [CrossRef] [PubMed]

61. Verhulst, C.; Coiffard, C.; Coiffard, L.J.M.; Rivalland, P.; De Roeck-Holtzhauer, Y. In vitro correlation between two colorimetric assays and the pyruvic acid consumption by fibroblasts cultured to determine the sodium laurylsulfate cytotoxicity. *J. Pharmacol. Toxicol. Methods* **1998**, *39*, 143–146. [CrossRef]

62. Wang, H.; Joseph, J.A. Quantifying cellular oxidative stress by dichlorofluorescein assay using microplate reader. *Free Radic. Biol. Med.* **1999**, *27*, 612–616. [CrossRef]

63. Hyun, Y.J.; Piao, M.J.; Zhang, R.; Choi, Y.H.; Chae, S.; Hyun, J.W. Photo-protection by 3-bromo-4, 5-dihydroxybenzaldehyde against ultraviolet B-induced oxidative stress in human keratinocytes. *Ecotoxicol. Environ. Saf.* **2012**, *83*, 71–78. [CrossRef] [PubMed]

64. Haruta-Ono, Y.; Ueno, H.; Ueda, N.; Kato, K.; Yoshioka, T. Investigation into the dosage of dietary sphingomyelin concentrate in relation to the improvement of epidermal function in hairless mice. *Anim. Sci. J.* **2012**, *83*, 178–183. [CrossRef] [PubMed]

65. Nishimori, Y.; Edwards, C.; Pearse, A.; Matsumoto, K.; Kawai, M.; Marks, R. Degenerative alterations of dermal collagen fiber bundles in photodamaged human skin and UVB-irradiated hairless mouse skin: Possible effect on decreasing skin mechanical properties and appearance of wrinkles. *Soc. Investig. Dermatol.* **2001**, *117*, 1458–1463.

66. Wang, Y.Y.; Hong, C.T.; Chiu, W.T.; Fang, J.Y. In vitro and in vivo evaluations of topically applied capsaicin and nonivamide from hydrogels. *Int. J. Pharm.* **2001**, *224*, 89–104. [CrossRef]

67. Bradford, M. A rapid and sensitive method for the quantitation of microgram quantities of protein utilizing the principle of protein-dye binding. *Anal. Biochem.* **1976**, *72*, 248–254. [CrossRef]

68. Talero, E.; Bolivar, S.; Ávila-Román, J.; Alcaide, A.; Fiorucci, S.; Motilva, V. Inhibition of chronic ulcerative colitis-associated adenocarcinoma development in mice by VSL#3. *Inflamm. Bowel Dis.* **2015**, *21*, 1027–1037. [PubMed]

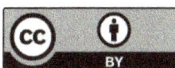

marine drugs

MDPI

Article

Protective Effects of Fucoxanthin on Ultraviolet B-Induced Corneal Denervation and Inflammatory Pain in a Rat Model

Shiu-Jau Chen [1,2,†], **Ching-Ju Lee** [3,4,†], **Tzer-Bin Lin** [5], **Hsien-Yu Peng** [2], **Hsiang-Jui Liu** [6], **Yu-Shan Chen** [4] and **Kuang-Wen Tseng** [2,7,*]

1   Department of Neurosurgery, Mackay Memorial Hospital, Taipei 10449, Taiwan; chenshiujau@gmail.com
2   Department of Medicine, Mackay Medical College, New Taipei 25245, Taiwan; hypeng@mmc.edu.tw
3   Internal Medicine, Taipei Hospital, Ministry of Health and Welfare, New Taipei 24213, Taiwan; lululee66@yahoo.com.tw
4   Department of Business Administration, National Taipei University, New Taipei 24741, Taiwan; yushan@gm.ntpu.edu.tw
5   Department of Physiology, School of Medicine, College of Medicine, Taipei Medical University, Taipei 11049, Taiwan; tblin2@tmu.edu.tw
6   Department of Optometry, Mackay Junior College of Medicine, Nursing and Management, New Taipei 11260, Taiwan; s458@eip.mkc.edu.tw
7   School of Life Science, National Taiwan Normal University, Taipei 10610, Taiwan
*   Correspondence: tseng@mmc.edu.tw; Tel.: +886-2-2636-0303 (ext. 1227)
†   These authors contributed equally to this work.

Received: 15 February 2019; Accepted: 28 February 2019; Published: 5 March 2019

Abstract: Fucoxanthin is a carotenoid with many pharmaceutical properties that is found in brown seaweed. However, the effects of fucoxanthin on corneal innervation and intense eye pain have not been extensively examined. To clarify the protective roles and underlying mechanisms of fucoxanthin on ocular lesions, we investigated the beneficial effects and mechanisms by which fucoxanthin ameliorates ultraviolet B (UVB)-induced corneal denervation and trigeminal pain. Treatment with fucoxanthin enhanced the expression of nuclear factor erythroid 2-related factor 2 in the cornea. Inhibition of typical denervation and epithelial exfoliation in the cornea were observed in rats treated with fucoxanthin following UVB-induced nerve disorders. Moreover, the active phosphorylated form of p38 MAP kinase (pp38) and the number of glial fibrillary acidic protein (GFAP)-positive neural cells were significantly reduced. Decreased expression of neuron-selective transient receptor potential vanilloid type 1 (TRPV1) in the trigeminal ganglia neurons was also demonstrated in rats treated with fucoxanthin after UVB-induced keratitis. Symptoms of inflammatory pain, including difficulty in opening the eyes and eye wipe behaviour, were also reduced in fucoxanthin-treated groups. Pre-treatment with fucoxanthin may protect the eyes from denervation and inhibit trigeminal pain in UVB-induced photokeratitis models.

Keywords: fucoxanthin; ultraviolet B; denervation

1. Introduction

Photokeratitis, a condition caused by exposure of the eyes to UV radiation, causes opacifications of the cornea, decreases visual acuity and induces inflammatory pain. UV-induced ocular damage has been demonstrated in previous human and animal studies [1,2]. The cornea absorbs about 90% of UVB radiation and is most sensitive to UVB impairment [3]. UVB rays irritate the superficial corneal epithelium, causing inhibition of mitosis, production of nuclear fragmentation and loosening of the epithelial layer, inducing an inflammatory response, such as stromal swelling and leukocyte infiltration [4]. UVB-induced corneal disorders could be caused by oxidative stress, as well as by the production of reactive oxygen species and inflammatory cytokines [5]. Oxidative stress may cause significant damage to cell structures and functions by increasing DNA mutations or inducing DNA damage and genome instability [6]. In addition, inflammatory cytokines have also been found to play an important role in promoting fibrosis, scarring and inflammatory pain in the cornea [7].

The transparent tissue of the cornea, which has about 2500 nerve endings per mm^2, is one of the most densely innervated avascular tissues in mammals [8]. Its dense innervation contributes to a wide range of corneal sensations and to the maintenance of corneal epithelial integrity; touching the cornea causes an involuntary reflex that closes the eyelid. The ophthalmic branch of the trigeminal ganglion afferent nerve fibres enters the corneal stroma through the limbus and innervates the corneal epithelium [9]. Corneal nerves penetrate the corneal periphery in a radial distribution to form the sub basal nerve plexus and influence signal transduction cascades involved in epithelial function, organization and homeostasis [10,11]. It is therefore essential to conserve the cooperative interplay between the corneal innervation and epithelial microenvironments.

The trigeminal ganglia comprise neuronal cells and two types of glial cells: satellite cells and Schwann cells. The cell bodies of the primary afferent neurons are surrounded completely by several satellite glial cells that form distinct functional units. Sensitization of nociceptor fibres alters the sensitivity and pain observed during eye surface inflammation [12]. Neuron-selective transient receptor potential vanilloid type 1 (TRPV1), the capsaicin receptor primarily expressed by nociceptive sensory ganglion neurons, is directly activated and sensitized by chemical mediators released during tissue injury [13]. Previous studies have shown that the active phosphorylated form of p38 MAP kinase (pp38) is involved in cellular responses to external signals such as pain, growth factors, stress and inflammatory mediators [14,15]. Activated satellite glial cells release several inflammatory and immune mediators in response to inflammation and nerve damage and influence other sensory neurons within the ganglion [16]. The immunoreactivity against glial fibrillary acidic protein (GFAP), an intermediate filament protein, is not readily detectable in satellite glial cells in the resting state or under normal physiological conditions. However, following nerve injury, inflammation or viral infection, GFAP is detectable in the satellite glial cells of the peripheral nervous system that are activated by these pathologies. Interestingly, neuron–glia interactions have been shown to be involved in all stages of inflammation and pain associated with several diseases [17,18].

Nuclear factor erythroid 2-related factor 2 (Nrf2), a basic leucine zipper transcription factor, mediates much of the protective anti-oxidant response, regulates a coordinated transcriptional program that maintains cellular redox homeostasis and protects the cell from oxidative injury [19]. Nrf2 regulates numbers of that play important roles in the anti-oxidant enzyme response, including "direct" and "indirect" enzymes [20]. The "direct" response enzymes include catalase or superoxide dismutase and the "indirect" enzymes include heme oxygenase-1, glutathione and thioredoxin generating enzymes. Nrf2 is an important mechanistic link between managing the anti-oxidant gene expression stress response and cell survival.

Fucoxanthin is an orange pigment present in brown seaweeds, such as *Hizikia fusiformis*, *Laminaria japonica* and *Sargassum fulvellum* and is responsible for their high anti-oxidant content [21]. It is metabolized to fucoxanthinol and amarouciaxanthin in vivo [22] and has therapeutic properties, such as anti-oxidant [23], anti-cancer [24], anti-inflammatory [25], anti-obese [26], anti-diabetic [27] and anti-angiogenic activities [28] and has a protective effect on the liver, blood vessels of the brain, bones and skin. We have previously demonstrated that pre-treatment with fucoxanthin inhibited the ultraviolet B-induced expression of pro-inflammatory cytokines in the cornea [29]. However, the effects of fucoxanthin on epithelial denervation and inflammatory pain in the avascular cornea have not been extensively examined. Studies examining the reduction of corneal irregularity and inflammatory pain during corneal wound healing are of great clinical value.

2. Results

2.1. Effect of Fucoxanthin on Nrf2 Expression

To investigate the effect of fucoxanthin on Nrf2 translocation in the cornea, experimental animals were first pre-treated with fucoxanthin ranging from 0.1 to 10 mg/kg for 6 days via oral administration. The Nrf2 protein levels were measured using western blotting analysis (Figure 1). Compared with the control group (no pre-treatment with fucoxanthin), the groups pre-treated with 0.1, 1 and 10 mg/kg fucoxanthin showed higher levels of Nrf2 protein. Moreover, Nrf2 expression increased with fucoxanthin pre-treatment.

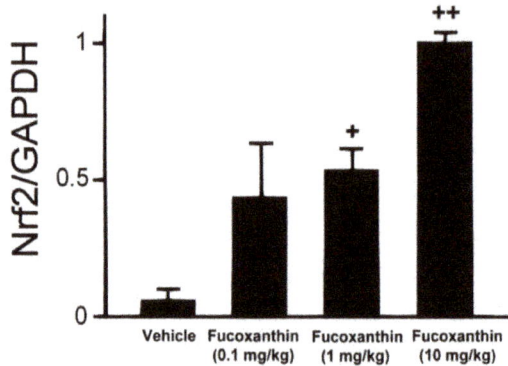

Figure 1. Fucoxanthin treatment enhanced the expression of Nrf2. Protein extraction was prepared and separated using SDS-PAGE, followed by western blot analysis with antibodies against Nrf2 and GAPDH. Increases in Nrf2 were observed following fucoxanthin treatment. Protein levels were measured using western blotting and band intensity was quantified using ImageJ software. The data are expressed as means ± standard deviation (SD) ($n = 5$ rats per group). + $p < 0.05$, ++ $p < 0.01$; one-way ANOVA followed by Dunnett's multiple comparison test.

2.2. Effect of Fucoxanthin on UVB-Induced Corneal Denervation

In an attempt to define the relationship between increased Nrf2 in the ocular tissues and degenerating corneal nerve endings in the groups treated with fucoxanthin, the general neuronal marker protein gene product (PGP) 9.5 was targeted for corneal tissue staining. In the control group, abundant epithelial nerves were found in the corneas and the nerve plexus had been arranged in a crisscrossed, dense and continuous pattern of immunoreactivity toward PGP 9.5 (Figure 2A). However, fewer, discontinuous and punctate-like degenerating nerves were observed in the epithelial layer of the cornea after UVB exposure (Figure 2B). In the 10 mg/kg fucoxanthin treatment group, the experimental animals showed a significant decrease in corneal denervation and an increase in nerve density (Figure 2E) compared with those treated with 0.1 or 1 mg/kg fucoxanthin groups after UVB irradiation (Figure 2C,D).

After statistical analysis of the corneal innervation, the reduction in corneal nerve density was statistically significant in the UVB group (25.3 ± 4.8%, $p < 0.05$) compared with the control. In contrast, the 10 mg/kg fucoxanthin treatment group displayed reduced denervation in the cornea (78.6 ± 5.5%, $p < 0.05$) compared with the UVB group. These findings suggest that the UVB-induced denervation in the cornea was effectively inhibited by treatment with 10 mg/kg fucoxanthin (Figure 3).

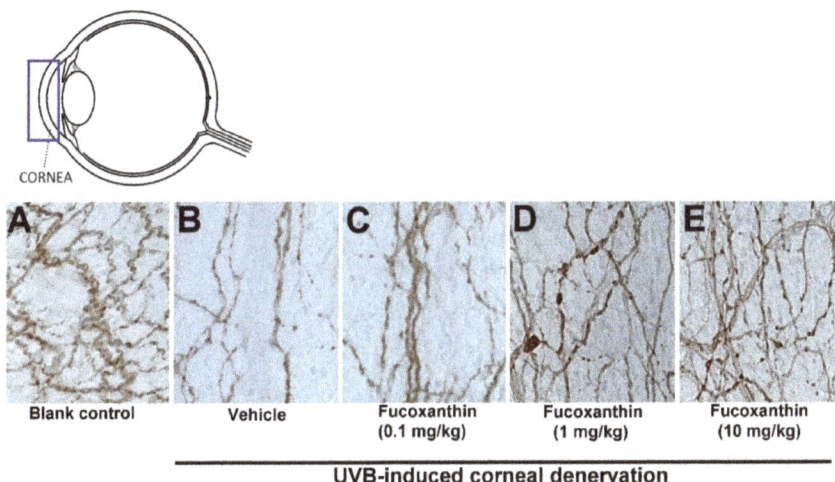

Blank control   Vehicle   Fucoxanthin   Fucoxanthin   Fucoxanthin
(0.1 mg/kg)   (1 mg/kg)   (10 mg/kg)

UVB-induced corneal denervation

Figure 2. Protective effects of fucoxanthin on nerve innervation after UVB-induced denervation in corneal tissues. Nerve innervation was evaluated via immunohistochemistry using a general neural marker PGP 9.5. Nerve innervation was compared between the following groups: blank control (**A**), UVB (**B**), UVB/0.1 mg/kg fucoxanthin (**C**), UVB/1 mg/kg fucoxanthin (**D**) and UVB/10 mg/kg fucoxanthin (**E**) groups. A significant reduction in the epithelial nerve innervation of the corneal tissues is evident after UVB-induced nerve injury (**B**) compared with the blank control group (**A**). Nerve innervation was significantly protected by 10 mg/kg fucoxanthin treatment and the corneal denervation was significantly decreased.

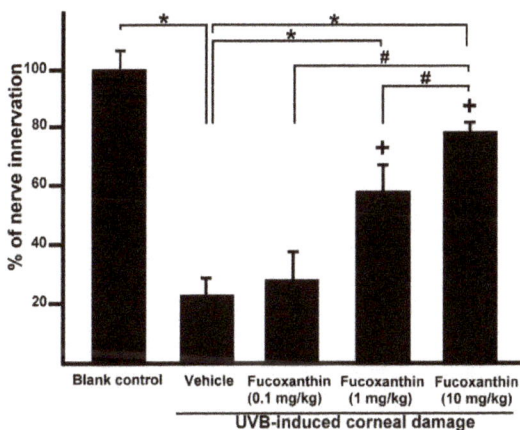

Figure 3. Effects of fucoxanthin on nerve innervation after UVB irradiation in the corneal tissues. Nerve innervation was compared with blank control, UVB, UVB/0.1 mg/kg fucoxanthin, UVB/1 mg/kg fucoxanthin and UVB/10 mg/kg fucoxanthin groups. A significant reduction in the nerve innervation of the corneal tissues and UVB-induced nerve injury is evident in the UVB-treated group compared with the blank control group. Nerve innervation was increased by treatment with fucoxanthin. The results are presented as means ±SD ($n = 5$ rats per group). The mean value was significantly different compared with the UVB/vehicle group (* $p < 0.05$; Student t test). The mean value was significantly different as UVB/0.1 and 1 mg/kg fucoxanthin groups compared with UVB/10 mg/kg fucoxanthin group (# $p < 0.05$; Student t test). The mean value was significantly different compared with UVB-exposed group (+ $p < 0.05$; one-way ANOVA followed by Bonferroni's multiple comparison test).

2.3. Effect of Fucoxanthin on UVB-Induced Corneal Epithelial Disorganization

Because of the protective effects of fucoxanthin treatment against UVB-induced corneal denervation, the relationship between corneal denervation and pathological examinations was applied to superficial corneal inspection. Analyses of corneal smoothness and corneal lissamine green staining were conducted. The corneas of the blank control rats were transparent, regular and neat and their reflecting ocular surface was intact (Figure 4A). UVB exposure caused severe damage to the corneal epithelial surface, including distortion and deformation (Figure 4C). In contrast, corneas treated with fucoxanthin showed mild corneal epithelial disorganizations following UVB irradiation. Moreover, significant enhancement of corneal epithelial organization was observed in the groups treated with 1 and 10 mg/kg fucoxanthin (Figure 4G,I) compared with the corneal damage detected in the UVB-treated experimental animals.

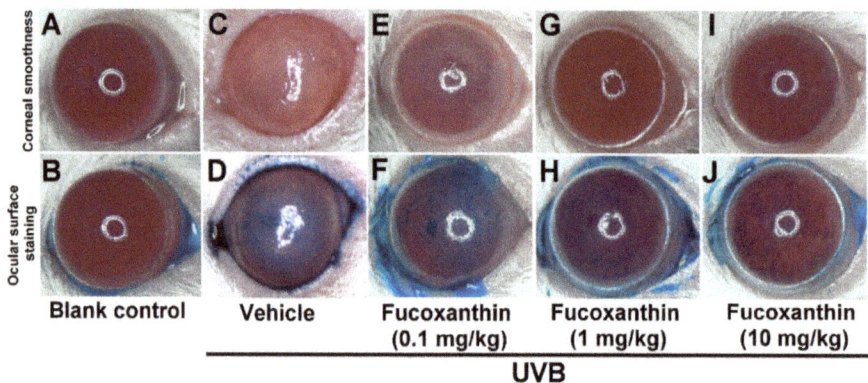

Figure 4. Effects of fucoxanthin on UVB-induced corneal disorders. Analyses of corneal smoothness and corneal lissamine green staining were conducted. The extent of corneal integrity and transparency was compared between the following groups: blank control (**A,B**), UVB (**C,D**), UVB/0.1 mg/kg fucoxanthin (**E,F**), UVB/1 mg/kg fucoxanthin (**G,H**) and UVB/10 mg/kg fucoxanthin. The cornea, which is normally transparent, becomes cloudy when damaged. UVB irradiation caused serious damage to the corneal tissue (**C,D**), including severe exfoliation, deteriorated smoothness, corneal opacity and intense staining with lissamine green, as compared with the blank controls (**A,B**). Corneal smoothness and surface staining analysis showed that fucoxanthin treatment preserved corneal integrity and transparency (**E–J**).

The epithelial cells lining the corneal surface were stained with lissamine green to evaluate the ocular surface damage. Corneas of the blank control group remained largely unstained by lissamine green (Figure 4B), whereas signs of corneal surface disorders, including a strikingly irregular ocular surface and intense staining with lissamine green, were present after UVB radiation (Figure 4D). Treatment with 1 and 10 mg/kg fucoxanthin led to decreased lissamine green staining (Figure 4H,J). Compared with the corneal injuries detected in the UVB-treated groups, significantly fewer punctate-stained areas were observed on the ocular surfaces of the group treated with 10 mg/kg fucoxanthin (Figure 4J).

Semi-quantitative analyses of corneal smoothness and lissamine green staining were scored (Figure 5) and significant differences were observed between all scores of the UVB-treated groups and those of the blank control. The corneas of the fucoxanthin-treated groups showed decreased corneal damage scores. Moreover, the analysis also revealed significantly decreased scores in the group treated with 10 mg/kg fucoxanthin as compared with the groups treated with 0.1 and 1 mg/kg fucoxanthin. Thus, the protective effects of fucoxanthin treatment against UVB-induced damage to the corneal innervation and epithelium were observed.

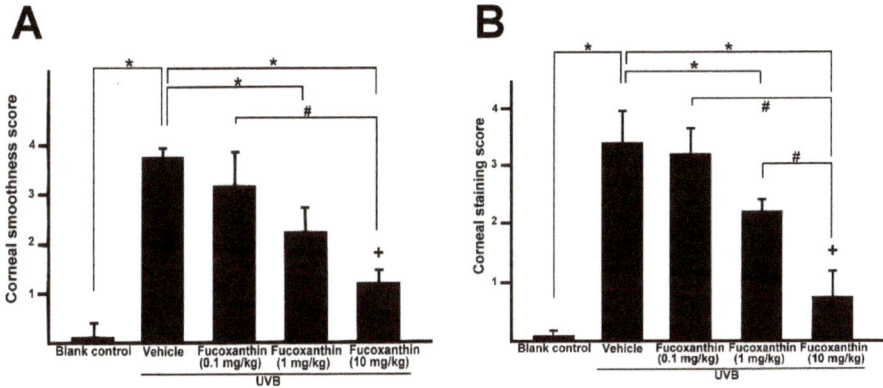

Figure 5. Semi-quantitative analyses of the effects of fucoxanthin on ocular surface irregularity (**A**) and lissamine green staining scores (**B**) following UVB-induced corneal damage. Data are shown as mean ± SD) (*n* = 5 rats per group). The mean value was significantly different compared with the UVB/vehicle group (* *p* < 0.05; Student *t* test). The mean value was significantly different as UVB/0.1 and 1 mg/kg fucoxanthin groups compared with UVB/10 mg/kg fucoxanthin group (# *p* <0.05; Student *t* test). The mean value was significantly different compared with UVB-exposed group (+ *p* < 0.05; one-way ANOVA followed by Bonferroni's multiple comparison test).

2.4. Effect of Fucoxanthin on UVB-Induced pp38, GFAP and TRPV1 Expression in the Trigeminal Ganglia

Neural activation results in increased levels of active pp38 MAP kinase, a key regulatory protein involved in signal transduction in response to inflammatory stimuli that result in changes in gene expression. To determine the relationship between UVB-induced corneal disorders and increased pp38 levels in vivo, the active levels of pp38 were monitored using immunohistochemistry. After UVB-induced photokeratitis, elevated levels of p38 were readily detected in both neurons and neighbouring satellite glial cells (Figure 6A). Moreover, the number of GFAP-immunopositive activated glial cells typically surrounding the neurons and TRPV1-positive neuronal cells were significantly increased in the trigeminal ganglion of the UVB/vehicle group (Figure 6B,C). In contrast, the number of pp38-positive neural cells, GFAP-positive activated glial cells and TRPV1-positive neuronal cells was limited in the UVB/10 mg/kg fucoxanthin group (Figure 6D–F) compared with the other UVB-treated group. These results imply that activation of satellite glial and neuronal cells was partially suppressed by fucoxanthin treatment.

2.5. Effect of Fucoxanthin on UVB-Induced Corneal Injury-Evoked Eye Wipe Behavior

To assess the impact of fucoxanthin-suppressed activation of satellite glial and neuronal cells, we evaluated the symptoms of inflammatory pain and eye wipe behaviour (Figure 7). Difficulty opening the eyes, the symptom of inflammatory pain, was observed in the UVB-irradiated group (Figure 7D). Moreover, a single drop of 5 M NaCl to the ocular surface evoked consistent increases in eye wiping after UVB irradiation compared with the blank control group during a 5-min test period on day 6. The frequency of the eye wipes evoked by UVB-induced photokeratitis was high. In contrast, the animals showed reduced eye wipe frequency in the UVB/10 mg/kg fucoxanthin group compared with the UVB/vehicle group. These results indicated that UVB-induced eye wipe behaviour was suppressed in the fucoxanthin-treated group (Figure 7G).

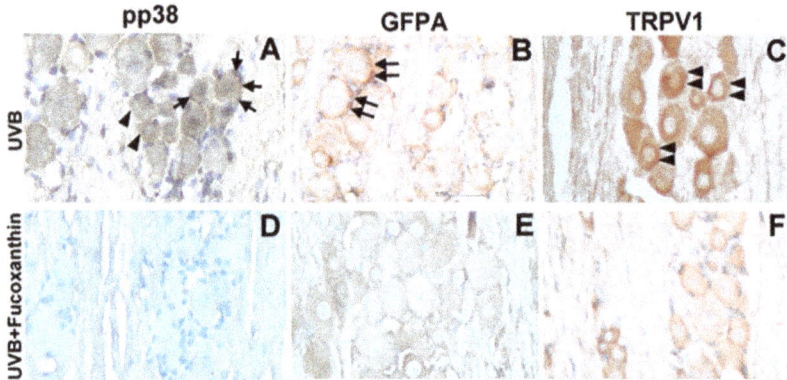

Figure 6. Characterization of pp38-, GFAP- and TRPV1-positive cells in the trigeminal ganglia of UVB/vehicle and UVB/10 mg/kg fucoxanthin groups. Sections were stained with haematoxylin and antibodies against pp38, GFAP and TRPV1. Expression of pp38 was increased in neuronal (arrowheads, **A**) and glial cells (arrows, **A**) in the trigeminal ganglion after UVB-induced photokeratitis. Note that the number of GFAP-immunopositive activated glial cells typically surrounding neurons (double arrows, **B**) and TRPV1-positive neuronal cells (double arrowheads, **C**) were significantly increased in the UVB/vehicle group. In contrast, the number of pp38-positive neural cells, GFAP-positive activated glial cells and TRPV1-positive neuronal cells were limited in the UVB/fucoxanthin group (**D–F**).

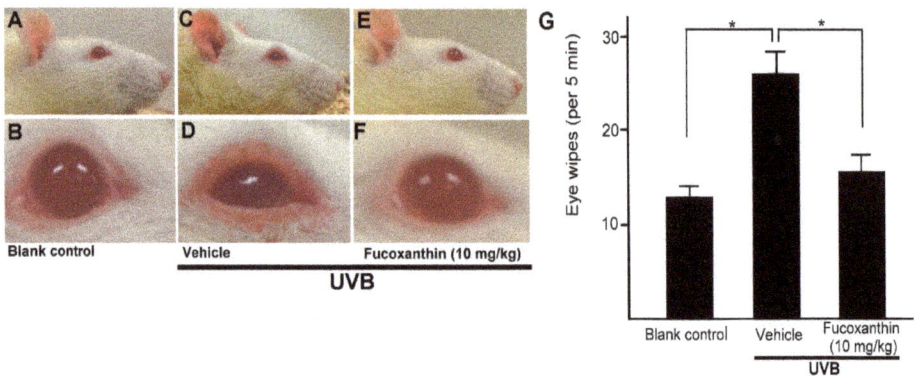

Figure 7. Effects of fucoxanthin on eye wipe behaviour after UVB-induced corneal damage. The cornea is composed of highly innervated tissue and pain caused by corneal damage is very intense. Photokeratitis caused inflammatory pain symptoms, including difficulty opening the eyes and eye wipe behaviour. Symptoms of inflammatory pain were compared between the following groups: blank control (**A,B**), UVB/vehicle (**C,D**) and UVB/10 mg/kg fucoxanthin treatment (**E,F**). Difficulty opening the eyes, the symptom of inflammatory pain, was reduced with fucoxanthin treatment (**E,F**). Eye wipe behaviour analysis showed a high frequency of eye wiping evoked by UVB-induced photokeratitis. In contrast, the animals showed reduced eye wiping in the UVB/10 mg/kg fucoxanthin group compared with the UVB group. The data are expressed as means $\pm$ SD (n = 5 rats per group). The mean value was significantly different compared with the UVB/vehicle group. (* $p < 0.05$; Student t test, **G**).

3. Discussions

UVB-induced corneal disorders could be caused by oxidative stress, as well as by the production of reactive oxygen species and inflammatory cytokines [5]. The main characteristic of an antioxidant is its ability to induce enzymes that snare free radicals. In this respect, Nrf2 and its interaction with anti-oxidant response element increase the transcription that play important roles in the anti-oxidant enzyme response, such as quinone oxidoreductase 1, heme oxygenase-1 and superoxide dismutase [20]. Fucoxanthin has been shown to be able to augment cellular antioxidant defence by inducing Nrf2-driven expression in in skin cells in vivo and in vitro [30,31]. In the present study, Nrf2 expression increased with fucoxanthin treatment in corneal tissues. It is possible that Nrf2 at higher expression interact with other mechanisms to increase the activity of antioxidant in corneal tissues.

Eye signs are often associated with corneal denervation and endocrinal disorders [32,33]. Nerve innervation anomalies affect epithelium metabolism, proliferation and wound healing, compromising the health of the cornea and visual axis [32]. The corneal epithelium preserves the intraepithelial corneal nerves and the intraepithelial nerve terminals that spread out toward the apical surface [34]. The corneal nerves typically release neuronal factors that promote corneal epithelial homeostasis and effect signal transduction cascades involved in epithelial function, organization and homeostasis [10,11]. In the present study, UVB radiation caused a significant reduction in the epithelial nerve innervation of corneal tissues, resulting in evident UVB-induced nerve injury. We demonstrated that UVB irradiation impairs the density and morphology of the sensory nerves within the corneal epithelium. In addition, serious damage to the corneal tissues, including severe exfoliation, deteriorated smoothness and corneal opacity, was detected more frequently in the UVB-irradiated groups than in the non-irradiated groups. In the present study, we observed that reduced corneal nerve density was significantly correlated with the disorganization of the corneal epithelium in UVB-irradiated eyes. In contrast, treatment with fucoxanthin inhibited UVB-induced corneal denervation and preserved the integrity of the corneal surface.

UVB radiation is non-invasive, produces localized inflammation and has been applied to humans in previous studies examining cutaneous pain [35–37]. Ocular itching and oedema are the most frequent symptoms complained by patients not only with photokeratitis but also with keratoconjunctivitis, due to the frequent corneal involvement [38]. The inflammatory responses involved in peripheral nerve damage also include the recruitment of immune cells to the site of injury. Immune cells, including neutrophils and macrophages, are involved in the release of various kinds of pro-inflammatory mediators that contribute to pain [39,40]. The corneal epithelium, the primary protector of the optic axis and the most densely innervated tissue in the body, changes after UVB exposure and corneal inflammation is a common clinical problem that causes ocular pain. Many studies on the mechanisms of neuropathic pain have used animal models of injury to the peripheral nerve, which involves multiple complex mechanisms. TRPV1 is an essential component of the cellular signalling mechanisms through which tissue damage or infection produces thermal hyperalgesia and pain hypersensitivity is primarily expressed on small, unmyelinated sensory neurons in the trigeminal ganglia [41,42]. Recent evidence suggests that activity of the satellite glial cells connected with gap junctions and reduces the pain threshold in the trigeminal ganglion. Furthermore, inhibition of satellite glial cell activation causes a significant reduction in neuronal excitability and nocifensive reflexes [43,44]. Otherwise, the proximity of satellite glial cells and neuronal cell bodies favours interactions through paracrine signalling and contributes to the sensitization of afferent neurons. Glia and neurons form an integrated network that modulates the excitability of pain pathways. Pp38 involves both the neuronal and glial activation during inflammatory for the trigeminal ganglia activation model [15]. In the present study, aside from sensory neurons, GFAP-positive activated glial cells that typically surround neurons in the trigeminal ganglia were limited and eye wipe behaviour evoked by UVB damage was suppressed in the UVB/10 mg/kg fucoxanthin-treated group. Thus, suppressive effects of fucoxanthin on pp38, TRPV-1 and GFAP may be important in avoid inflammatory pain following photokeratitis in the trigeminal ganglia.

Previous studies have reported that neuropathic pain involves the modulation of motor activity. Neuropathic orofacial pain leads to difficulties in mandibular movements of the orofacial region, including mastication, swallowing, speaking and toothbrushing [45,46]. Following injury to the sensory branch of trigeminal nerve, not only are the number of activated satellite glial cells in the trigeminal ganglia and microglia cells in the trigeminal sensory increased but the activity of the glial cells in the trigeminal motor nuclei is also evoked [47–49]. It remains unclear how hyperactive glial cells interact with motor neurons. It is possible that pro-inflammatory mediators released from activated glial cells affect the excitability of motor neurons. The blink reflex is mediated by sensory fibres of the trigeminal nerve (cranial nerve V 1) and the efferent limb via the motor fibres of the facial nerve (cranial nerve VII). Anatomically, the afferent corneal V1 fibres may synapse within the main sensory nucleus and facial motor neurons in turn provide input to close the eyelids. Various ganglia and sensory and motor nuclei are involved in the feedback loops between the cornea surface and orbicularis oculi muscles. UVB-induced disorders of the cornea cause inflammatory pain and may alter the wink function. In the present study, we observed that the eyelids appeared closer together in the UVB irradiation groups than in the blank control group and that fucoxanthin treatment restored the distance between the eyelids.

Nrf2 is a transcription factor with potent antioxidant effects against cellular damage and may serve an essential role in the protection against various inflammatory diseases [50]. Otherwise, pp38 signalling pathways are associated in the regulation of the Nrf2-mediated cytoprotective effect [51]. In the present study, we demonstrated that oral pre-treatment with fucoxanthin promoted the expression of Nrf2. Exposure of the ocular surface to UVB-induced changes in corneal innervation, epithelial organization and neural activity in the trigeminal ganglia matched well with increases in the frequency of eye wipe behaviour. By contrast, significant suppression of corneal denervation and epithelial disorganization was observed in the groups treated with fucoxanthin compared with the corneal damage detected in the UVB-treated experimental animals. Activated neural cells in the trigeminal ganglia and eye wipe behaviour were also reduced and UVB-induced inflammatory pain was suppressed in fucoxanthin-treated groups. These results demonstrated that fucoxanthin treatment upregulated the expression of Nrf2, inhibited the denervation of corneal tissue and activated neural cells of the trigeminal ganglia. These findings suggested that fucoxanthin has a protective effect against UVB-induced corneal denervation and inflammatory pain and the mechanism may be associated with regulation by Nrf2 pathway in rats.

4. Materials and Methods

4.1. Experimental Animals

Fifty male SD rats (6–8 weeks old) were obtained from the Animal Department of BioLASCO Taiwan Co (Taipei, Taiwan, ROC). Experimental rats were quarantined and allowed to acclimate for 1 week before beginning experimentation. Experimental rats were housed 3–4 per cage under standard laboratory conditions with a 12-h light/dark cycle. Care and treatment of animals were conducted in accordance with standard laboratory animal protocols (IACUC-A1050023) approved by the Animal Care Committee (Mackay Medical College). Food and water were available *ad libitum*. The experimental protocols for the present study were approved by the Institutional Animal Care and Use Committee and the animals were cared for in accordance with the institutional ethical guidelines.

4.2. UVB-Induced Photokeratitis and Fucoxanthin Treatment

Rats were randomly divided into five groups: Group I, blank control (no UVB exposure or fucoxanthin treatment); Group II, UVB (exposure to UVB irradiation without treatment); Group III, UVB/0.1 mg/kg fucoxanthin (exposure to UVB irradiation and pre-treatment with fucoxanthin (Sigma-Aldrich, St. Louis, MO, USA) oral administration at 0.1 mg/kg body weight); Group IV, UVB/1 mg/kg fucoxanthin (exposure to UVB irradiation and pre-treatment with fucoxanthin oral administration at 1 mg/kg body weight); and Group V, UVB/10 mg/kg fucoxanthin (exposure to UVB irradiation and pre-treatment fucoxanthin oral administration at 10 mg/kg body weight). To induce corneal damage in vivo, the eyes of the rats in Groups II, III, IV and V were exposed to UVB irradiation using the procedures reported in our previous study [29]. The wavelength of the UVB source peaked at 308 nm (range, 280–315 nm). After anaesthesia with intraperitoneal injection of sodium pentobarbital

(60 mg/kg bodyweight), the oculus was exposed to 550 μW/cm^2 of UVB light (UVGL-58; UVP Inc., San Gabriel, CA) for 4 min in a darkroom. Group II (UVB) was exposed to UVB irradiation daily for a period of 5 days (Day 2 to Day 6). Groups III, IV and V (UVB/fucoxanthin at various concentrations per kg body weight) were exposed to UVB irradiation daily for a period of 5 days and treated daily with their respective concentrations of fucoxanthin (1 day before UVB exposure) for a period of 6 days (Day 1 to Day 6).

4.3. Tissue Fractionation and Western Blot

Rats were sacrificed by cervical dislocation after deeply anaesthesia with chloral hydrate (400 mg/kg of body weight, intraperitoneally). Corneas were rinsed once with ice-cold phosphate buffered saline (PBS) and then lysed with PBS containing 1% Triton X-100, 0.1% SDS, 0.5% sodium deoxycholate, 1 μg/mL leupeptin, 10 μg/mL aprotinin and 1 mM phenylmethylsulphonyl fluoride on ice for 15 min. After sonication for 30 s using microprobe sonicator, crude extracts were subjected to centrifugation at 4 °C. All protein concentrations were measured by a protein assay (Bio-Rad laboratories, Richmond, CA, USA). Equal amounts (50 μg) of protein extracts were separated electrophoresed on 8% SDS-polyacrylamide gel and then transblotted onto the ImmobilonTM-P membrane. After being blocked with 10% non-fat milk in Tween-20/PBS, blots were incubated with rabbit anti-Nrf2 antibody (SAB4501984; Sigma-Aldrich, St. Louis, MO, USA) and then incubated with horseradish peroxidase-conjugated secondary antibodies. The signal of specific proteins was detected using enhanced chemiluminescence kit (ECL; PerkinElmer Life Sciences, Inc. Boston, MA, USA).

4.4. Immunohistochemistry for Nerve Innervations in Corneal Tissues

Experimental rats were deeply anesthetized using chloral hydrate and intracardially perfused with a fixative containing 4% paraformaldehyde. A 2-mm circular corneal epithelial defect was made in each rat using a scalpel blade. For immunocytochemistry, whole-mount tissues or 50-μm cryostat sections were collected. The floating sections were rinsed in PBS, incubated in 1.5% hydrogen peroxide for 45 min to eliminate endogenous peroxidase activity and finally blocked for 1 h in PBS containing 5% goat serum and 0.5% Triton X-100 (Sigma-Aldrich, St. Louis, MO, USA). Nerve innervation was evaluated via immunohistochemistry using antibodies against general neural marker protein PGP 9.5 (AB1761, Chemicon, Temecula, CA, USA). The reaction products of nerve profiles in the cornea were evaluated using a Vector ABC kit and the 3,3-diaminobenzidine (DAB) reaction (Vector Labs, Burlingame, CA, USA). PGP 9.5-immnopositive nerve fibres in the epithelium of each cornea were counted at a magnification of 400$\times$ with a light microscope. Nerves were traced and the total length calculated with commercial software (Adobe Illustrator; Adobe Systems, San Jose, CA, USA) using an object-length function was reported in a previous protocol [52], with slight modifications. The density of the nerves was then charted as a percentage of the control.

4.5. Determination of Corneal Injuries

Rat corneal damage was appraised as in our previous study [29]. A circular illumination source was attached to a stereoscopic microscope (Stemi DV4 Stereo Microscope, Carl Zeiss, Oberkochen, Germany), which was then used to evaluate the corneas. Ocular surface irregularity was graded on a scale of 0–4 as follows: grade 0, absent; grade 1, mild; grade 2, moderate; grade 3, severe with a twisted circle shape; and grade 4, severe with an undistinguished shape. After corneal smoothness was scored, the ocular surface was stained with 1% lissamine green (Sigma-Aldrich, St. Louis, MO, USA) and washed three times with PBS. Images of the corneal surface after lissamine green staining were taken and scored according to the grading system based on the proportion of staining noted in the damaged cornea. The severity of corneal damage was graded on a scale from 0 to 4. Briefly, the total area without dot staining was designated as grade 0; grade 1, less than 25% of the corneal surface was stained with dotted punctuate staining; grade 2, 25–50% of the corneal surface was stained with diffuse punctuate staining; grade 3, 50–75% of the corneal surface was stained with punctuate staining and apparent corneal defects; and grade 4, more than 75% of the corneal surface was stained with profuse punctuate staining and more serious corneal defects. Corneal scoring was performed by three observers who had no prior knowledge of photokeratitis.

4.6. Immunohistochemistry of pp38, TRPV1 and GFAP in Trigeminal Ganglia

Whole trigeminal ganglia were fixed in 4% paraformaldehyde for 45 min, embedded in media (Miles, Elkhart, IN, USA), maintained at the optimal cutting temperature and frozen in isopentane supercooled with liquid nitrogen. Using a cryostat (Leica Microsystems, Heidelberg, Germany), 8-μm cryosections were cut and collected on silanized slides (DAKO, Tokyo, Japan). For immunohistochemical staining of the trigeminal ganglion, serial sections were reacted with rabbit anti-activated pp38 MAP kinase anti-serum (ab47363; Abcam, Cambridge, MA, USA), rabbit anti-GFAP (ab7260; Abcam, Cambridge, MA, USA) or rabbit anti-TRPV1 anti-serum (ab6166; Abcam, Cambridge, MA, USA) after dilution in PBS containing 4% normal goat serum and 0.3% Triton X-100 (Sigma-Aldrich, St. Louis, MO, USA). Sections were then reacted with biotinylated goat anti-rabbit IgG (Vector Laboratories, Burlingame, CA, USA), avidin and biotin-peroxidase complex (Vector Laboratories) and visualized with 0.1% DAB.

4.7. Eye Wipe Behavior Test

The eye wipe test was performed using hypertonic saline as the inducing stimulus following a previous protocol [53], with modifications. This is a sensitive test for acute ocular irritation-related behaviour in conscious rats that is non-invasive and non-inflammatory. A single drop of NaCl (5 M, 20 μL) was placed on the ocular surface with a micropipette and the number of eye wipes with the ipsilateral forelimb that occurred in 30 s was counted on day 6. Means and standard deviations were calculated for all parameters determined in this study. Comparison analyses between any two groups were performed using Student's t-test. A p-value < 0.05 was considered statistically significant.

4.8. Statistical Analysis

Statistics were analysed using the SPSS program (SPSS, Inc., Chicago, IL, USA). Means and standard deviations were calculated for all parameters determined in this study. In all samples, Kolmogorov-Smirnov test was used to verify the normality of the data. The non-parametric values were analysed by Mann–Whitney test. The parametric values groups were analysed by one-way analysis of variance (ANOVA) followed by Dunnett's or Bonferroni's multiple comparison test. Statistically significant differences between groups were defined as $p < 0.05$.

Author Contributions: S.-J.C., C.-J.L. and K.-W.T. conceived and designed the experiments. S.-J.C., C.-J.L., T.-B.L., H.-Y.P., H.-J.L. performed the experiments. Y.-S.C. analysed the statistical data. K.-W.T. wrote the drafted the manuscript. All authors commented and approved the submitted manuscript.

Funding: This work was supported by grants to K.-W.T. (MOST 106-2320-B-715-002-MY2) from the Ministry of Science and Technology, Taiwan and (1061B20 and 1071B30) from Mackay Medical College, Taiwan and to S.-J.C. (MMH-MM-10717 and MMH-MM-10805) from Mackay Memorial Hospital, Taiwan.

Conflicts of Interest: The authors declare no conflict of interest.

References

1. Willmann, G. Ultraviolet Keratitis: From the Pathophysiological Basis to Prevention and Clinical Management. *High Alt. Med. Biol.* **2015**, *16*, 277–282. [CrossRef] [PubMed]
2. Podskochy, A.; Fagerholm, P. Cellular response and reactive hyaluronan production in UV-exposed rabbit corneas. *Cornea* **1998**, *17*, 640–645. [CrossRef] [PubMed]
3. Schein, O.D. Phototoxicity and the cornea. *J. Natl. Med. Assoc.* **1992**, *84*, 579–583. [PubMed]
4. Mureşan, S.; Filip, A.; Mureşan, A.; Şimon, V.; Moldovan, R.; Gal, A.F.; Miclăuş, V. Histological findings in the Wistar rat cornea following UVB irradiation. *Rom. J. Morphol. Embryol.* **2013**, *54*, 247–252. [PubMed]

5. Pauloin, T.; Dutot, M.; Joly, F.; Warnet, J.M.; Rat, P. High molecular weight hyaluronan decreases UVB-induced apoptosis and inflammation in human epithelial corneal cells. *Mol. Vis.* **2009**, *15*, 577–583. [PubMed]

6. Visconti, R.; Grieco, D. New insights on oxidative stress in cancer. *Curr. Opin. Drug Discov. Dev.* **2009**, *12*, 240–245.

7. Yamanaka, O.; Liu, C.Y.; Kao, W.W. Fibrosis in the anterior segments of the eye. *Endocr. Metab. Immune Disord. Drug Targets* **2010**, *10*, 331–335. [CrossRef] [PubMed]

8. De Castro, F.; Silos-Santiago, I.; De Armentia, M.L.; Barbacid, M.; Belmonte, C. Corneal innervation and sensitivity to noxious stimuli in trkA knockout mice. *Eur. J. Neurosci.* **1998**, *10*, 146–152. [CrossRef] [PubMed]

9. De Leeuw, A.M.; Chan, K.Y. Corneal nerve regeneration. Correlation between morphology and restoration of sensitivity. *Investig. Ophthalmol. Vis. Sci.* **1989**, *30*, 1980–1990.

10. Garcia-Hirschfeld, J.; Lopez-Briones, L.G.; Belmonte, C. Neurotrophic influences on corneal epithelial cells. *Exp. Eye Res.* **1994**, *59*, 597–605. [CrossRef] [PubMed]

11. Kim, S.Y.; Choi, J.S.; Joo, C.K. Effects of nicergoline on corneal epithelial wound healing in rat eyes. *Investig. Ophthalmol. Vis. Sci.* **2009**, *50*, 621–625. [CrossRef] [PubMed]

12. Belmonte, C.; Aracil, A.; Acosta, M.C.; Luna, C.; Gallar, J. Nerves and sensations from the eye surface. *Ocul. Surf.* **2004**, *2*, 248–253. [CrossRef]

13. Davis, J.B.; Gray, J.; Gunthorpe, M.J.; Hatcher, J.P.; Davey, P.T.; Overend, P.; Harries, M.H.; Latcham, J.; Clapham, C.; Atkinson, K.; et al. Vanilloid receptor-1 is essential for inflammatory thermal hyperalgesia. *Nature* **2000**, *405*, 183–187. [CrossRef] [PubMed]

14. Jin, S.X.; Zhuang, Z.Y.; Woolf, C.J.; Ji, R.R. p38 mitogen-activated protein kinase is activated after a spinal nerve ligation in spinal cord microglia and dorsal root ganglion neurons and contributes to the generation of neuropathic pain. *J. Neurosci.* **2003**, *23*, 4017–4022. [CrossRef] [PubMed]

15. Csáti, A.; Edvinsson, L.; Vécsei, L.; Toldi, J.; Fülöp, F.; Tajti, J.; Warfvinge, K. Kynurenic acid modulates experimentally induced inflammation in the trigeminal ganglion. *J. Headache Pain* **2015**, *16*, 99. [CrossRef] [PubMed]

16. Komiya, H.; Shimizu, K.; Ishii, K.; Kudo, H.; Okamura, T.; Kanno, K.; Shinoda, M.; Ogiso, B.; Iwata, K. Connexin 43 expression in satellite glial cells contributes to ectopic tooth-pulp pain. *J. Oral Sci.* **2018**, *60*, 493–499. [CrossRef] [PubMed]

17. Hanani, M. Satellite glial cells in sensory ganglia: From form to function. *Brain Res. Rev.* **2005**, *48*, 457–476. [CrossRef] [PubMed]

18. Liu, H.; Zhao, L.; Gu, W.; Liu, Q.; Gao, Z.; Zhu, X.; Wu, Z.; He, H.; Huang, F.; Fan, W. Activation of satellite glial cells in trigeminal ganglion following dental injury and inflammation. *J. Mol. Histol.* **2018**, *49*, 257–263. [CrossRef] [PubMed]

19. Nguyen, T.; Sherratt, P.J.; Pickett, C.B. Regulatory mechanisms controlling gene expression mediated by the antioxidant response element. *Annu. Rev. Pharmacol. Toxicol.* **2003**, *43*, 233–260. [CrossRef] [PubMed]

20. Osburn, W.O.; Yates, M.S.; Dolan, P.D.; Chen, S.; Liby, K.T.; Sporn, M.B.; Taguchi, K.; Yamamoto, M.; Kensler, T.W. Genetic or pharmacologic amplification of nrf2 signaling inhibits acute inflammatory liver injury in mice. *Toxicol. Sci.* **2008**, *104*, 218–227. [CrossRef] [PubMed]

21. Nomura, T.; Kikuchi, M.; Kubodera, A.; Kawakami, Y. Proton-donative antioxidant activity of fucoxanthin with 1,1-diphenyl-2-picrylhydrazyl (DPPH). *Biochem. Mol. Biol. Int.* **1997**, *42*, 361–370. [CrossRef] [PubMed]

22. Asai, A.; Sugawara, T.; Ono, H.; Nagao, A. Biotransformation of fucoxanthinol into amarouciaxanthin A in mice and HepG2 cells: Formation and cytotoxicity of fucoxanthin metabolites. *Drug Metab. Dispos.* **2004**, *32*, 205–211. [CrossRef] [PubMed]

23. Gammone, M.A.; Riccioni, G.; D'Orazio, N. Marine Carotenoids against Oxidative Stress: Effects on Human Health. *Mar. Drugs* **2015**, *13*, 6226–6246. [CrossRef] [PubMed]

24. Rengarajan, T.; Rajendran, P.; Nandakumar, N.; Balasubramanian, M.P.; Nishigaki, I. Cancer preventive efficacy of marine carotenoid fucoxanthin: Cell cycle arrest and apoptosis. *Nutrients* **2013**, *5*, 4978–4989. [CrossRef] [PubMed]

25. Tan, C.P.; Hou, Y.H. First evidence for the anti-inflammatory activity of fucoxanthin in high-fat-diet-induced obesity in mice and the antioxidant functions in PC12 cells. *Inflammation* **2014**, *37*, 443–450. [CrossRef] [PubMed]

26. Woo, M.N.; Jeon, S.M.; Shin, Y.C.; Lee, M.K.; Kang, M.A.; Choi, M.S. Anti-obese property of fucoxanthin is partly mediated by altering lipid-regulating enzymes and uncoupling proteins of visceral adipose tissue in mice. *Mol. Nutr. Food Res.* **2009**, *53*, 1603–1611. [CrossRef] [PubMed]

27. Beppu, F.; Hosokawa, M.; Yim, M.J.; Shinoda, T.; Miyashita, K. Down-regulation of hepatic stearoyl-CoA desaturase-1 expression by fucoxanthin via leptin signaling in diabetic/obese KK-A(y) mice. *Lipids* **2013**, *48*, 449–455. [CrossRef] [PubMed]

28. Sugawara, T.; Matsubara, K.; Akagi, R.; Mori, M.; Hirata, T. Antiangiogenic activity of brown algae fucoxanthin and its deacetylated product, fucoxanthinol. *J. Agric. Food Chem.* **2006**, *54*, 9805–9810. [CrossRef] [PubMed]

29. Chen, S.J.; Lee, C.J.; Lin, T.B.; Liu, H.J.; Huang, S.Y.; Chen, J.Z.; Tseng, K.W. Inhibition of Ultraviolet B-Induced Expression of the Proinflammatory Cytokines TNF-α and VEGF in the Cornea by Fucoxanthin Treatment in a Rat Model. *Mar. Drugs* **2016**, *14*, 13. [CrossRef] [PubMed]

30. Rodríguez-Luna, A.; Ávila-Román, J.; González-Rodríguez, M.L.; Cózar, M.J.; Rabasco, A.M.; Motilva, V.; Talero, E. Fucoxanthin-containing cream prevents epidermal hyperplasia and UVB-induced skin erythema in mice. *Mar. Drugs* **2018**, *16*, 378. [CrossRef] [PubMed]

31. Yang, Y.; Yang, I.; Cao, M.; Su, Z.Y.; Wu, R.; Guo, Y.; Fang, M.; Kong, A.N. Fucoxanthin elicits epigenetic modifications, Nrf2 activation and blocking transformation in mouse skin JB6 P+ Cells. *AAPS J.* **2018**, *20*, 32. [CrossRef] [PubMed]

32. Muller, L.J.; Marfurt, C.F.; Kruse, F.; Tervo, T.M. Corneal nerves: Structure, contents and function. *Exp. Eye Res.* **2003**, *76*, 521–542. [CrossRef]

33. Chen, Y.; Liu, Z.H.; Lin, Z.H.; Shi, X.Z. Eyes in pituitary disorders. *J. Biol. Regul. Homeost. Agents* **2018**, *32*, 97–99. [PubMed]

34. Stepp, M.A.; Tadvalkar, G.; Hakh, R.; Pal-Ghosh, S. Corneal epithelial cells function as surrogate Schwann cells for their sensory nerves. *Glia* **2017**, *65*, 851–863. [CrossRef] [PubMed]

35. Bishop, T.; Hewson, D.W.; Yip, P.K.; Fahey, M.S.; Dawbarn, D.; Young, A.R.; McMahon, S.B. Characterisation of ultraviolet-B-induced inflammation as a model of hyperalgesia in the rat. *Pain* **2007**, *131*, 70–82. [CrossRef] [PubMed]

36. Bishop, T.; Marchand, F.; Young, A.R.; Lewin, G.R.; McMahon, S.B. Ultraviolet-B-induced mechanical hyperalgesia: A role for peripheral sensitisation. *Pain* **2010**, *50*, 141–152. [CrossRef] [PubMed]

37. Davies, E.K.; Boyle, Y.; Chizh, B.A.; Lumb, B.M.; Murrell, J.C. Ultraviolet B-induced inflammation in the rat: A model of secondary hyperalgesia? *Pain* **2011**, *152*, 2844–2851. [CrossRef] [PubMed]

38. Sacchetti, M.; Abicca, I.; Bruscolini, A.; Cavaliere, C.; Nebbioso, M.; Lambiase, A. Allergic conjunctivitis: Current concepts on pathogenesis and management. *J. Biol. Regul. Homeost. Agents* **2018**, *32*, 49–60. [PubMed]

39. Moalem, G.; Tracey, D.J. Immune and inflammatory mechanisms in neuropathic pain. *Brain Res. Rev.* **2006**, *51*, 240–264. [CrossRef] [PubMed]

40. Shepherd, A.J.; Mickle, A.D.; Golden, J.P.; Mack, M.R.; Halabi, C.M.; de Kloet, A.D.; Samineni, V.K.; Kim, B.S.; Krause, E.G.; Gereau, R.W., 4th; et al. Macrophage angiotensin II type 2 receptor triggers neuropathic pain. *Proc. Natl. Acad. Sci. USA* **2018**, *115*, E8057–E8066. [CrossRef] [PubMed]

41. Karai, L.; Brown, D.C.; Mannes, A.J.; Connelly, S.T.; Brown, J.; Gandal, M.; Wellisch, O.M.; Neubert, J.K.; Olah, Z.; Iadarola, M.J. Deletion of vanilloid receptor 1-expressing primary afferent neurons for pain control. *J. Clin. Investig.* **2004**, *113*, 1344–1352. [CrossRef] [PubMed]

42. Julius, D. TRP channels and pain. *Annu. Rev. Cell Dev. Biol.* **2013**, *29*, 355–384. [CrossRef] [PubMed]

43. Kaji, K.; Shinoda, M.; Honda, K.; Unno, S.; Shimizu, N.; Iwata, K. Connexin 43 contributes to ectopic orofacial pain following inferior alveolar nerve injury. *Mol. Pain* **2016**, *12*, 1–12. [CrossRef] [PubMed]

44. Retamal, M.A.; Riquelme, M.A.; Stehberg, J.; Alcayaga, J. Connexin43 hemichannels in satellite glial cells, can they influence sensory neuron activity? *Front. Mol. Neurosci.* **2017**, *10*, 374. [CrossRef] [PubMed]

45. Murray, H.; Locker, D.; Mock, D.; Tenenbaum, H.C. Pain and the quality of life in patients referred to a craniofacial pain unit. *J. Orofac. Pain* **1996**, *10*, 316–323. [PubMed]

46. Hodges, P.W.; Tucker, K. Moving differently in pain: A new theory to explain the adaptation to pain. *Pain* **2011**, *152*, S90–S98. [CrossRef] [PubMed]

47. Piao, Z.G.; Cho, I.H.; Park, C.K.; Hong, J.P.; Choi, S.Y.; Lee, S.J.; Lee, S.; Park, K.; Kim, J.S.; Oh, S.B. Activation of glia and microglial p38 MAPK in medullary dorsal horn contributes to tactile hypersensitivity following trigeminal sensory nerve injury. *Pain* **2006**, *121*, 219–231. [CrossRef] [PubMed]

48. Xie, Y.F.; Zhang, S.; Chiang, C.Y.; Hu, J.W.; Dostrovsky, J.O.; Sessle, B.J. Involvement of glia in central sensitization in trigeminal subnucleus caudalis (medullary dorsal horn). *Brain Behav. Immun.* **2007**, *21*, 634–641. [CrossRef] [PubMed]

49. Zhu, L.; Lu, J.; Tay, S.S.; Jiang, H.; He, B.P. Induced NG2 expressing microglia in the facial motor nucleus after facial nerve axotomy. *Neuroscience* **2010**, *166*, 842–851. [CrossRef] [PubMed]

50. Ryu, J.; Kwon, M.J.; Nam, T.J. Nrf2 and NF-κB signaling pathways contribute to porphyra-334-mediated inhibition of UVA-induced inflammation in skin fibroblasts. *Mar. Drugs* **2015**, *13*, 4721–4732. [CrossRef] [PubMed]

51. Chen, H.H.; Wang, T.C.; Lee, Y.C.; Shen, P.T.; Chang, J.Y.; Yeh, T.K.; Huang, C.H.; Chang, H.H.; Cheng, S.Y.; Lin, C.Y.; et al. Novel Nrf2/ARE activator, trans-coniferylaldehyde, induces a HO-1-mediated defense mechanism through a dual p38α/MAPKAPK-2 and PK-N3 signaling pathway. *Chem. Res. Toxicol.* **2015**, *28*, 1681–1692. [CrossRef] [PubMed]

52. Yu, C.Q.; Zhang, M.; Matis, K.I.; Kim, C.; Rosenblatt, M.I. Vascular endothelial growth factor mediates corneal nerve repair. *Investig. Ophthalmol. Vis. Sci.* **2008**, *49*, 3870–3878. [CrossRef] [PubMed]

53. Farazifard, R.; Safarpour, F.; Sheibani, V.; Javan, M. Eye-wiping test: A sensitive animal model for acute trigeminal pain studies. *Brain Res. Protoc.* **2005**, *16*, 44–49. [CrossRef] [PubMed]

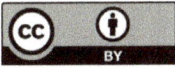

marine drugs

MDPI

Article

Fucoxanthin and Rosmarinic Acid Combination Has Anti-Inflammatory Effects through Regulation of NLRP3 Inflammasome in UVB-Exposed HaCaT Keratinocytes

Azahara Rodríguez-Luna [1,‡], Javier Ávila-Román [1,*,†,‡], Helena Oliveira [2], Virginia Motilva [1] and Elena Talero [1]

1. Department of Pharmacology, Faculty of Pharmacy, Universidad de Sevilla, 41012 Seville, Spain
2. Department of Biology, Faculty of Biology, University of Aveiro, 3810-193 Aveiro, Portugal
* Correspondence: javieravila@us.es or franciscojavier.avila@urv.cat; Tel.: +34 977558486
† Current position: Department of Biochemistry and Biotechnology, Faculty of Chemistry, Universitat Rovira i Virgili, 43007 Tarragona, Spain.
‡ Both authors contributed equally to this work.

Received: 16 July 2019; Accepted: 29 July 2019; Published: 1 August 2019

Abstract: Excessive exposure to ultraviolet (UV) radiation is the main risk factor to develop skin pathologies or cancer because it encourages oxidative condition and skin inflammation. In this sense, strategies for its prevention are currently being evaluated. Natural products such as carotenoids or polyphenols, which are abundant in the marine environment, have been used in the prevention of oxidative stress due to their demonstrated antioxidant activities. Nevertheless, the anti-inflammatory activity and its implication in photo-prevention have not been extensively studied. Thus, we aimed to evaluate the combination of fucoxanthin (FX) and rosmarinic acid (RA) on cell viability, apoptosis induction, inflammasome regulation, and anti-oxidative response activation in UVB-irradiated HaCaT keratinocytes. We demonstrated for the first time that the combination of FX and RA (5 μM RA plus 5 μM FX, designated as M2) improved antioxidant and anti-inflammatory profiles in comparison to compounds assayed individually, by reducing UVB-induced apoptosis and the consequent ROS production. Furthermore, the M2 combination modulated the inflammatory response through down-regulation of inflammasome components such as NLRP3, ASC, and Caspase-1, and the interleukin (IL)-1β production. In addition, Nrf2 and HO-1 antioxidant genes expression increased in UVB-exposed HaCaT cells pre-treated with M2. These results suggest that this combination of natural products exerts photo-protective effects by down-regulating NRLP3-inflammasome and increasing Nrf2 signalling pathway.

Keywords: fucoxanthin; rosmarinic acid; NRLP3; inflammasome; anti-oxidative; anti-inflammatory; photo-protection; UVB

---

1. Introduction

Skin is considered as the outmost protective barrier in the body, protecting from detrimental substances, mechanical damage, pathological invasion and radiation that could cause perturbations to the skin structure. In this sense, skin is a well-known essential piece of the immune system. Several factors can contribute to the initiation and development of cutaneous alterations. In this line, the excessive exposure to UV radiation remains the main risk factor for the skin cancer [1]. Solar UV radiation consists of three broad ranges of wavelength: UVC (100–280 nm), UVB (280–315 nm) and UVA (315–400 nm). UVB causes dermal changes, affects epidermal function and is the main factor responsible for the development of melanoma and non-melanoma skin cancer [2]. In this regard, a high dose of UVB exposure promotes cutaneous inflammation, which is traduced in sunburn, photo-aging, DNA damage, immunosuppression and induction of skin cancer [3].

It has been extensively studied that UVB-induced ROS production leads to activation of mitogen-activated protein kinase (MAPK) and nuclear factor-κB (NF-κB), among others, which further promote inflammation and apoptosis in cells and increase skin aging [4]. Furthermore, this type of inflammation results in the production of cytokines as tumour necrosis factor alpha (TNF-α), IL-6 and IL-1β, which are released by keratinocytes after UVB irradiation [5]. In this sense, it has been reported the relation between IL-1β secretion and activation of protein complexes called inflammasome [6]. Inflammasome is a wide cytosolic multiprotein complex that acts as mediator of the innate immune system, which is activated by multiple types of tissue damages. The nucleotide-binding domain, leucine-rich-repeat-containing family, pyrin domain-containing 3 (NLRP3) is the most studied inflammasome. NLRP3 gen induction results in activation of caspase-1, which by cleavage catalyses the processing of pro-IL-1β in cytosol to mature form, leading to IL-1β production in the extracellular medium [7]. In the last years, some authors have demonstrated the implication of NLRP3 inflammasome in tumorigenesis and cancer development, specifically in basal cell carcinomas [8,9].

Nowadays, non-melanoma skin cancer (NMSC) remains the most frequently diagnosed cancer in Caucasian people worldwide and strategies for its prevention are being developed [10]. At this regards, photo-chemoprevention by natural products is one of the most studied alternatives for skin protection, due to their anti-oxidative actions [1]. Although the anti-inflammatory properties of natural compounds have not been extensively investigated yet, in recent years, different studies have evaluated the beneficial effects of these compounds in photoprotection through their anti-inflammatory activity [1].

In last years, microalgae have been employed as a vast source of bioactive molecules with potential activity in inflammation and cancer [11]. Specifically, carotenoids have shown antioxidant, anti-inflammatory or anti-carcinogenic properties in several skin inflammatory models [12,13]. The orange carotenoid fucoxanthin (FX) is not exclusive from marine environmental [14] but it is an extensive compound produced by microalgae and brown seaweeds, as previously published [15] and it is known for its potent antioxidant properties. Nevertheless, its effect on NRLP3-inflammasome regulation has been little explored.

Polyphenols are the most popular antioxidant molecules in our diet, and exhibit other properties as anti-inflammatory or anti-neoplastic agents. For this reason, these compounds are also proposed as an important key for the management of skin protection [16]. In this regard, rosmarinic acid (RA) is a phenolic ester that has been traditionally isolated from some terrestrial plants as *Rosmarinus officinalis* L. or *Melissa officinalis* L. [17]. Moreover, this polyphenol has been abundantly found in *Zostera marina* seagrass beds [18,19]. This aspect is very interesting since *Zostera* has a rapid generation time and similar requirements to microalgae; thus it could be a great source to obtain a traditional phenolic compound like this. RA has been widely studied due to its remarkable biological and pharmacological activities, including anti-microbial, antioxidant and anti-inflammatory properties [20]. Until now, only a limited number of studies have dealt with the effect of RA on NLRP3-inflammasome [21–23], and none of them on human immortalized HaCaT keratinocytes.

These antecedents led us to evaluate the effects of a combination of FX and RA on ROS production, apoptosis prevention, cell cycle alterations, inflammasome regulation and Nrf2 pathway activation, in UVB-exposed human keratinocytes.

2. Results

2.1. Effects of RA and FX on Cell Viability

The UVB intensity was selected in a preliminary study in which three different intensities (100, 150 and 225 mJ/cm^2) were tested. To study the cell viability was used MTT assay (3-(4,5-dimethylthiazol-2-yl)-2,5-diphenyltetrazolium bromide). As expected, a UVB dose-dependent effect on cell death and morphology was observed. The intensity of 100 mJ/cm^2 was chosen for further assays since it allowed over 50% of cell survival and showed a significant difference in comparison with non-irradiated control group (Figure 1A). In addition, MTT results showed that the treatment with RA or FX at 5 μM, M1 (2.5 μM RA + 5 μM FX) and M2 (5 μM RA + 5 μM FX) significantly increased cell viability in UVB-exposed cells, being more effective M1 and M2 treatments (Figure 1B).

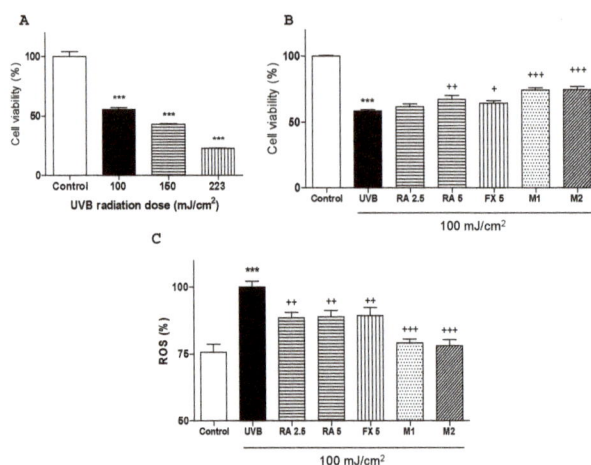

Figure 1. Selection of UVB dose and effect of rosmarinic acid (RA), fucoxanthin (FX) and combinations on cell viability and ROS production in UVB-irradiated HaCaT cells. (**A**) Effect of different UVB doses on cell viability determined by MTT assay. Results are expressed as percentage respect to untreated control cells and bars represents mean ± SEM of four independent experiments ($n = 4$) in duplicate. (*** $p < 0.001$ vs. untreated cells; Student t test) (**B**) Effect of RA, FX and their combinations on cell viability in human HaCaT keratinocytes was measured by MTT assay after 24 h of UVB exposition. (**C**) Intracellular ROS generation was evaluated 30 min after UVB irradiation by relative fluorescence intensity using 2′,7′-dichlorodihydrofluorescein diacetate (DCF-DA) assay. For experiments B and C, cells were pre-treated with RA (2.5 and 5 μM), FX (5 μM) and two combinations M1 (2.5 RA plus 5 μM FX) and M2 (5 μM RA plus 5 μM FX), for 1 h. Then, cells were irradiated with selected UVB dose (100 mJ/cm^2) and incubated for the required times. Results are expressed as percentage respect to untreated control cells (**B**) or UVB-exposed control cells (**C**), and bars represents mean ± SEM of at least six independent experiments ($n = 6$) in duplicate. The mean was significantly different compared to control cells (*** $p < 0.001$; Student t test). The mean was significantly different compared to UVB-irradiated cells (+ $p < 0.05$, ++ $p < 0.01$ and +++ $p < 0.001$; one-way ANOVA followed by Bonferroni's multiple comparison test).

2.2. Effect of RA and FX on UVB-induced ROS Production.

It is well known that intracellular ROS levels can be increased by UVB exposure [24]. In this sense, HaCaT cells were treated with the compounds for 1 h and then were irradiated with UVB (100 mJ/cm^2). Cells exposed to UVB showed a significant increase in ROS production in comparison with non-exposed control cells ($p < 0.001$). The pre-treatment with either RA at the concentration of 2.5 or 5 μM or FX at 5 μM notably reduced intracellular ROS levels by 12%, 12% and 10%, respectively ($p < 0.01$). Nevertheless, concomitant administration of RA and FX (M1 or M2) showed a more marked decrease in ROS production, by 21% and 22%, respectively ($p < 0.001$) than the single treatments (Figure 1C).

2.3. Effect of RA and FX on Apoptosis

It is well reported that apoptosis is the most important type of programmed cell death in response to cell damage induced by UVB exposure [25]. In this sense, Annexin V (annexin family of intracellular protein)-FITC assay allows to differentiate cell subpopulations in different stages as necrotic (R1), viable (R2), early apoptosis (R3) or late apoptosis (R4). For this assay, only the adherent cells were considered, which means that the dead cells in suspension after UVB irradiation were not analysed and thus significant changes were not observed in this phase [26]. Our results showed that UVB exposure, in comparison with non-irradiated cells, significantly decreased the percentage of viable cells from 88% to 20%, increased the number of cells in early apoptosis from 1% to 5% and strongly augmented the percentage of cells in late apoptosis from 8% to 72% (Figure 2A). Regarding to pre-treatments, neither RA nor FX exhibited percentages changes in the different subpopulations, respect to UVB-exposed cells. Nevertheless, the treatment with M1 or M2 allowed a significant reduction of the percentage of late apoptotic cells and a marked increase of viable cells in comparison with irradiated control cells (Figure 2A).

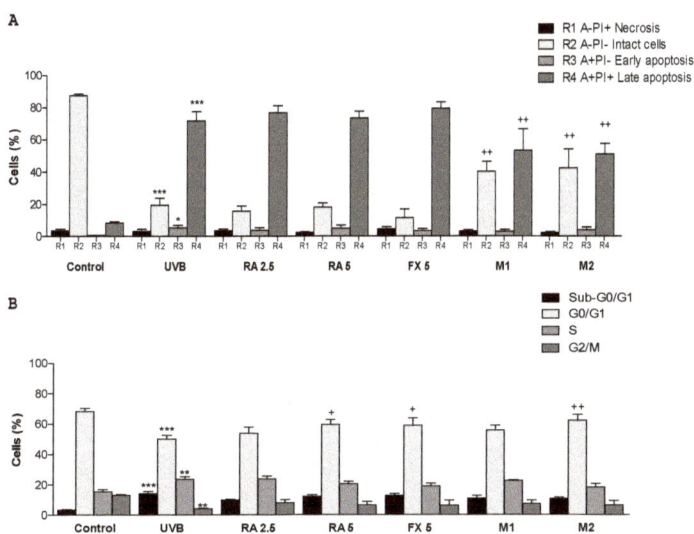

Figure 2. Effect of rosmarinic acid (RA), fucoxanthin (FX) and combinations on apoptosis and cell cycle arrest by using flow cytometry. (**A**) Results of Annexin V-FITC assay as percentage of cells in different apoptotic phases; R1: necrotic cells (Annexin V-FITC negative, PI positive), R2: viable cells (Annexin V-FITC negative, PI negative), R3: early apoptotic cells (Annexin V-FITC positive, PI negative), R4: late apoptotic cells (Annexin V-FITC positive, PI positive). Cells were pre-treated with RA (2.5 and 5 μM), FX (5 μM) and two combinations M1 (2.5 RA plus 5 μM FX) and M2 (5 μM RA plus 5 μM FX), then were irradiated with selected UVB dose (100 mJ/cm^2) and incubated for 24 h. (**B**) Cell cycle phase distribution of UVB-exposed HaCaT cells. Cells were incubated with treatments for 48 h. Data are expressed as percentage and bars represents mean ± SEM of four independent experiments (n = 4) in duplicate. Results are expressed as percentage and bars represents mean ± SEM of four independent experiments (n = 4) in duplicate. The mean value was significantly different compared with control group (*** $p < 0.001$, ** $p < 0.01$, * $p < 0.05$ vs. untreated cells; Mann–Whitney U-test). The mean value was significantly different compared with UVB-irradiated cells $^+$ $p < 0.05$, $^{++}$ $p < 0.01$ vs. UVB-irradiated cells; Kruskal–Wallis test followed by Dunn's multiple comparison test).

2.4. Effect of RA and FX on Cell Cycle

It is well known that UV light exposure promotes skin photo-damage such as cell death and DNA damage and, consequently, cell cycle arrest [27]. Our results indicated that UVB-exposure highly affects the percentage of cells at G0/G1 phase, showing a reduction in this percentage from 68% to 50%, accompanied by an increase in apoptotic sub-G1 subpopulations from 3% to 14%, compared with non-exposed cells (Figure 2B). Moreover, UVB-exposed control group showed a significant increase in the percentage of cells in S phase, from 16% to 24%, and a marked decrease of cells in G2/M phase from 13% to 3% in comparison with non-irradiated control group. Pre-treatment with RA or FX at 5 μM, as well as concomitant administration of RA and FX at 5 μM (M2) significantly augmented the number of cells at G0/G1 phase in comparison with UVB-exposed cells. However, the percentage of cells in S phase was only reduced by M2, reaching similar values that those in control group (Figure 2B).

2.5. Effect of RA and FX on Inflammasome Regulation

It has been well documented that inflammasome can be activated by several factors, among them UVB exposure [8]. In the present study, we demonstrated that UVB irradiation led to up-regulation of NLRP3, ASC and caspase-1 expression and, consequently, promoted a significant increase in IL-1β production in comparison with non-exposed cells (Figure 3A–D). Pre-treatment with either RA or FX at 5 μM did not significantly modify the expression levels of inflammasome-related proteins. Nevertheless, combination of RA and FX at 5 μM (M2) significantly down-regulated NLRP3 and ASC expression levels ($p < 0.01$) as well as caspase-1 levels ($p < 0.05$) in comparison with UVB-exposed cells. Furthermore, pre-treatment with M2 reduced IL-1β production in a significant manner ($p < 0.01$) (Figure 3D).

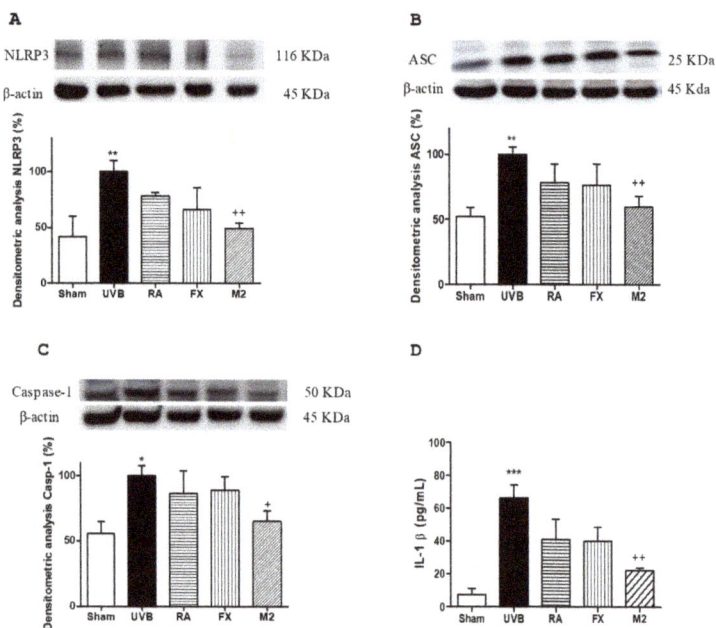

Figure 3. Effect of rosmarinic acid (RA), fucoxanthin (FX) and concomitant administration of RA and FX (M2) on inflammasome components expression and IL-1β levels in UVB-exposed HaCaT keratinocytes. Cells were pre-treated with RA (5 μM), FX (5 μM) and M2 (5 μM RA plus 5 μM FX) for 1h, then were UVB-irradiated (100 mJ/cm^2) and incubated for 24 h. Densitometry analysis of (**A**) nucleotide-binding domain, leucine-rich-repeat-containing family, pyrin domain- containing 3 (NLRP3), (**B**) inflammasome adaptor protein (ASC) and (**C**) caspase-1 positivity were performed following normalization to the control (β-actin housekeeping gene). (**D**) IL-1β production was evaluated by ELISA assay. Results are expressed as percentage respect to UVB-irradiated control and bars represents mean ± SEM of four independent experiments ($n = 4$). The mean value was significantly different compared with control group (* $p < 0.05$, ** $p < 0.01$ and *** $p < 0.001$; Mann–Whitney U-test). The mean value was significantly different compared with UVB-irradiated cells ([+] $p < 0.05$ and [++] $p < 0.01$; Kruskal–Wallis test followed by Dunn's multiple comparison test).

2.6. Effect of RA and FX on Nrf-2 Antioxidant Signaling Pathway

To further elucidate the photo-protective mechanism of the combination of RA and FX, we evaluated the capacity to activate antioxidant pathways as Nrf2, which promotes the transcription of antioxidant genes and detoxification of enzymes such as heme-oxygenase 1 (HO-1) to protect against an oxidative damage as UVB exposure [28]. Our results showed that UVB irradiation prevented the increase of Nrf2 and HO-1 expression (Figure 4A–B). Non-irradiated control cells (sham) did not exhibit the highest expression levels of these antioxidant proteins because these cells were not exposed to any stress. Nevertheless, UVB-exposed HaCaT cells and pre-treated with FX at 5 μM or the combination of RA and FX at 5 μM (M2) significantly up-regulated Nrf2 expression levels ($p < 0.05$ and $p < 0.01$, respectively), reaching higher values that those in control cells. Regarding HO-1 expression, only M2 was able to significantly enhance this protein levels ($p < 0.05$).

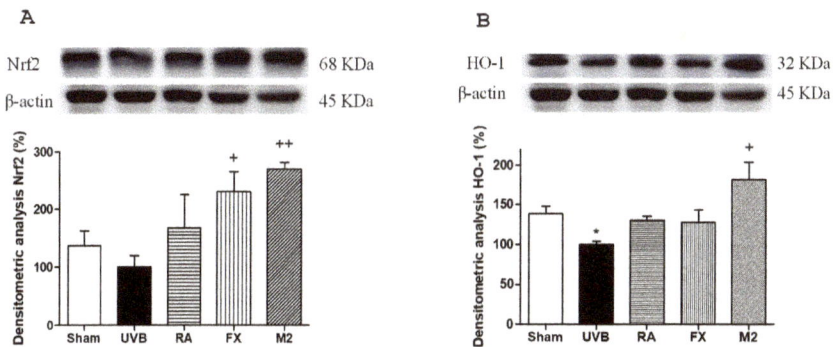

Figure 4. Effect of rosmarinic acid (RA), fucoxanthin (FX) and concomitant administration of RA and FX (M2) on Nrf2 and HO-1 expression in UVB-exposed HaCaT keratinocytes. Cells were pre-treated with RA (5 μM), FX (5 μM) and M2 (5 μM RA plus 5 μM FX) for 1 h, then were UVB-irradiated (100 mJ/cm^2) and incubated for 24 h. Densitometry analysis of (**A**) Nrf2 and (**B**) HO-1 were performed following normalization to the control (β-actin housekeeping gene). Data shown are expressed as percentage respect to UVB-irradiated control and bars represents mean ± SEM of four independent experiments ($n = 4$). The mean value was significantly different compared with control group (* $p < 0.05$; Mann–Whitney U-test). The mean value was significantly different compared with UVB-irradiated cells ($^+$ $p < 0.05$ and $^{++}$ $p < 0.01$; Kruskal–Wallis test followed by Dunn's multiple comparison test.

3. Discussion

Skin represents the first barrier that protects us from the deleterious effects of solar UV radiation, which is the main cause for skin cancer. Nevertheless, human skin is normally exposed to UV irradiation in a non-controlled way. Whereas a short-term UV exposure might suppress immune function or trigger an inflammatory response, chronic UV exposition conduces to photo-aging, DNA damage, or carcinoma [29]. Skin has an antioxidant system, composed by enzymatic and non-enzymatic antioxidants, to prevent against toxic exogenous/endogenous ROS levels. Nowadays, it is well known the importance of natural substances that support the endogenous antioxidant systems of the skin via diet or dermatological preparations [30]. To develop new skin photo-protective agents it is necessary to understand the molecular mechanism of UV-induced cellular responses and determine how these products may act in the skin cells. In this sense, many treatments with a unique compound have demonstrated successful results against photo-damage, but a more hopeful impact was obtained when a combination of several compounds was used [31]. The efficacy of combinations could be due to the synergistic effect of their components. In this regard, natural products may be good candidates for skin photo-protection due to their low toxicity and high antioxidant capacity [32]. Thus, the present study aimed to evaluate the preventive effect of a combination of RA and FX in UVB-exposed human HaCaT keratinocytes.

It is well reported that UVB radiation increases ROS production and DNA damage as well as promotes a strong inflammatory response characterized by pro-inflammatory mediator production [33]. In this condition, apoptosis activation can eliminate the irreversibly damaged cells that could harbour oncogenic mutation [25]. In this line, FX has demonstrated antioxidant activity offering protection against DNA damage and preventing cellular apoptosis in HaCaT human keratinocytes [34,35]. In a similar way, several studies have reported that RA reduces ROS production, protects against DNA damage and regulates apoptotic markers in vitro [31,36]. According to these findings, our results showed that the pre-treatment with FX or RA at 5 μM significantly attenuated UVB-induced damage by increasing cell viability and inhibiting ROS production in human HaCaT keratinocytes, but did not modify the number of apoptotic cells after UVB exposure. Nevertheless, the selected combination of RA and FX at 5 μM at equal dose (M2) not only improved cell viability and ROS levels in comparison with FX and RA administered separately, but also enhanced the cellular protection, reducing the number of cells in apoptosis after UVB irradiation. In addition to cellular responses previously detailed, UVB exposure also affected cell cycle dynamics. Previous studies have reported that UV exposure activates cell cycle arrest in both G1 and G2 phases [37]. At this respect, our results reported that UVB irradiation significantly reduced cells at G0/G1 phase when compared with non-exposed cells. Furthermore, a S-phase delay was observed in UVB-exposed cells although it did not show to be highly affected by the treatments. The pre-treatment with FX, RA and concomitant administration of RA and FX (M2) significantly increased the percentage of cells at G0/G1 and reduced the percentage of cells at sub-G1. In this sense, our observations are in accordance with the results obtained in apoptosis assay. M2 prevented cell damage, reducing the percentage of cells under apoptosis 24 h after UVB exposure. In consequence, this combination promoted a higher percentage of viable cells at 48 h in UVB-exposed cells.

In terms of inflammation, it has been reported that pro-IL-1β is cleaved and IL-1β is released from cells as a pro-inflammatory cytokine after NLRP3 inflammasome activation [38]. Thus, it could be concluded that IL-1β production in keratinocytes is inflammasome-dependent [6]. Moreover, NLRP3 inflammasome activation by UVB increases not only IL-1β but also other pro-inflammatory cytokines such as IL-1α, IL-6, TNF-α or the mediator PGE2 [7]. In this line, NLRP3 inflammasome plays an important role in UVB-induced skin inflammatory responses and has a critical function in skin pathologies initiation such as cancer [8]. In addition, the inflammasome adaptor protein ASC has shown anti-tumour activity by activation of tumour suppressor protein p53 in UVB-irradiated keratinocytes [39]. Due to the high connection between inflammasome, inflammation and cancer, the therapeutic strategies targeting inflammasome-related products are currently in development and suppose a pivotal tool for skin pathologies and cancer prevention [40]. In previous studies, FX has shown anti-inflammatory activity through NF-κB and MAPKs signalling pathways regulation [41], and consequently the down-regulation of IL-1β, TNF-α, inducible nitric oxide synthase, and cyclooxygenase-2 expression [42–44]. On the other hand, the polyphenol RA has been previously reported to inhibit pro-inflammatory cytokines production, including IL-1β, and to down-regulate NF-κB signalling pathway in skin cells [45]. In addition, this polyphenol has shown to modulate inflammasome activation, through down-regulation of caspase-1, NLRP3 and ASC expression in a poly(I:C)-induced inflammation in an infectious model by using epidermal keratinocytes [21]. Moreover, due to its anti-inflammatory properties, RA has been proposed to ameliorate allergic reactions in allergic rhinitis and rhinoconjunctivitis [46]. Furthermore, this compound has shown to prevent cisplatin-induced apoptosis in chemotherapy by down-regulating the caspase-1 expression [47]. However, the role of FX or RA on NLRP3 inflammasome regulation in human keratinocytes has not been studied yet. In this line, our findings reported for the first time that the combination of RA and FX notably reduced inflammasome-related proteins such as NLRP3, ASC and caspase-1 in

UVB-irradiated HaCaT keratinocytes. Interestingly, this effect was not detected when both compounds were administered separately, suggesting the beneficial effect of concomitant treatment with RA and FX.

The antioxidant role of FX and RA has been well-described. FX has shown to promote AKT/Nrf2/GSH-dependent antioxidant response in keratinocytes [48,49], as well as reduce wrinkles formation and epidermal hypertrophy in mice [50] and supress melanogenesis and prostaglandin synthesis [51]. In this line, due to its antioxidant activity, this carotenoid has been proposed as a photo-protective compound by stimulating skin barrier restoration in UVA-induced sunburn [52]. Furthermore, a previous study by our group evidenced that FX increased Nrf2 and HO-1 expression in UVB-induced acute erythema in SKH-1 hairless mice [44]. These results are in line with other authors that suggest that this compound could be an interesting strategy to counteract UVB-induced oxidative damage in skin [53]. At this regard, similar properties have been demonstrated with RA applications, confirming the antioxidant activity of this polyphenol via activation of Nrf2-antioxidant system [54,55]. In accordance with these findings, the combination between FX and RA (M2) used in this study showed an up-regulation of Nrf2 transcriptional factor and its main target gene HO-1. These data indicate that the protective activity of M2 may be due to the reduction of oxidative stress through modulation of Nrf2 signalling pathway.

4. Materials and Methods

4.1. Compounds

RA and FX were obtained from Sigma-Aldrich (St. Louis, MO, USA). RA and FX stocks were prepared in DMSO at 10 mM and diluted to the desired concentration with culture medium. Controls were incubated with the corresponding quantity of DMSO, which was always below 1% and did not affect cell viability

4.2. Cell Line

Human immortalized keratinocytes HaCaT were obtained from the American Type Culture Collection (ATCC) and maintained in high glucose Dulbecco's modified Eagle's medium (DMEM, GIBCO, Grand Island, NY, USA) containing 2 mM L-glutamine. The culture media was supplemented with 10% heat-inactivated fetal bovine serum, 100 U/mL penicillin and 100 mg/mL streptomycin (PAA Laboratories, Pasching, Austria). Cultures were incubated in an atmosphere of 5% CO_2 at 37 °C.

4.3. UVB-Irradiation

The CL-1000M UV Crosslinker system (UVP, Upland, CA, USA), formed by 5 UVB tubes (8 W), was used to submit an energy spectrum of UVB radiation (peak intensity 302 nm, inside of the spectrum of UVB light 280–315 nm). To prevent UVB light absorption by the cell culture medium the medium was replaced by a thin layer of phosphate buffer solution (PBS) to cover the cells during irradiation. Three UVB intensities were evaluated (100, 150 and 225 mJ/cm^2) to determine the most suitable to evaluate cell cycle alterations and apoptosis [22]. In this sense, 100 mJ/cm^2 was selected for the study.

4.4. Cell Proliferation Assay

Cell viability was evaluated by the colorimetric 3-(4,5-dimethyl-2-thiazolyl)-2,5-diphenyl tetrazolium bromide (MTT) (Sigma-Aldrich, St. Louis, MO, USA) assay, which determines the formation of purple formazan in viable cells and allows estimate cellular viability [56]. MTT assay was performed according to protocol described with slight modifications. Briefly, HaCaT cells were seeded at a density of 10^4 cells/well in a 96-well plate for 24 h. Cells were pre-treated with different doses either RA (2.5, 5, 7.5 and 10 µM) or FX (5, 10, 15 and 20 µM) and the sixteen possible combinations between RA and FX, for 1 h. Then, the culture medium was replaced with a thin layer of PBS and exposed to a single dose of UVB radiation at 100 mJ/cm^2. Cells were supplied with fresh culture medium and incubated for 24 h. Absorbance was measured at 570 nm using a Synergy HT Multi-mode Microplate Reader (BioTek Instruments, Winooski, VT, USA).

4.5. Intracellular ROS Scavenging Activity

The 2′,7′-dichlorodihydrofluorescein diacetate (DCF-DA) assay was used to detect intracellular ROS levels in HaCaT keratinocytes [57]. Briefly, keratinocytes were seeded at 10^4 cells/well in 96-well plates and were treated with RA (2.5 and 5 μM), FX (5 μM) and the combinations M1 (2.5 RA plus 5 μM FX) and M2 (5 μM RA plus 5 μM FX) for 1 h. After UVB exposure (100 mJ/cm^2), cells were incubated with 2′,7′-dichlorodihydrofluorescein diacetate (DCFH-DA) solution (5 mg/mL) in PBS for 30 min at 37 °C. Then, the medium was discarded and the cells were washed with PBS. The fluorescence of the 2′,7′-dichlorofluorescein (DCF) product was determined by using a fluorescence plate reader (Sinergy HT, Biotek®, Bad Friedrichshall, Germany) at 485 nm for excitation and 535 nm for emission.

4.6. Apoptosis Determination

Apoptosis was evaluated by flow cytometry using Annexin V-FITC Apoptosis detection kit from BD Pharmingen (Franklin Lakes, NJ, USA), as previously reported [26]. Briefly, HaCaT cells were seeded at 5×10^5 cells/well in 6-well plates and incubated for complete adhesion. The day after seeding, cells were treated with RA (2.5 and 5 μM), FX (5 μM) and mixtures M1 (2.5 RA plus 5 μM FX) and M2 (5 μM RA plus 5 μM FX) for 1 h. After that, treatments were removed and cells were irradiated at 100 mJ/cm^2, and then incubated with fresh medium for 24 h. Cells were harvested and suspended in binding buffer at 10^5 cells/mL. Then, annexin V-FITC and propidium iodide (PI) were added as indicated in the manufacture's protocol. Subsequently, samples were kept in darkness for 15 min and 400 μL of binding buffed were added. Fluorescence intensity of PI and FITC-Annexin-V-stained cells was determined on a Coulter Epics XL Flow Cytometer (Beckman Coulter, Hialeah, FL, USA). Data were obtained using the SYSTEM II (v.2.5.) software examining 10^4 events. The cytogram of FITC fluorescence in log scale versus PI fluorescence in log scales allows the identification of viable cells (Annexin V-FITC negative, PI negative), early apoptotic cells (Annexin V-FITC positive, PI negative), late apoptotic cells (Annexin V-FITC positive, PI positive) and necrotic cells (Annexin V-FITC negative, PI positive). Flow cytometry data were analysed by FlowJo software (Tree Star Inc., Ashland, OR, USA).

4.7. Cell Cycle Determination

For cell cycle determination, a similar procedure to apoptosis evaluation was carried out, with the difference of that after irradiation, cells were incubated with fresh medium for 48 h. After incubation, keratinocytes were harvested by trypsinization as previously detailed [26], fixed in 85% cold ethanol (5×10^5 cells/mL) and kept at −20 °C until further analysis. Ethanol was eliminated, cells were resuspended in PBS, and the cell suspension was filtered through a 35 μm nylon mesh to separate aggregated cells. Then, 50 μL RNase (1 mg/mL) and 50 μL PI (1 mg/mL) were added to each sample, which was then incubated for 20 min in darkness at room temperature until analysis. DNA content was determined on a Coulter Epics XL Flow Cytometer (Beckman Coulter, Hialeah, FL, USA). Data were acquired using the SYSTEM II (v. 2.5.) software examining 10^4 events. Percentages of cells in apoptotic-sub G1, G0/G1, S and G2/M were calculated using CXP software.

4.8. Determination of IL-1β Production

HaCaT cells were seeded at 5×10^5 cells/well in 6-well plates, incubated for 24 h and treated with either RA (5 μM), FX (5 μM) or M2 (5 μM RA plus 5 μM FX), for 1 h. Then, the cells were irradiated at 100 mJ/cm^2, and incubated with fresh medium for 24 h. Supernatant fluids were collected and stored at −80 °C until use. Commercial enzyme-linked immunosorbent assay (ELISA) kits (Diaclone GEN-PROBE, Besançon cedex, France) was used to quantify IL-1β production according to the manufacturer's protocol. The absorbance at 450 nm was read by a microplate reader (Sinergy HT, Biotek®, Bad Friedrichshall,

Germany). To calculate the concentration of IL-1β (pg/mL), a standard curve was constructed using serial dilutions of cytokine standards provided with the kit.

4.9. Western Blot Analysis

The cell culture and treatments were similar to those carried out for cytokine production. Then, HaCaT cells were harvested by trypsinization, centrifuged and resuspended in lysis buffer (50 mM HEPES, 150 mM NaCl, 1 mM EDTA, 1 mM EGTA, 10% glycerol, 1% Triton-X-100, 1 mM phenylmethylsulphonyl fluoride, protease inhibitor cocktail tablet, 0.5 mM sodium orthovanadate, 20 mM sodium pyrophosphate). The homogenates were centrifuged (12,000 g, 15 min, 4 °C), and the supernatants were collected and stored at −80 °C. Bradford colorimetric method was utilized to determine the protein concentration of the homogenates [58]. Samples of the supernatants with equal amounts of protein (20 µg) were separated on 10% acrylamide gel by sodium dodecyl sulphate polyacrylamide gel electrophoresis. Next, the proteins were electrophoretically transferred onto a nitrocellulose membrane and incubated with specific primary antibodies: rabbit anti-ASC (Bio-Rad, Hercules, CA, USA) (1:1000), rabbit anti-NLRP3 (1:1000), rabbit anti-Nrf2 (1:1000), rabbit anti-HO-1 (1:1000), rabbit anti-caspase-1 (1:1000) (Cell Signaling, Danvers, MA, USA) overnight at 4 °C. After rising, the membranes were incubated with the horseradish peroxidase-linked (HRP) secondary antibody anti-rabbit (Cayman Chemical®, Ann Arbor, MI, USA) (1:1000) or anti-mouse (Dako®, Atlanta, GA, USA) (1:1000) containing blocking solution for 1 h at room temperature. To prove equal loading, the blots were analysed for β-actin expression using an anti-β-actin antibody (Sigma Aldrich®, St. Louis, MO, USA). Immunodetection was performed employing an enhanced chemiluminescence light-detecting kit (SuperSignal West Pico Chemiluminescent Substrate, Pierce, IL, USA). Then, the immunosignals were monitored by using an Amersham Imaging 600 (GE Healthcare Life Sciences, Barcelona, Spain) and densitometric data were analysed after normalization to the control (housekeeping gene). The signals were analysed and quantified with a Scientific Imaging Systems (Biophotonics ImageJ Analysis Software, National Institute of Mental Health, Bethesda, MD, USA) and expressed as total percentage respect to UVB-exposed control group.

4.10. Statistical Analysis

All values in the figures and text are expressed as arithmetic means ± standard error of the mean (S.E.M.). Data were evaluated with GraphPad Prism® Version 5.00 software (San Diego, CA, USA). In all cases, the Shapiro–Wilk test was used to verify the normality of the data. The Mann–Whitney U-test was chosen for non-parametric values. The parametric values groups were analysed by one-way analysis of variance (ANOVA) followed by Bonferroni's multiple comparison test. p values < 0.05 were considered statistically significant.

5. Conclusions

In conclusion, we have demonstrated for the first time that the combination of RA and FX shows additional benefits in comparison with the compounds administered separately on UVB-irradiated keratinocytes. The studied combination (M2) increased cell viability by reducing UVB-induced apoptosis and decreased intracellular ROS production. Moreover, the concomitant administration of RA and FX showed anti-inflammatory activity through NLRP3 inflammasome modulation, as well as antioxidant properties via up-regulation of Nrf2/HO-1 antioxidant system. Overall, we propose the combination of RA and FX as a natural promising tool in prevention of UVB-induced skin alterations as photo-aging, skin inflammation and its derivation to pre-cancerous lesions and skin carcinomas.

Author Contributions: Conceptualization, J. A-R, E.T. and V.M.; methodology, A.R-L and H.O; formal analysis A R-L, J. A-R, H.O, V-M and E.T; and E.T, J. A-R and H.O analysed the data; writing—original draft preparation A.R-L., J.A.-R., H.O, V.M., and E.T; writing—review and editing J.A.-R, E.T; funding acquisition, V.M. All the authors critically reviewed and approved the final version of the manuscript.

Funding: This work was supported by grants from the Consejería de Innovación, Ciencia y Empresa-Junta de Andalucía POLFANAT-P12-AGR-430 and from University of Seville "V Plan Propio US-PPI2015-1.5". Thanks are due to FCT/MCTES for the financial support to CESAM (UID/AMB/50017/2019), through national funds. FCT is also acknowledged for the research contract under Stimulus of Scientific Employment 2017 to H. Oliveira (CEECIND/04050/2017). We thank "Centro de Investigación, Tecnología e Innovación (CITIUS)" at University of Seville for providing technical assistance.

Conflicts of Interest: The authors have no conflicts of interest to declare.

Abbreviations

ASC	apoptosis-attached-speck-like protein containing a CARD
DCFH-DA	2′,7′-dichlorodihydrofluorescein diacetate
FX	Fucoxanthin
HO-1	heme oxygenase 1
IL	Interleukin
NMSC	non-melanoma skin cancer
NLRP3	nucleotide-binding domain, leucine-rich-repeat-containing family, pyrin domain- containing 3
Nrf2	nuclear factor E2-related factor 2
ROS	reactive oxygen species
SRB	sulforhodamine B
TNF-α	tumour necrosis factor alpha
TPA	12-O-tetradecanoylphorbol-13-acetate
UV	ultraviolet

References

1. Alam, S.; Pal, A.; Singh, D.; Ansari, K.M. Topical Application of Nexrutine Inhibits UVB-induced Cutaneous Inflammatory Responses in SKH-1 Hairless Mouse. *Photodermatol. Photoimmunol. Photomed.* **2018**, *34*, 82–90. [CrossRef] [PubMed]

2. Katiyar, S.K.; Pal, H.C.; Prasad, R. Dietary Proanthocyanidins Prevent Ultraviolet Radiation-Induced Non-Melanoma Skin Cancer Through Enhanced Repair of Damaged DNA-Dependent Activation of Immune Sensitivity. *Semin. Cancer Biol.* **2017**, *46*, 138–145. [CrossRef] [PubMed]

3. Hatakeyama, M.; Fukunaga, A.; Washio, K.; Taguchi, K.; Oda, Y.; Ogura, K.; Nishigori, C. Anti-Inflammatory Role of Langerhans Cells and Apoptotic Keratinocytes in Ultraviolet-B-Induced Cutaneous Inflammation. *J. Immunol.* **2017**, *199*, 2937–2947. [CrossRef] [PubMed]

4. Subedi, L.; Lee, T.H.; Wahedi, H.M.; Baek, S.H.; Kim, S.Y. Resveratrol-Enriched Rice Attenuates UVB-ROS-Induced Skin Aging Via Downregulation of Inflammatory Cascades. *Oxid. Med. Cell. Longev.* **2017**, *2017*, 8379539. [CrossRef] [PubMed]

5. Kondo, S.; Sauder, D.N.; Kono, T.; Galley, K.A.; McKenzie, R.C. Differential Modulation of Interleukin-1 Alpha (IL-1α) and Interleukin-1 beta (IL-1β) in Human Epidermal Keratinocytes by UVB. *Exp. Dermatol.* **1994**, *3*, 29–39. [CrossRef] [PubMed]

6. Feldmeyer, L.; Keller, M.; Niklaus, G.; Hohl, D.; Werner, S.; Beer, H.D. The Inflammasome Mediates UVB-Induced Activation and Secretion of Interleukin-1β by Keratinocytes. *Curr. Biol.* **2007**, *17*, 1140–1145. [CrossRef]

7. Hasegawa, T.; Nakashima, M.; Suzuki, Y. Nuclear DNA Damage-Triggered NLRP3 Inflammasome Activation Promotes UVB-Induced Inflammatory Responses in Human Keratinocytes. *Biochem. Biophys. Res. Commun.* **2016**, *477*, 329–335. [CrossRef]

8. Ahmad, I.; Muneer, K.M.; Chang, M.E.; Nasr, H.M.; Clay, J.M.; Huang, C.C.; Yusuf, N. Ultraviolet Radiation-Induced Downregulation of SERCA2 Mediates Activation of NLRP3 Inflammasome in Basal Cell Carcinoma. *Photochem. Photobiol.* **2017**, *93*, 1025–1033. [CrossRef]

9. Huang, C.F.; Chen, L.; Li, Y.C.; Wu, L.; Yu, G.T.; Zhang, W.F.; Sun, Z.J. NLRP3 Inflammasome Activation Promotes Inflammation-Induced Carcinogenesis in Head and Neck Squamous Cell Carcinoma. *J. Exp. Clin. Cancer Res.* **2017**, *36*, 116. [CrossRef]

10. Zink, A.; Koch, E.; Seifert, F.; Rotter, M.; Spinner, C.D.; Biedermann, T. Non-Melanoma Skin Cancer in Mountain Guides: High Prevalence and Lack of Awareness Warrant Development of Evidence-Based Prevention Tools. *Swiss Med. Wkly.* **2016**, *146*, w14380.

11. Talero, E.; García-mauriño, S.; Ávila-román, J.; Rodríguez-Luna, A.; Alcaide, A.; Motilva, V. Bioactive Compounds Isolated from Microalgae in Chronic Inflammation and Cancer. *Mar. Drugs* **2015**, *13*, 6152–6209. [CrossRef] [PubMed]

12. Oh, J.; Kim, J.H.; Park, J.G.; Yi, Y.S.; Park, K.W.; Rho, H.S.; Lee, M.S.; Yoo, J.W.; Kang, S.H.; Hong, Y.D.; et al. Radical Scavenging Activity-Based and AP-1-Targeted Anti-Inflammatory Effects of Lutein in Macrophage-Like and Skin Keratinocytic Cells. *Mediat. Inflamm.* **2013**, *2013*, 787042. [CrossRef] [PubMed]

13. Yoshihisa, Y.; Andoh, T.; Matsunaga, K.; Rehman, M.U.; Maoka, T.; Shimizu, T. Efficacy of Astaxanthin for the Treatment of Atopic Dermatitis in a Murine Model. *PLoS ONE* **2016**, *11*, e0152288. [CrossRef] [PubMed]

14. Amicucci, A.; Barbieri, E.; Sparvoli, V.; Gioacchini, A.M.; Calcabrini, C.; Palma, F.; Stocchi, V.; Zambonelli, A. Microbial and Pigment Profile of the Reddish Patch Occurring within Tuber Magnatum Ascomata. *Fungal Biol.* **2018**, *122*, 1134–1141. [CrossRef] [PubMed]

15. D'Orazio, N.; Gemello, E.; Gammone, M.A.; de Girolamo, M.; Ficoneri, C.; Riccioni, G. Fucoxantin: A Treasure from the Sea. *Mar. Drugs* **2012**, *10*, 604–616. [CrossRef] [PubMed]

16. Saric, S.; Sivamani, R. Polyphenols and Sunburn. *Int. J. Mol. Sci.* **2016**, *17*, 1521. [CrossRef] [PubMed]

17. Petersen, M. Rosmarinic Acid: New Aspects. *Phytochem. Rev.* **2013**, *12*, 207–227. [CrossRef]

18. Wang, J.; Pan, X.; Han, Y.; Guo, D.; Guo, Q.; Li, R. Rosmarinic Acid from Eelgrass Shows Nematicidal and Antibacterial Activities Against Pine Wood Nematode and Its Carrying Bacteria. *Mar. Drugs* **2012**, *10*, 2729–2740. [CrossRef]

19. Guan, C.; Parrot, D.; Wiese, J.; Sönnichsen, F.D.; Saha, M.; Tasdemir, D.; Weinberger, F. Identification of Rosmarinic Acid and Sulfated Flavonoids as Inhibitors of Microfouling on the Surface of Eelgrass *Zostera* Marina. *Biofouling* **2017**, *33*, 867–880. [CrossRef]

20. Amoah, S.K.S.; Sandjo, L.P.; Kratz, J.M.; Biavatti, M.W. Rosmarinic Acid-Pharmaceutical and Clinical Aspects. *Planta Med.* **2016**, *82*, 388–406. [CrossRef]

21. Zhou, M.W.; Jiang, R.H.; Kim, K.D.; Lee, J.H.; Kim, C.D.; Yin, W.T.; Lee, J.H. Rosmarinic Acid Inhibits Poly(I:C)-Induced Inflammatory Reaction of Epidermal Keratinocytes. *Life Sci.* **2016**, *155*, 189–194. [CrossRef]

22. Wei, Y.; Chen, J.; Hu, Y.; Lu, W.; Zhang, X.; Wang, R.; Chu, K. Rosmarinic Acid Mitigates Lipopolysaccharide-Induced Neuroinflammatory Responses through the Inhibition of TLR4 and CD14 Expression and NF-κB and NLRP3 Inflammasome Activation. *Inflammation* **2018**, *41*, 732–740. [CrossRef]

23. Yao, Y.; Mao, J.; Xu, S.; Zhao, L.; Long, L.; Chen, L.; Li, D.; Lu, S. Rosmarinic Acid Inhibits Nicotine-Induced C-Reactive Protein Generation by Inhibiting NLRP3 Inflammasome Activation in Smooth Muscle Cells. *J. Cell. Physiol.* **2019**, *234*, 1758–1767. [CrossRef]

24. Kovacs, D.; Raffa, S.; Flori, E.; Aspite, N.; Briganti, S.; Cardinali, G.; Torrisi, M.R.; Picardo, M. Keratinocyte Growth Factor Down-Regulates Intracellular ROS Production Induced by UVB. *J. Dermatol. Sci.* **2009**, *54*, 106–113. [CrossRef]

25. Feehan, R.P.; Shantz, L.M. Molecular Signaling Cascades Involved in Nonmelanoma Skin Carcinogenesis. *Biochem. J.* **2016**, *473*, 2973–2994. [CrossRef]

26. Ascenso, A.; Pedrosa, T.; Pinho, S.; Pinho, F.; de Oliveira, J.M.; Cabral-Marques, H.; Oliveira, H.; Simões, S.; Santos, C. The Effect of Lycopene Preexposure on UV-B-Irradiated Human Keratinocytes. *Oxid. Med. Cell. Longev.* **2016**, *2016*, 8214631. [CrossRef]

27. Lee, J.J.; Kim, K.B.; Heo, J.; Cho, D.H.; Kim, H.S.; Han, S.H.; Ahn, K.J.; An, I.S.; An, S.; Bae, S. Protective Effect of *Arthrospira platensis* Extracts Against Ultraviolet B-Induced Cellular Senescence Through Inhibition of DNA Damage and Matrix Metalloproteinase-1 Expression in Human Dermal Fibroblasts. *J. Photochem. Photobiol. B Biol.* **2017**, *173*, 196–203. [CrossRef]

28. Furue, M.; Uchi, H.; Mitoma, C.; Hashimoto-Hachiya, A.; Chiba, T.; Ito, T.; Nakahara, T.; Tsuji, G. Antioxidants for Healthy Skin: The Emerging Role of Aryl Hydrocarbon Receptors and Nuclear Factor-Erythroid 2-Related Factor-2. *Nutrients* **2017**, *9*, 223. [CrossRef]

29. Sajo, M.E.J.; Kim, C.S.; Kim, S.K.; Shim, K.Y.; Kang, T.Y.; Lee, K.J. Antioxidant and Anti-Inflammatory Effects of Shungite Against Ultraviolet B Irradiation-Induced Skin Damage in Hairless Mice. *Oxid. Med. Cell. Longev.* **2017**, *2017*, 7340143. [CrossRef]

30. Chen, L.; Hu, J.Y.; Wang, S.Q. The Role of Antioxidants in Photoprotection: A Critical Review. *J. Am. Acad. Dermatol.* **2012**, *67*, 1013–1024. [CrossRef]

31. Psotova, J.; Svobodova, A.; Kolarova, H.; Walterova, D. Photoprotective Properties of Prunella vulgaris and Rosmarinic Acid on Human Keratinocytes. *J. Photochem. Photobiol. B Biol.* **2006**, *84*, 167–174. [CrossRef]

32. Dreher, F.; Gabard, B.; Schwindt, D.; Maibach, H.I. Topical Melatonin in Combination with Vitamins E and C Protects Skin from Ultraviolet-Induced Erythema: A Human Study In Vivo. *Br. J. Dermatol.* **1998**, *139*, 332–339. [CrossRef]

33. Leerach, N.; Yakaew, S.; Phimnuan, P.; Soimee, W.; Nakyai, W.; Luangbudnark, W.; Viyoch, J. Effect of Thai Banana (Musa AA group) in Reducing Accumulation of Oxidation End Products in UVB-Irradiated Mouse Skin. *J. Photochem. Photobiol. B Biol.* **2017**, *168*, 50–58. [CrossRef]

34. Heo, S.J.; Jeon, Y.J. Protective Effect of Fucoxanthin Isolated from Sargassum Siliquastrum on UV-B Induced Cell Damage. *J. Photochem. Photobiol. B Biol.* **2009**, *95*, 101–107. [CrossRef]

35. Zheng, J.; Piao, M.J.; Keum, Y.S.; Kim, H.S.; Hyun, J.W. Fucoxanthin Protects Cultured Human Keratinocytes Against Oxidative Stress by Blocking free Radicals and Inhibiting Apoptosis. *Biomol. Ther. (Seoul)* **2013**, *21*, 270–276. [CrossRef]

36. Vostálová, J.; Zdařilová, A.; Svobodová, A. Prunella Vulgaris Extract and Rosmarinic Acid Prevent UVB-Induced DNA Damage and Oxidative Stress in HaCaT Keratinocytes. *Arch. Dermatol. Res.* **2010**, *302*, 171–181. [CrossRef]

37. Pavey, S.; Russell, T.; Gabrielli, B. G2 Phase Cell Cycle Arrest in Human Skin Following UV Irradiation. *Oncogene* **2001**, *20*, 6103–6110. [CrossRef]

38. Jang, Y.; Lee, A.Y.; Jeong, S.H.; Park, K.H.; Paik, M.K.; Cho, N.J.; Kim, J.E.; Cho, M.H. Chlorpyrifos Induces NLRP3 Inflammasome and Pyroptosis/Apoptosis Via Mitochondrial Oxidative Stress in Human Keratinocyte HaCaT Cells. *Toxicology* **2015**, *338*, 37–46. [CrossRef]

39. Drexler, S.K.; Bonsignore, L.; Masin, M.; Tardivel, A.; Jackstadt, R.; Hermeking, H. Tissue-Specific Opposing Functions of the Inflammasome Adaptor ASC in the Regulation of Epithelial Skin Carcinogenesis. *Proc. Natl. Acad. Sci. USA* **2012**, *109*, 18384–18389. [CrossRef]

40. Lin, C.; Zhang, J. Inflammasomes in Inflammation-Induced Cancer. *Front. Immunol.* **2017**, *8*, 271. [CrossRef]

41. Choi, J.H.; Kim, N.H.; Kim, S.J.; Lee, H.J.; Kim, S. Fucoxanthin Inhibits the Inflammation Response in Paw Edema Model Through Suppressing MAPKs, Akt, and NFκB. *J. Biochem. Mol. Toxicol.* **2016**, *30*, 111–119. [CrossRef]

42. Tan, C.; Hou, Y. First Evidence for the Anti-Inflammatory Activity of Fucoxanthin in High-Fat-Diet-Induced Obesity in Mice and the Antioxidant Functions in PC12 Cells. *Inflammation* **2014**, *37*, 443–450. [CrossRef]

43. Gong, D.; Chu, W.; Jiang, L.; Geng, C.; Li, J.; Ishikawa, N.; Kajima, K.; Zhong, L. Effect of Fucoxanthin Alone and in Combination with D-Glucosamine Hydrochloride on Carrageenan/Kaolin-Induced Experimental Arthritis in Rats. *Phyther. Res.* **2014**, *28*, 1054–1063. [CrossRef]

44. Rodríguez-Luna, A.; Ávila-Román, J.; González-Rodríguez, M.L.; Cózar, M.J.; Rabasco, A.M.; Motilva, V.; Talero, E. Fucoxanthin-Containing Cream Prevents Epidermal Hyperplasia and UVB-Induced Skin Erythema in Mice. *Mar. Drugs* **2018**, *16*, 378. [CrossRef]

45. Lee, J.; Jung, E.; Kim, Y.; Lee, J.; Park, J.; Hong, S.; Hyun, C.G.; Park, D.; Kim, Y.S. Rosmarinic Acid as a Downstream Inhibitor of IKK-Beta in TNF-Alpha-Induced Upregulation of CCL11 and CCR3. *Br. J. Pharmacol.* **2006**, *148*, 366–375.

46. Oh, H.A.; Park, C.S.; Ahn, H.J.; Park, Y.S.; Kim, H.M. Effect of Perilla Frutescens Var. Acuta Kudo and Rosmarinic Acid on Allergic Inflammatory Reactions. *Exp. Biol. Med. (Maywood)* **2011**, *236*, 99–106. [CrossRef]

47. Jeong, H.J.; Choi, Y.; Kim, M.H.; Kang, I.C.; Lee, J.H.; Park, C.; Park, R.; Kim, H.M. Rosmarinic Acid, Active Component of Dansam-Eum Attenuates Ototoxicity of Cochlear Hair Cells Through Blockage of Caspase-1 Activity. *PLoS ONE* **2011**, *6*, e18815. [CrossRef]

48. Zheng, J.; Piao, M.J.; Kim, K.C.; Yao, C.W.; Cha, J.W.; Hyun, J.W. Fucoxanthin Enhances the Level of Reduced Glutathione Via the Nrf2-Mediated Pathway in Human Keratinocytes. *Mar. Drugs* **2014**, *12*, 4214–4230. [CrossRef]

49. Liu, Y.; Zheng, J.; Zhang, Y.; Wang, Z.; Yang, Y.; Bai, M.; Dai, Y. Fucoxanthin Activates Apoptosis Via Inhibition of PI3K/Akt/mTOR Pathway and Suppresses Invasion and Migration by Restriction of p38-MMP-2/9 Pathway in Human Glioblastoma Cells. *Neurochem. Res.* **2016**, *41*, 2728–2751. [CrossRef]

50. Urikura, I.; Sugawara, T.; Hirata, T. Protective Effect of Fucoxanthin Against UVB-Induced Skin Photoaging in Hairless Mice. *Biosci. Biotechnol. Biochem.* **2011**, *75*, 757–760. [CrossRef]

51. Shimoda, H.; Tanaka, J.; Shan, S.J.; Maoka, T. Anti-Pigmentary Activity of Fucoxanthin and Its Influence on Skin mRNA Expression of Melanogenic Molecules. *J. Pharm. Pharmacol.* **2010**, *62*, 1137–1145. [CrossRef]

52. Matsui, M.; Tanaka, K.; Higashiguchi, N.; Okawa, H.; Yamada, Y.; Tanaka, K.; Taira, S.; Aoyama, T.; Takanishi, M.; Natsume, C.; et al. Protective and Therapeutic Effects of Fucoxanthin Against Sunburn Caused by UV Irradiation. *J. Pharmacol. Sci.* **2016**, *132*, 55–64. [CrossRef]

53. Sun, Z.; Park, S.Y.; Hwang, E.; Park, B.; Seo, S.A.; Cho, J.G.; Zhang, M.; Yi, T.H. Dietary Foeniculum Vulgare Mill Extract Attenuated UVB Irradiation-Induced Skin Photoaging by Activating of Nrf2 and Inhibiting MAPK Pathways. *Phytomedicine* **2016**, *23*, 1273–1284. [CrossRef]

54. Sun, Z.; Park, S.Y.; Hwang, E.; Zhang, M.; Seo, S.A.; Lin, P.; Yi, T.H. Thymus Vulgaris Alleviates UVB Irradiation Induced Skin Damage Via Inhibition of MAPK/AP-1 and Activation of Nrf2-ARE Antioxidant System. *J. Cell. Mol. Med.* **2016**, *21*, 336–348. [CrossRef]

55. Lu, C.; Zou, Y.; Liu, Y.; Niu, Y. Rosmarinic Acid Counteracts Activation of Hepatic Stellate Cells Via Inhibiting the ROS-Dependent MMP-2 Activity: Involvement of Nrf2 Antioxidant System. *Toxicol. Appl. Pharmacol.* **2017**, *318*, 69–78. [CrossRef]

56. Twentyman, P.R.; Luscombe, M. A Study of Some Variables in a Tetrazolium Dye (MTT) Based Assay for Cell Growth and Chemosensitivity. *Br. J. Cancer* **1987**, *56*, 279–285. [CrossRef]

57. Wang, H.; Joseph, J.A. Quantifying Cellular Oxidative Stress by Dichlorofluorescein Assay Using Microplate Reader. *Free Radic. Biol. Med.* **1999**, *27*, 612–616. [CrossRef]

58. Bradford, M. A Rapid and Sensitive Method for The Quantitation of Microgram Quantities of Protein Utilizing the Principle of Protein-Dye Binding. *Anal. Biochem.* **1976**, *72*, 248–254. [CrossRef]

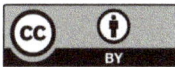

marine drugs

MDPI

Article

Frondanol, a Nutraceutical Extract from *Cucumaria frondosa*, Attenuates Colonic Inflammation in a DSS-Induced Colitis Model in Mice

Sandeep B. Subramanya [1,*], Sanjana Chandran [1], Saeeda Almarzooqi [2], Vishnu Raj [1], Aisha Salem Al Zahmi [1], Radeya Ahmed Al Katheeri [1], Samira Ali Al Zadjali [1], Peter D. Collin [3] and Thomas E. Adrian [1,*]

[1]   Department of Physiology, College of Medicine and Health Sciences, United Arab Emirates University, P.O. Box–17666, Al Ain, UAE; sanjanachandran25@gmail.com (S.C.); rajvishnu@uaeu.ac.ae (V.R.); 201400107@uaeu.ac.ae (A.S.A.Z.); 201304934@uaeu.ac.ae (R.A.A.K.); 201304302@uaeu.ac.ae (S.A.A.Z.)
[2]   Department of Pathology, College of Medicine and Health Sciences, United Arab Emirates University, P.O. Box–17666, Al Ain, UAE; saeeda.almarzooqi@uaeu.ac.ae
[3]   Coastside Bio Resources, Deer Isle, ME 04627, USA; pcollin48@gmail.com
*   Correspondence: sandeep.bs@uaeu.ac.ae (S.B.S.); tadrian@uaeu.ac.ae (T.E.A.); Tel.: +971-3-713-7534 (S.B.S. & T.E.A.); Fax: +971-3-7671966/2033 (S.B.S. & T.E.A.)

Received: 18 March 2018; Accepted: 27 April 2018; Published: 30 April 2018

Abstract: Frondanol is a nutraceutical lipid extract of the intestine of the edible Atlantic sea cucumber, *Cucumaria frondosa*, with potent anti-inflammatory effects. In the current study, we investigated Frondanol as a putative anti-inflammatory compound in an experimental model of colonic inflammation. C57BL/6J male black mice (C57BL/6J) were given 3% dextran sodium sulfate (DSS) in drinking water for 7 days to induce colitis. The colitis group received oral Frondanol (100 mg/kg body weight/per day by gavage) and were compared with a control group and the DSS group. Disease activity index (DAI) and colon histology were scored for macroscopic and microscopic changes. Colonic tissue length, myeloperoxidase (MPO) concentration, neutrophil and macrophage marker mRNA, pro-inflammatory cytokine proteins, and their respective mRNAs were measured using ELISA and real-time RT-PCR. The tissue content of leukotriene B4 (LTB4) was also measured using ELISA. Frondanol significantly decreased the DAI and reduced the inflammation-associated changes in colon length as well as macroscopic and microscopic architecture of the colon. Changes in tissue MPO concentrations, neutrophil and macrophage mRNA expression (F4/80 and MIP-2), and pro-inflammatory cytokine content (IL-1β, IL-6 and TNF-α) both at the protein and mRNA level were significantly reduced by Frondanol. The increase in content of the pro-inflammatory mediator leukotriene B4 (LTB4) induced by DSS was also significantly inhibited by Frondanol. It was thus found that Frondanol supplementation attenuates colon inflammation through its potent anti-inflammatory activity.

Keywords: Frondanol; *Cucumaria frondosa*; DSS colitis; colon inflammation

1. Introduction

Inflammatory bowel disease (IBD) refers to Crohn's disease (CD) or ulcerative colitis (UC), which involve both small and large intestines. IBD is characterized by chronic inflammation with mucosal ulceration in the intestinal tract [1]. The prevalence of IBD is increasing (150–250/100,000) in developed nations [2], and greatly diminishes quality of life because of the morbidity associated with it such as pain, vomiting, and diarrhea. IBD also increases the risk of colorectal cancer [2]. The current mainstream therapies for IBD are sulfasalazine, corticosteroids, immunosuppressive agents such as azatriopine, and anti-tumor necrosis factor-α antibodies, either as single agents or in combination, to inhibit aberrant immune response and inflammation. However, the adverse effects associated with these treatments over prolonged periods as well as the concomitant high relapse rate of the disease limits their use [3]. With the lack of effective treatment, in addition to the associated side effects and costs, many IBD patients turn to complementary and alternate therapy [4].

The marine environment has been of great interest for drug discovery in the last several decades, as researchers acknowledge its promising potential for new drug leads. To date, only a few drugs from marine sources have been isolated, developed, and approved to treat diseases such as cancer, but the search continues [5]. Sea cucumbers have been used for hundreds of years as food and folk medicine in the communities of Asia and the Middle East [6]. Sea cucumbers are also referred to as 'marine ginseng', and they contain numerous useful specific compounds that could have broad applications in agricultural, nutraceutical, pharmaceutical, and cosmeceutical products [7]. Frondanol is a US-patented nutraceutical lipid extract of the intestines of the edible Atlantic sea cucumber *Cucumaria frondosa*. Frondanol has potent anti-inflammatory activity. It has been purported to suppress inflammation in the adjuvant arthritis rat model and ear edema mice model when it is administered either orally or applied topically [8]. Frondanol exhibits potent inhibitory activity on both 5-lipoxygenase (5-LOX) and 12-lipoxygenase (12-LOX) pathways, suppressing the production of 12-hydroxyeicosatetraenoic acid (12-HETE), 5-hydroxyeicosatetraenoic acid (5-HETE), and leukotriene B4 (LTB4) in human polymorphonuclear cells [8]. There is considerable evidence for the involvement of the 5-LOX pathway in colitis. The products of 5-LOX, 5-HETE, and LTB4 are markedly increased in the dextran sodium sulfate (DSS) model [9–11]. When DSS-treated animals are given a 5-LOX inhibitor or an LTB4 antagonist, colonic shortening as well as histological and inflammatory scores were improved in the mouse model of colonic inflammation [9,11–13]. Therefore, we hypothesized that Frondanol may attenuate the inflammatory responses seen in IBD. Various experimental animal models of IBD have been developed to mimic the pathophysiological processes that characterize UC [14,15]. Perhaps the most accepted model of colon inflammation is the murine model of colitis that utilizes oral administration of DSS, a murine chemical colitogen to induce UC [16]. In the present study, we investigated the efficacy of Frondanol in attenuating the colonic inflammation induced by DSS in mice.

2. Results

2.1. Effect of Frondanol on Disease Activity Index (DAI) and Colon Length

In C57BL/6J mice, 3% DSS in drinking water induced distinct features of ulcerative colitis. There was a marked and significant increase in the DAI score in the DSS-treated group ($p < 0.001$). Frondanol administration significantly prevented the increase in the DAI score in DSS-treated animals ($p < 0.05$, Figure 1). However, Frondanol alone had no significant effect on the DAI score compared with the control. DSS treatment significantly reduced colon length (cm) when compared to the control ($p < 0.001$). Frondanol treatment in of the DSS group significantly prevented the shortening of colon length ($p < 0.05$, Figure 2a,b). However, Frondanol alone did not affect colon length compared to the control.

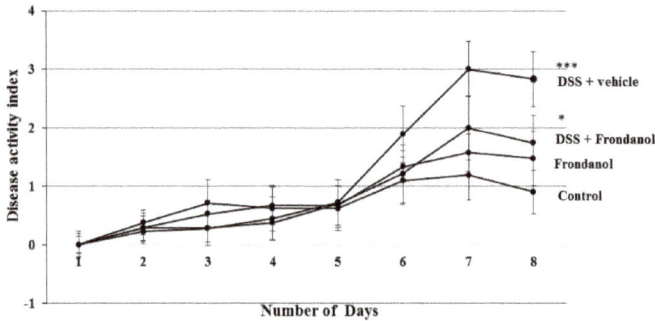

Figure 1. Effect of Frondanol on disease activity index (DAI) and colon length. Dextran sodium sulfate (DSS) treatment significantly increased the DAI score. Frondanol treatment significantly decreased the DAI score compared to the DSS-treated group. Data were obtained from n = 8 animals in each group and are expressed as means ± SEM (control vs. DSS, *** $p < 0.001$ and DSS vs. Frondanol + DSS. * $p < 0.05$, was obtained by one-way ANOVA followed by Tukey's multiple comparison test).

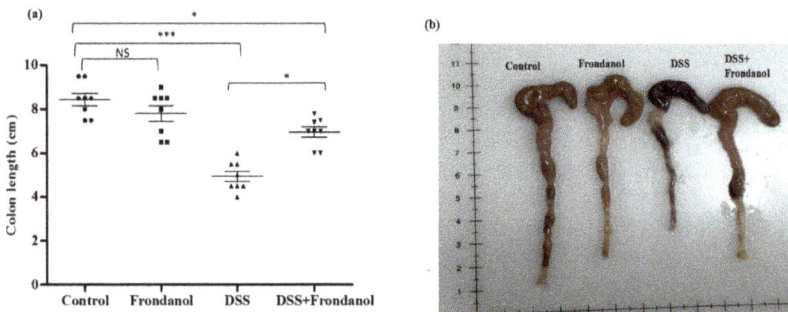

Figure 2. Effect of Frondanol on colon length. The average colon length (cm) (**a,b**) was significantly decreased in the DSS-treated group. Frondanol treatment significantly prevented the shortening of colon length compared to the DSS-treated group. Data were obtained from n = 8 animals in each group and are expressed as means ± SEM (control vs. DSS *** $p < 0.001$, DSS vs. DSS + Frondanol, and control vs. DSS + Frondanol * $p < 0.05$. NS indicate not significant was obtained by one-way ANOVA followed by Tukey's multiple comparison test).

2.2. Effect of Frondanol on Microscopic Architecture

The healthy normal control colon section depicted typical architecture of a colon with normal thickness of the submucosa and muscle layer, as well as regular crypt structure in the mucosa. In the DSS-treated control group, colonic inflammation reached up into the submucosa with focal loss of crypts and surface epithelium. In contrast, the Frondanol-treated DSS group had intact epithelium with minimal loss of crypt and inflammation compared the normal control group (Figure 3a).

The most reproducible histological abnormality in the DSS-treated control group was excessive crypt damage with edema, collapse, or complete destruction (Figure 3a). Crypt damage score was significantly worse in DSS-mice compared with untreated controls and Frondanol-treated DSS animals ($p < 0.0001$ and $p < 0.001$, respectively, Figure 3a,b). However, the crypt damage score was still significantly higher in the Frondanol-treated DSS group compared with healthy controls ($p < 0.001$). Frondanol alone had no effect on the crypt damage score. The colonic inflammation score was markedly and significantly increased in the DSS-treated mice compared to untreated control animals ($p < 0.0001$, Figure 3c). Frondanol treatment in the DSS-treated group significantly prevented the increase in colonic inflammation score compared to DSS treatment alone ($p < 0.001$, Figure 3c). The inflammation score was still significantly elevated in the Frondanol-treated DSS group compared to healthy controls, indicating only partial, but significant protection of both colonic crypt damage and inflammation by Frondanol ($p < 0.001$, Figure 3c). Frondanol alone (without DSS) had no significant effect on the colon inflammation score compared to controls. These results confirm that Frondanol has a protective effect on the colonic micro architecture, damaged by DSS treatment.

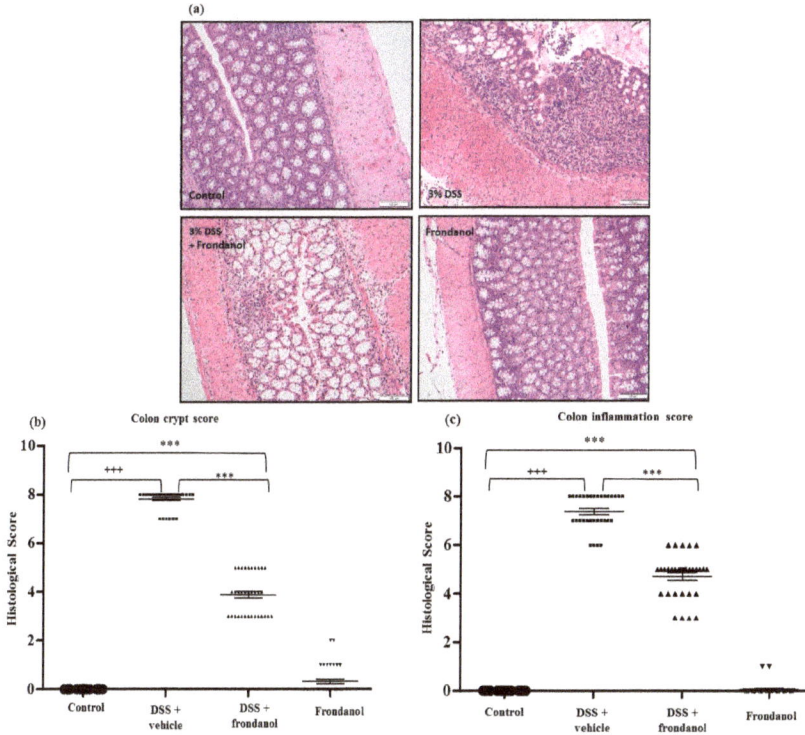

Figure 3. Effect of Frondanol on colon histology. (**a**) Hematoxylin and Eosin (H&E) staining was carried out to provide material for microscopic scoring (Scale Bars: 100 μm). Microscopic analysis shows typical architecture of the colon with normal thickness of the submucosa, muscle layer, and regular crypt structure in the mucosa in the control. The DSS-treated colon section shows focal loss of crypts and surface epithelium with inflammation reaching up to the submucosa. Frondanol protected the microscopic architectures in the DSS-treated group. Crypt distortion score and colon inflammation score (**b,c**) were significantly higher in the DSS-treated group. Frondanol treatment significantly lowered both crypt distortion and colon inflammation scores. All of the histology pictures are represented at 20× magnification. Data were obtained from $n = 8$ animals in each group and are expressed as means $\pm$ SEM. (control vs. DSS +++ $p < 0.0001$, DSS vs. DSS + Frondanol, and control vs. DSS + Frondanol *** $p < 001$, obtained by one-way ANOVA followed by Tukey's multiple comparison test).

2.3. Effect of Frondanol on the Expression of Myeloperoxidase (MPO) Protein, F4/80 Macrophage Marker mRNA, and Macrophage Inflammatory Protein-2 (MIP-2) mRNA Concentrations

Myeloperoxidase (MPO) is an enzyme secreted from activated neutrophils and is commonly used a marker to assess the level of neutrophil infiltration at a site of inflammation. MPO concentrations were measured in colon homogenates using an ELISA assay. MPO concentrations were markedly and significantly increased in the DSS group compared to the control ($p < 0.001$, Figure 4a). Frondanol administration significantly prevented the DSS-induced increase in MPO concentrations ($p < 0.01$), indicating the role of Frondanol in mitigating inflammatory response induced by DSS. Frondanol alone did not significantly affect MPO concentrations (Figure 4a). In DSS-induced colitis, both neutrophil and macrophage infiltration was significantly increased. We measured mRNA expression of F4/80 protein as a marker of macrophage infiltration. F4/80 mRNA was significantly increased in the DSS-treated group compared to the control ($p < 0.001$). Frondanol treatment in the DSS-treated animals significantly ($p < 0.01$) prevented F4/80 mRNA expression ($p < 0.001$, Figure 4b). However, Frondanol alone had no effect on F4/80 mRNA expression. MIP-2 mRNA expression massively and significantly increased in the DSS-treated group compared to the control ($p < 0.001$, Figure 4c). Frondanol administration in the DSS-treated group significantly prevented the increase in MIP-2 mRNA expression ($p < 0.001$, Figure 4c). However, the group receiving Frondanol treatment following DSS still had an MIP-2 mRNA level higher than that of the control ($p < 0.05$, Figure 4c). Frondanol alone had no effect on MIP-2 mRNA expression. These results confirm that Frondanol limits the infiltration of macrophages and neutrophils due to damage induced by DSS.

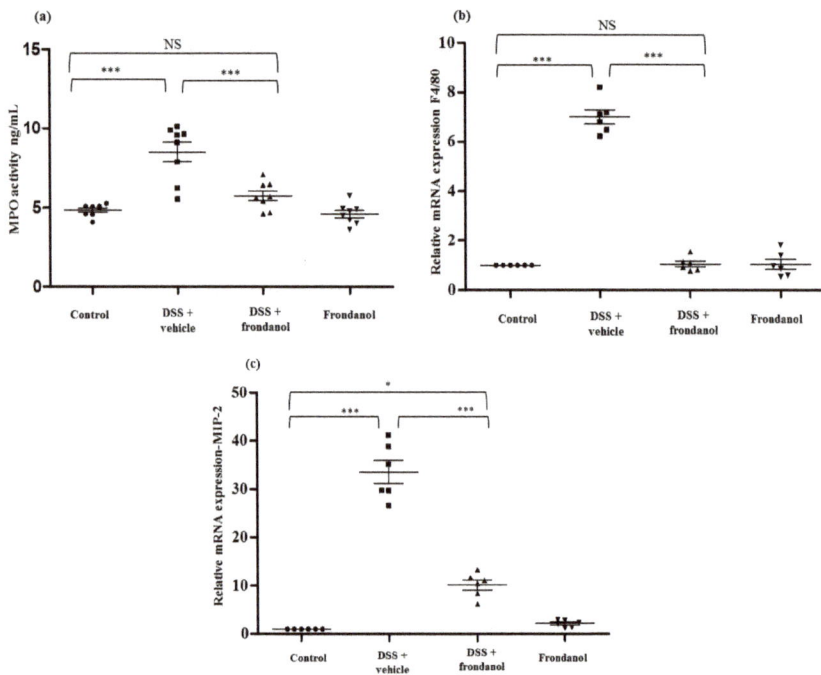

Figure 4. Effect of Frondanol on MPO concentration, F4/80 neutrophil markers, and MIP-2 mRNA expression. DSS treatment significantly enhanced neutrophil infiltration, as marked by an increase in (**a**) MPO concentration and (**b,c**) F4/80 and MPI-2 mRNA expression compared to the control. Frondanol administration significantly decreased (**a**) MPO activity, F4/80, and MIP-2 mRNA expression in the DSS-treated group. Frondanol alone did not affect (**a**) MPO concentration, (**b**) F4/80, or (**c**) MIP-2 mRNA expression. MPO concentrations were quantitated using ELISA. F4/80 and MIP-2 mRNA expression studies were carried out using real-time RT-PCR. Data were obtained from $n = 8$ animals for MPO concentration and $n = 6$ animals for mRNA expression studies in each group, and are expressed as means ± SEM (control vs. DSS, and DSS vs. DSS + Frondanol, *** $p < 0.001$; control vs. DSS + Frondanol, * $p < 0.05$. NS indicate not significant was obtained by one-way ANOVA followed by Tukey's multiple comparison test).

2.4. Effect of Frondanol on Pro-Inflammatory Cytokine Protein and mRNA Concentrations

DSS treatment caused massive increases in protein concentrations of the pro-inflammatory cytokines interleukin-1β (IL-1β), interleukin-6 (IL-6) ($p < 0.001$, Figure 5a,b), and tumor necrosis factor-α (TNF-α), ($p < 0.01$, Figure 5c), as well as the relative expression of the mRNAs for these respective cytokines (IL-6 and IL-1β, $p < 0.001$; TNF-α, $p < 0.01$, Figure 5d–f). Frondanol administration prevented increases in pro-inflammatory cytokines and their respective mRNA expression in response to DSS treatment ($p < 0.001$ for IL-6, IL-1β and $p < 0.01$ for TNF-α cytokines. $p < 0.001$ for IL-6, and $p < 0.05$ Il-1β and TNF-α mRNAs). In control animals, Frondanol alone had no effect on the expression of the cytokines or their respective mRNAs. These results indicate that Frondanol strongly inhibits the pro-inflammatory cytokine response induced by DSS.

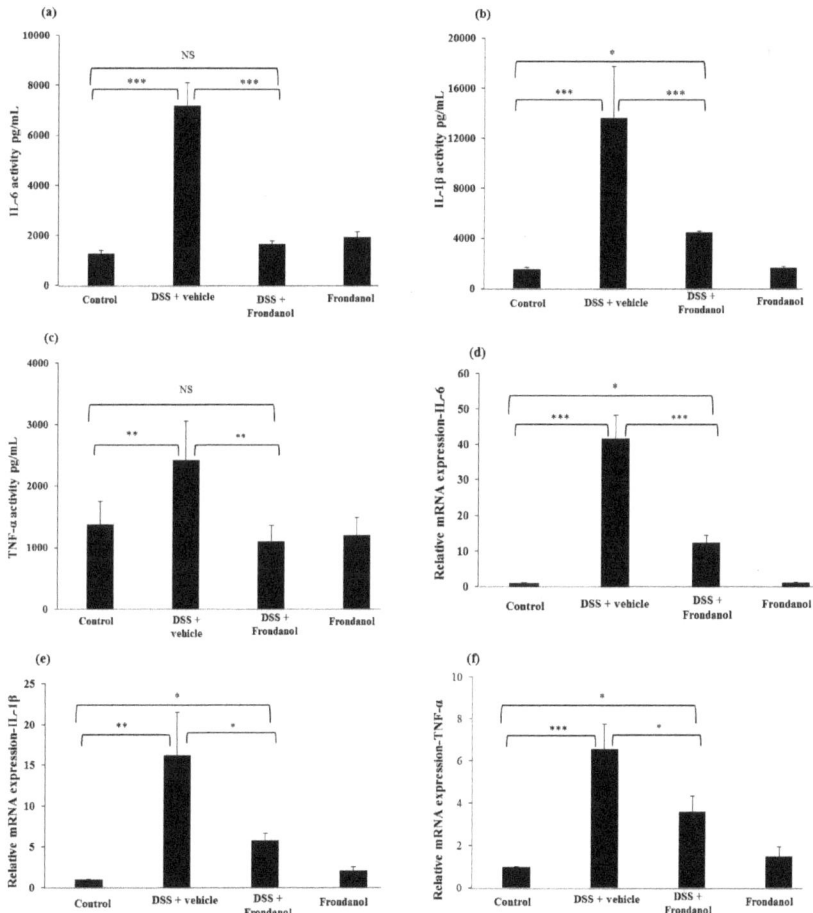

Figure 5. Effect of Frondanol on pro-inflammatory cytokine protein and mRNA expression. Frondanol significantly inhibits pro-inflammatory cytokines both at the protein level (IL-6 (**a**), IL-1β (**b**) and the TNF-α (**c**)) and mRNA expression level in the DSS-treated group (Il-6 (**d**), IL-1β (**e**), TNF-α (**f**)). Pro-inflammatory cytokine proteins were measured using ELISA and the expression of their respective mRNAs were measured in using real-time RT-PCR. Data were obtained from $n = 8$ animals for ELISA and $n = 6$ animals for mRNA expression studies in each group, and are expressed as means ± SEM. (ELISA

results of IL-6 and IL-1β: control vs. DSS, and DSS vs. DSS + Frondanol, *** $p < 0.001$; control vs. DSS + Frondanol, * $p < 0.05$. ELISA of TNF-α: control vs. DSS, and control vs. DSS + Frondanol, ** $p < 0.001$. mRNA expression of IL-6: control vs. DSS, and DSS vs. DSS + Frondanol, *** $p < 0.001$. IL-1β: control vs. DSS ** $p < 0.01$; DSS vs. DSS + Frondanol, and control vs. DSS + Frondanol, * $p < 0.05$. TNF-α: control vs. DSS *** $p < 0.001$; DSS vs. DSS + Frondanol, and control vs. DSS + Frondanol, * $p < 0.05$. NS indicate not significant was obtained by one-way ANOVA followed by Tukey's multiple comparison test).

2.5. Effect of Frondanol on Leukotriene B4 (LTB4)

LTB4 is secreted from neutrophils, and a markedly increased response is seen in inflammatory conditions. Frondanol is reported to inhibit the function of 5-lipoxygensase, which is upstream of leukotriene B4 synthase [8]. In our DSS model, LTB4 concentrations were measured using a commercially available ELISA kit. DSS administration markedly increased LTB4 concentrations compared with the control ($p < 0.01$). Frondanol treatment completely prevented this increase ($p < 0.001$) in DSS-treated animals, reflecting its inhibitory effect on LTB4 production. As expected, Frondanol alone had no effect on the LTB4 level in control animals (Figure 6).

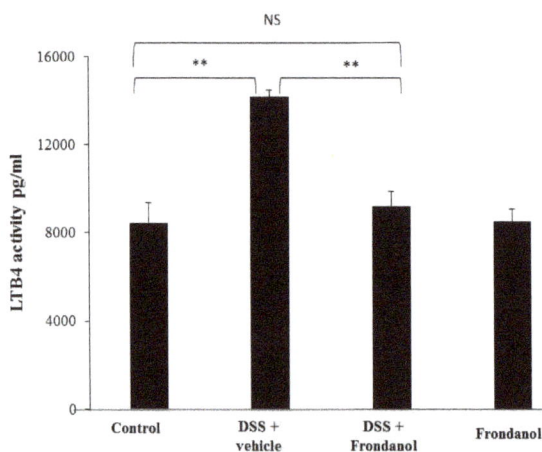

Figure 6. Effect of Frondanol on LTB4 concentrations. Frondanol administration significantly reduced LTB4 level in the DSS-treated group. Data were obtained from $n = 8$ animals in each group and are expressed as means ± SEM (control vs. DSS and DSS vs. DSS + Frondanol, ** $p < 0.01$. NS indicate not significant was obtained by one-way ANOVA followed by Tukey's multiple comparison test).

3. Discussion

In the current study, we investigated the effects of Frondanol on DSS-induced experimental colitis. The DSS-induced colitis model is a widely accepted model of colon inflammation for both understanding the disease process as well as screening the efficacy of various anti-inflammatory natural and dietary compounds because of its clinical relevancy to human ulcerative colitis [17].

Frondanol is a US-patented nutraceutical non-polar extract of the intestines of the edible Atlantic sea cucumber, *Cucumaria frondosa*, which has potent anti-inflammatory properties. This extract should not be confused with Frondanol A5, which is a polar extract of skin from the same animal that has been shown to have potent anti-cancer properties [18]. Frondanol suppresses inflammation in the adjuvant-induced arthritis model [18], developed in rats as a model for screening compounds that might prove useful in the treatment of rheumatoid arthritis in humans. In this model, Frondanol (10 mg/kg by gavage) was reported to be at least as effective as phenylbutazone (10 mg/kg) and more effective than hydrocortisone (10 mg/kg) [8]. In the mouse ear inflammatory edema model using croton oil (containing phorbol esters and arachidonic acid) Frondanol was applied topically and suppressed the edematous response by 84% [8]. Frondanol was also reported to reduce the proliferation of peripheral blood mononuclear cells stimulated by the mitogen concanavalin A. Frondanol at 0.1% suppressed concanavalin A-induced proliferation by 85% in human and 95% in sheep mononuclear cells [19]. In the mixed lymphocyte reaction (MLR), Frondanol reduced thymidine incorporation by 40–52% at 0.025% and by 82–98% at 0.05%; this was similar to the inhibition caused by the cyclosporin A control, which reduced the MLR by 37–75% at 100 ng/mL and by 81–90% at 500 ng/mL [8,19]. Cell viability was maintained by these concentrations of Frondanol, indicating the lack of toxicity of the compound.

With regard to the mechanism of action of the effects of Frondanol, the extract has reported potent inhibitory activity on 5-LOX, 12-LOX, and cyclooxygenase pathways. Frondanol suppressed the production of 5-HETE and LTB4 from human polymorphonuclear cells by 53% and 62%, respectively, at a concentration of 0.01% [8]. Similarly, Frondanol suppressed the production of 12-HETE by 44% at the same concentration [8]. Frondanol also caused a concentration-dependent reduction of PGE2 production. In separate studies on the effect of Frondanol on 5-LOX activity, dose-responsive effects were seen. Frondanol at 0.01% inhibited the production of 5-HETE and LTB4 by $84.7 \pm 0.8\%$ and $75.2 \pm 7.2\%$, respectively. At 0.1% Frondanol inhibited the production of 5-HETE and LTB4 by $98.4 \pm 0.8\%$ and $91.9 \pm 0.6\%$, respectively (unpublished results). While Frondanol suppresses the production of pro-inflammatory eicosanoids, it increases the activity of the anti-inflammatory 15-LOX, as evidenced by a concentration-dependent increase in the production of 15-HETE (Personal Communication, Peiying Yang, MD Anderson Cancer Center, Houston, TX, USA).

The inhibitory effects of Frondanol on 5-LOX and 12-LOX activity could be explained, at least in part, by some of the known constituent fatty acids in the extract. For example, 12-methyl tetradecanoic (12-MTA) acid is a major constituent of Frondanol (20–30% by weight) and this branched chain fatty acid has potent 5-LOX and 12-LOX inhibitory activity [20]. Topical administration of 12-MTA has been reported to reduce MPO activity by inhibiting neutrophil infiltration at the site of injury when the cornea was damaged by chemical injury [21]. Another fatty acid constituent of Frondanol is myristoleic acid, which also potently inhibits 5-LOX activity [22]. Myristoleic acid is found at lower concentrations in Frondanol, but has potent 5-LOX inhibitory effects. These fatty acids are likely to contribute to the anti-inflammatory effects of Frondanol. Astaxanthin is a carotenoid present in Frondanol that has marked anti-inflammatory effects, and has also been shown to suppress inflammation in the DSS colitis model [23].

In the present study, Frondanol markedly suppressed the inflammation driven by oral DSS administration. This was evidenced by marked decreases in the disease activity index (DAI), reduction in colon length, and macroscopic and microscopic architecture changes that reflected the inflammation. Frondanol also attenuated the increases in MPO concentrations, neutrophil and macrophage mRNA expression (F4/80 and MIP-2), and pro-inflammatory cytokine production (IL-1β, IL-6 and TNF-α) at both at the protein and mRNA levels, as well as the increase in the expression of the pro-inflammatory mediator LTB4.

Prevention of the DSS-induced increase in MPO concentrations indicates that Frondanol prevents the accumulation of polymorphonuclear granulocytes in DSS-induced colitis tissue, since MPO activity reflects the increase in neutrophil accumulation in the submucosa due to the severity of colitis [24]. The increased levels of LTB4 in colonic tissue from DSS-treated mice are strongly implicated in attracting both neutrophils and macrophages to the site of injury, thus amplifying the inflammatory cascade in IBD [10].

Along with neutrophils, the infiltration of macrophages also increases during the course of colitis, indicating its involvement in the inflammatory process [25,26]. To determine the level of macrophage infiltration, we quantitated the F4/80 mRNA expression level. F4/80 is considered a surrogate biomarker for infiltrating macrophages, suggesting the role of innate immune cells in DSS-induced colitis [27]. Frondanol significantly decreased F4/80 mRNA expression, thus suggesting its role in preventing the further recruitment of macrophages in colitis. MIP-2 is a chemoattractant secreted by both neutrophils and macrophages, and plays a central role in recruiting an increased number of neutrophils and macrophages at the site of injury [28]. Furthermore, in the DSS-induced model of colitis, MIP-2 plays an integral role in the recruitment of neutrophils and macrophages [28]. Additionally, it has also been shown that overexpression of MIP-2 enhances the severity of DSS-induced colitis, Ohtsuka et al. [29] suggesting its crucial role in the development of DSS-induced colitis. Thus, we quantitated the expression of MIP-2 mRNA by real time PCR. The MIP-2 mRNA level was significantly upregulated in DSS-induced mice, and Frondanol beneficially and significantly decreased the MIP-2 mRNA expression level. These studies suggest that Frondanol prevents the upregulation of MIP-2, thereby decreasing neutrophil accumulation as reflected by MPO concentration. These data reflecting macrophage statuses in the treated animals could partially explain Frondanol's anti-inflammatory role in protecting against DSS-mediated colitis.

Frondanol significantly suppressed the DSS-induced production of pro-inflammatory cytokines (IL-6, IL-1β, and TNF-α) both at the protein and mRNA levels. When Frondanol was administered by oral gavage (10 mg/kg weight) in the adjuvant arthritis model, it was as effective as phenylbutazone and much more effective than hydrocortisone at a similar dose [8]. In another model of inflammation, mouse ear edema was induced by croton oil, which contains phorbol esters and arachidonic acid (potent mediators of inflammation), and was subsequently reduced by 84% when Frondanol was applied topically [8].

There is considerable evidence for the involvement of the 5-LOX pathway and COX-2 in the DSS model of colitis [9,11–13,30,31]. A recent study reported the measurement of lipid inflammatory mediators throughout the different phases of inflammation [9]. In the induction phase, prostaglandin E2 (PGE2) and thromboxane A2 (TBA2) increased 2-fold [9]. In the acute phase, the production of n-6 fatty acid-derived leukotrienes increased by more than 10-fold, while that of the anti-inflammatory n-3 fatty acid-derived leukotrienes decreased [9]. In the recovery phase, the production of protectin D1 increased 3-fold [9]. The 5-LOX inhibitor B-98 reduced the colonic shortening and histological inflammatory score in DSS-treated mice [11]. In the DSS model, a peroxisome proliferator-activated receptor gamma (PPARγ) agonist, 5-ASA (that blocks nuclear factor kappa B-induced production of pro-inflammatory eicosanoids), a LOX inhibitor (AA-861), or an LTB4 receptor antagonist all prevented erosions in the large bowel [12]. The anti-inflammatory agent 5-ASA and the LTB4 receptor antagonist also prevented the shortening of the colon [12]. The COX inhibitor indomethacin and the thromboxane A2 inhibitor OKY-046 were ineffective [12]. This study indicates the importance of lipoxygenase products in this model [12]. Intracolonic administration of a selective 5-LOX inhibitor, zileuton, accelerated healing in a rat model of colitis [32]. In a DSS study using a LOX inhibitor (AA-861) and linolenic acid supplementation, the combination was able to suppress the excessive chloride secretion that results in diarrhea. Linolenic acid is metabolized to the anti-inflammatory eicosanoids PGE1 and TBA1 and prevents the formation of leukotrienes, while AA-861 is a selective 5-LOX and LTB4 inhibitor [13]. In another study, DSS caused a marked inflammatory response in the colon and a subsequent 5-fold increase in eicosanoid production [31]. This increase was completely prevented by treatment with olsalazine (a prodrug that delivers 5-ASA directly into the colon) [31]. In a study investigating the production of eicosanoids in patients with relapsing ulcerative colitis, luminal PGE2 and LTB4 concentrations were positively correlated with disease activity and were reduced to near normal levels by successful treatment with specific inhibitors of the prostaglandin and leukotriene pathways [33]. Indeed, as surrogate biomarkers, prostaglandin and leukotriene expressions appear to be better indicators of treatment outcomes for relapsing ulcerative colitis than the traditional clinical indices of disease activity [33].

In addition to its inflammatory role, the 5-LOX pathway also appears to be involved in colitis-associated neoplasia. 5-lipoxygenase is overexpressed in all adenomatous colonic polyps and in colonic carcinomas, but it is not expressed in normal mucosal cells or hyperplastic polyps [34]. Indeed, 5-LOX has been proposed as a marker for early pancreatic intraepithelial neoplastic lesions [35].

Lipoxygenase inhibitors block the growth of human colonic cancer cells in culture and induce apoptosis in these cells [34]. Other proteins in the 5-LOX pathway are also expressed in colonic cancer cells, including LTB4 receptors [36]. Furthermore, the LTB4 receptor antagonist etalocib blocks cancer cell growth both in vitro and in vivo and enhances the effect of gemcitabine on colon cancer growth in a mouse xenograft model [36]. Finally, the reported observation that Fondanol activates 15-LOX is interesting since, when overexpressed, this enzyme suppresses colitis-associated colon cancer through inhibition of the IL-6/STAT3 signaling pathway [37,38].

4. Materials and Methods

4.1. Chemicals and Reagents

Dextran Sulfate Sodium (DSS), molecular weight 36,000–50,000 Da, was purchased from Sigma-Aldrich (St. Louis, MO, USA). Frondanol was supplied by Coastside Bio Resources (Deer Isle, ME, USA). Enzyme-linked immunosorbent assay (ELISA) kits for the measurement of concentrations of myeloperoxidase (MPO), interleukin-6 (IL-6), interleukin-1β (IL-1β), tumor necrosis factor-α (TNF-α), and leukotriene B4 (LTB4) in colon tissues were obtained from R&D systems (Minneapolis, MN, USA). RNA extraction was performed using RNeasy kits obtained from Qiagen (Hilden, Germany). SYBR green and reverse transcription kit to convert mRNA into cDNA was purchased from Applied Biosystems (Foster City, CA, USA). Primers for the real time (RT-PCR) quantification of mRNA expression were supplied by Macrogen Inc. (Seoul, Korea).

4.2. Experimental Animals

C57BL/6J male mice (10–12 weeks old) were used for the study. Mice were housed individually in controlled environmental conditions at a room temperature 23 ± 2 °C, with a 12-h light-dark cycle and ad libitum access to food and water. Animal experiments were performed in accordance with protocols approved by the UAEU Animal Care and Research Ethical Committee on 6 June 2017 (ERA_2017_5567).

4.3. Experimental Design, Induction of Colitis and Tissue Collection

The mice were randomly assigned to four groups. Group 1: control untreated, Group 2: control treated with Frondanol, Group 3: DSS-induced colitis untreated, and Group 4: DSS-induced colitis treated with Frondanol. Fresh 3% DSS solutions were made every morning in autoclaved drinking water. The two DSS groups of mice were given 3% DSS for 8 days (day 0–day 7) as previously described, while the control groups received only autoclaved tap water [24]. The two treated groups were given Frondanol (100 mg/kg body weight/per day) using refined sunflower oil as a vehicle by gavage, for a total volume of 150 μL. The control groups were administered only 150 μL of refined sunflower oil. Mice were euthanized on the eighth day by intraperitoneal (IP) injection of pentobarbital (80 mg/kg body weight). After laparotomy, the colon was excised, and the length of each colon was measured carefully and photographed to determine colonic shortening induced by DSS treatment. Subsequently, each colon was flushed thoroughly with ice-cold normal saline (0.9% NaCl) several times to remove remnant DSS and then the colon was cut into several circular pieces. For histology, a small circular piece of tissue (5 mm) was taken, measuring 5 cm from distal to caecum, from all animals and fixed in 4% buffered formalin for histology (hematoxylin and eosin staining). Remaining pieces of tissue were snap-frozen in liquid nitrogen and then stored at −80 °C for subsequent extraction for ELISA and mRNA expression studies.

4.4. Macroscopic Assessment or Disease Activity Index (DAI)

To establish disease activity index (DAI), body weight, stool consistency, and rectal bleeding were monitored in each mouse daily to score the severity of colitis using a previously described scoring system (Table 1) [39]. The sum of the three values constitutes the DAI, resulting in a total clinical score ranging from a minimum of 0 to a maximum of 12.

Table 1. Disease activity index score.

Weight Loss	Score	Stool Consistency	Score	Rectal Bleeding	Score
No loss	0	Normal	0	No Blood	0
1–5%	1	Loose stool	2	Heme occult + ve and visual pellet bleeding	2
5–10%	2	Diarrhea	4	Gross bleeding and blood around anus	4
10–20%	3				
>20%	4				

4.5. ELISA

Concentrations of MPO and cytokines (IL-6, IL-1β, and TNF-α) and LTB4 were quantified using ELISA assays, according to the manufacturer's protocol. Briefly, approximately 100 mg pieces of colon tissue were weighed and homogenized using a T-25 digital Ultra TURRAX homogenizer (Staufen, Germany) at 14,000 RPM in 1 ml ice-cold phosphate-buffered saline solution (PBS, pH = 7.2) containing a proteases cocktail (St. Louis, MO, USA) at 4 °C. The homogenate was centrifuged at $12,000 \times g$ for 10 min. The supernatant was used for the measurement of MPO, IL-6, IL-1β, TNF-α, and LTB4. The results were calculated as pg/mg tissue.

4.6. Colonic Cytokine mRNA Content Determined by Real-Time PCR

Total RNA was extracted from frozen pieces of colon using the RNeasy Mini-Kit. The quality and the quantity of total RNA were assessed using a NanoDrop 2000 spectrophotometer (Thermo Fisher Scientific Inc., Waltham, MA, USA). Reverse transcription was carried out using a high capacity cDNA Reverse Transcription kit. Real-time polymerase chain reaction (PCR) was performed using the QuantStudio 7 Flex Real-Time PCR System (Applied Biosytems, Culver City, CA, USA) with SYBR Select Master Mix (Applied Biosystems). The obtained data was normalized using 18s RNA as a reference gene and the $2^{-\Delta\Delta CT}$ method was used as a relative quantification method for mRNA expression [40]. Primer sequences for each mRNA are shown in Table 2 [41,42].

Table 2. Real time PCR primer sequence.

Name	Forward	Reverse
IL-6	5′-ACAACCACGGCCTTCCCTACTT-3′	5′-CACGATTTCCCAGAGAACATGTG-3′
IL-1β	5′-ACCTGCTGGTGTGTGACGTT-3′	5′-TCGTTGCTTGGTTCTCCTTG-3′
TNF-α	5′-CACGTCCGTAGCAAACCACCAA-3′	5′-GTTGGTTGTCTTTGAGATCCAT-3′
F4/80	5′-TGTGTCGTGCTGTTCAGAACC-3′	5′-AGGAATCCCGCAATGATGG-3′
MIP-2	5′-GGATGGCTTTCATGGAAGGAG-3′	5′-TTGCTAAGCAAGGCACTGTGC-3′
18S	5′-AAATCAGTTATGGTTCCTTTGGTC-3′	5′-GCTCTAGAATTACCACAGTTATCCAA-3′

4.7. Histological Scoring

After overnight fixation in 4% buffered formalin, tissues were placed in 100% ethanol overnight. Tissues were then embedded in paraffin for routine histology. Four transverse sections (2 μm) taken from each colonic sample were stained with hematoxylin and eosin (H&E) and examined by light microscopy (Zeiss, Stuttgart, Germany). Colonic crypt distortion and inflammation were evaluated microscopically. The histological scoring was performed by an experienced pathologist (SAM) in a blinded fashion. Histological examination of tissues from DSS-treated animals involved a scoring system that includes the evaluation of the severe disruption of tissue architecture, the severity of edema, the massive immune cell infiltration indicating inflammation, crypt damage, and any significant area of complete epithelial denudation. Colonic crypt distortion and inflammation were scored out of 8. The histology scoring system is indicated in Tables 3 and 4 [39]. All the histology pictures are represented at 20× magnification.

Table 3. Crypt score = product of percentage of crypt change and crypt distortion, graded out of a maximum score of 8.

Crypt Grade		Quantification of the Percentage of Crypt Change		Crypt Distortion—Graded Based on the Extent of Involvement	
Grade 0:	Intact crypt	1	1–25%	0	No crypt distortion
Grade 1:	Shortening and loss of basal 1/3 of crypts	2	26–50%	1	1–25%
Grade 2:	Loss of basal 2/3 of crypts	3	51–75%	2	26–50%
Grade 3:	Loss of entire crypt with intact surface epithelium	4	76–100%	3	51–75%
Grade 4:	Loss of both entire crypt and surface epithelium (erosion)			4	76–100%

Table 4. Score of inflammation = grade of inflammation × percentage of involvement, graded out of a maximum score of 8.

Inflammation Graded	Percentage of Inflammation Involvement of Mucosal Surface Area		Hyperplastic Epithelium—Graded Based on the Extent of Involvement	
0	0	No inflammation	0	None
1	1	1–25%	1	1–25%
2	2	26–50%	2	26–50%
3	3	51–75%	3	51–75%
4	4	76–100%	4	76–100%

4.8. Statistics

All statistical analysis was carried out using SPSS Software (Armonk, NY, USA). Comparisons between groups were performed by one-way analysis of variance (ANOVA), followed by Tukey's post-hoc test for multiple comparisons. Data are plotted as means ± SEM in the figures. p values < 0.05 were considered statistically significant.

5. Conclusions

These studies demonstrate that Frondanol, a non-polar extract from the edible Atlantic sea cucumber *Cucumaria frondosa*, has marked anti-inflammatory properties in a mouse model of colitis. These anti-inflammatory effects are most likely attributable to the inhibitory effects of the extract on 5-LOX, 12-LOX, and cyclooxygenase enzymes, with perhaps a contribution from activation of the 15-LOX pathway. This nutraceutical may be of value in the treatment of this condition. Furthermore, since both the LOX and COX pathways were implicated in the development of precancerous colonic polyps, the use of such broad-spectrum LOX and COX inhibitors together with the activation of 15-LOX may be valuable in the chemoprevention of colitis-associated colon cancer.

Author Contributions: Conceptualized the study (S.B.S. and T.E.A.), performed the experiments (S.B.S., S.C., V.R., A.S.A.Z., R.A.A.K., and S.A.A.Z.), analyzed the data (S.B.S., T.E.A., S.A., S.C., and V.R.), S.A. helped with histology and scoring. Preparation of first draft (S.B.S. and T.E.A.), editing the manuscript (S.B.S., T.E.A., and P.D.C.).

Funding: This research was funded by United Arab Emirates University, SURE + grant, grant number: 31M346; and UAEU start up grant, grant number: 31M178.

Acknowledgments: Sandeep B Subramanya. was supported by United Arab Emirates University, SURE + grant, 31M346 and UAEU start up grant 31M178.

Conflicts of Interest: Peter Collin is the holder of a patent for the preparation and use of Frondanol. Thomas E Adrain is a joint holder with Peter Collin of other patents regarding marine-derived compounds, unrelated to Frondanol. The other authors declare no conflict of interest.

References

1. Lee, S.H.; Kwon, J.E.; Cho, M.L. Immunological pathogenesis of inflammatory bowel disease. *Intest. Res.* **2018**, *16*, 26–42. [CrossRef] [PubMed]

2. Ananthakrishnan, A.N. Epidemiology and risk factors for IBD. *Nat. Rev. Gastroenterol. Hepatol.* **2015**, *12*, 205–217. [CrossRef] [PubMed]

3. Duijvestein, M.; Battat, R.; Vande Casteele, N.; D'Haens, G.R.; Sandborn, W.J.; Khanna, R.; Jairath, V.; Feagan, B.G. Novel therapies and treatment strategies for patients with inflammatory bowel disease. *Curr. Treat. Options Gastroenterol.* **2018**, *16*, 129–146. [CrossRef] [PubMed]

4. Zezos, P.; Nguyen, G.C. Use of complementary and alternative medicine in inflammatory bowel disease around the world. *Gastroenterol. Clin. N. Am.* **2017**, *46*, 679–688. [CrossRef] [PubMed]

5. Malve, H. Exploring the ocean for new drug developments: Marine pharmacology. *J. Pharm. Bioallied Sci.* **2016**, *8*, 83–91. [CrossRef] [PubMed]

6. Bordbar, S.; Anwar, F.; Saari, N. High-value components and bioactives from sea cucumbers for functional foods—A review. *Mar. Drugs* **2011**, *9*, 1761–1805. [CrossRef] [PubMed]

7. Bahrami, Y.; Zhang, W.; Franco, C. Discovery of Novel Saponins from the Viscera of the Sea Cucumber Holothuria lessoni. *Mar. Drugs* **2014**, *12*, 2633–2667. [CrossRef] [PubMed]

8. Collin, P.D. Sea Cucumber Carotenoid Lipid Fraction Products and Methods of Use. U.S. Patent 6,399,105B1, 4 June 2002.

9. Hamabata, T.; Nakamura, T.; Masuko, S.; Maeda, S.; Murata, T. Production of lipid mediators across different disease stages of dextran sulfate sodium-induced colitis in mice. *J. Lipid Res.* **2018**, *59*, 586–595. [CrossRef] [PubMed]

10. Singh, V.P.; Patil, C.S.; Kulkarni, S.K. Effect of 5-lipoxygenase inhibition on events associated with inflammatory bowel disease in rats. *Indian J. Exp. Biol.* **2004**, *42*, 667–673. [PubMed]

11. Song, E.M.; Jung, S.A.; Lee, J.S.; Kim, S.E.; Shim, K.N.; Jung, H.K.; Yoo, K.; Park, H.Y. Benzoxazole derivative B-98 ameliorates dextran sulfate sodium-induced acute murine colitis and the change of T cell profiles in acute murine colitis model. *Korean J. Gastroenterol.* **2013**, *62*, 33–41. [CrossRef] [PubMed]

12. Kimura, I.; Nagahama, S.; Kawasaki, M.; Kataoka, M.; Sato, M. Study on the experimental ulcerative colitis (UC) model induced by dextran sulfate sodium (DSS) in rats (3). *Nihon Yakurigaku Zasshi* **1996**, *108*, 259–266. [CrossRef] [PubMed]

13. Shimizu, T.; Kitamura, T.; Suzuki, M.; Fujii, T.; Shoji, H.; Tanaka, K.; Igarashi, J. Effects of alpha-linolenic acid on colonic secretion in rats with experimental colitis. *J. Gastroenterol.* **2007**, *42*, 129–134. [CrossRef] [PubMed]

14. Low, D.; Nguyen, D.D.; Mizoguchi, E. Animal models of ulcerative colitis and their application in drug research. *Drug Des. Dev. Ther.* **2013**, *7*, 1341–1357.

15. Eichele, D.D.; Kharbanda, K.K. Dextran sodium sulfate colitis murine model: An indispensable tool for advancing our understanding of inflammatory bowel diseases pathogenesis. *World J. Gastroenterol.* **2017**, *23*, 6016–6029. [CrossRef] [PubMed]

16. Chassaing, B.; Aitken, J.D.; Malleshappa, M.; Vijay-Kumar, M. Dextran sulfate sodium (DSS)-induced colitis in mice. *Curr. Protoc. Immunol.* **2014**, *104*, 15–25.

17. Mizoguchi, A. Animal models of inflammatory bowel disease. *Prog. Mol. Biol. Transl. Sci.* **2012**, *105*, 263–320. [PubMed]

18. Roginsky, A.B.; Ding, X.Z.; Woodward, C.; Ujiki, M.B.; Singh, B.; Bell, R.H., Jr.; Collin, P.; Adrian, T.E. Anti-pancreatic cancer effects of a polar extract from the edible sea cucumber, Cucumaria frondosa. *Pancreas* **2010**, *39*, 646–652. [CrossRef] [PubMed]

19. Krishnan, R.; Collin, P.D. Method of Inhibiting Rejection of Transplanted Material. World Patent Application No. WO200309267281, 13 November 2003.

20. Collin, P.D.; Yang, P.; Newman, R. Methods and Compositions for Treating Lipoxygenase-Medaited Disease States. U.S. Patent 6541519B2, 1 April 2003.

21. Cole, N.; Hume, E.B.; Jalbert, I.; Vijay, A.K.; Krishnan, R.; Willcox, M.D. Effects of topical administration of 12-methyl tetradecanoic acid (12-mta) on the development of corneal angiogenesis. *Angiogenesis* **2007**, *10*, 47–54. [CrossRef] [PubMed]

22. Ding, X.-Z.; Collin, P.D.; Adrian, T.E. Myristoleic acid inhibits pancreatic cancer growth Via 5-lipoxygenase inhibition. *Pancreas* **2009**, *38*, 993.

23. Yasui, Y.; Hosokawa, M.; Mikami, N.; Miyashita, K.; Tanaka, T. Dietary astaxanthin inhibits colitis and colitis-associated colon carcinogenesis in mice via modulation of the inflammatory cytokines. *Chem. Biol. Interact.* **2011**, *193*, 79–87. [CrossRef] [PubMed]

24. Kim, J.J.; Shajib, M.S.; Manocha, M.M.; Khan, W.I. Investigating intestinal inflammation in DSS-induced model of IBD. *J. Vis. Exp.* **2012**, *60*, e3678. [CrossRef] [PubMed]

25. Ohkusa, T.; Okayasu, I.; Tokoi, S.; Araki, A.; Ozaki, Y. Changes in bacterial phagocytosis of macrophages in experimental ulcerative colitis. *Digestion* **1995**, *56*, 159–164. [CrossRef] [PubMed]

26. Okayasu, I.; Hatakeyama, S.; Yamada, M.; Ohkusa, T.; Inagaki, Y.; Nakaya, R. A novel method in the induction of reliable experimental acute and chronic ulcerative colitis in mice. *Gastroenterology* **1990**, *98*, 694–702. [CrossRef]

27. Ohkawara, T.; Mitsuyama, K.; Takeda, H.; Asaka, M.; Fujiyama, Y.; Nishihira, J. Lack of macrophage migration inhibitory factor suppresses innate immune response in murine dextran sulfate sodium-induced colitis. *Scand. J. Gastroenterol.* **2008**, *43*, 1497–1504. [CrossRef] [PubMed]

28. Carr, M.W.; Roth, S.J.; Luther, E.; Rose, S.S.; Springer, T.A. Monocyte chemoattractant protein 1 acts as a T-lymphocyte chemoattractant. *Proc. Natl. Acad. Sci. USA* **1994**, *91*, 3652–3656. [CrossRef] [PubMed]

29. Ohtsuka, Y.; Sanderson, I.R. Dextran sulfate sodium-induced inflammation is enhanced by intestinal epithelial cell chemokine expression in mice. *Pediatr. Res.* **2003**, *53*, 143–147. [PubMed]

30. Sklyarov, A.Y.; Panasyuk, N.B.; Fomenko, I.S. Role of nitric oxide-synthase and cyclooxygenase/lipooxygenase systems in development of experimental ulcerative colitis. *J. Physiol. Pharmacol.* **2011**, *62*, 65–73. [PubMed]

31. Zijlstra, F.J.; Garrelds, I.M.; van Dijk, A.P.; Wilson, J.H. Experimental colitis in mice: Effects of olsalazine on eicosanoid production in colonic tissue. *Agents Actions* **1992**, *36*, C76–C78. [CrossRef]

32. Bertran, X.; Mane, J.; Fernandez-Banares, F.; Castella, E.; Bartoli, R.; Ojanguren, I.; Esteve, M.; Gassull, M.A. Intracolonic administration of zileuton, a selective 5-lipoxygenase inhibitor, accelerates healing in a rat model of chronic colitis. *Gut* **1996**, *38*, 899–904. [CrossRef] [PubMed]

33. Lauritsen, K.; Laursen, L.S.; Bukhave, K.; Rask-Madsen, J. Effects of topical 5-aminosalicylic acid and prednisolone on prostaglandin e2 and leukotriene b4 levels determined by equilibrium in vivo dialysis of rectum in relapsing ulcerative colitis. *Gastroenterology* **1986**, *91*, 837–844. [CrossRef]

34. Melstrom, L.G.; Bentrem, D.J.; Salabat, M.R.; Kennedy, T.J.; Ding, X.Z.; Strouch, M.; Rao, S.M.; Witt, R.C.; Ternent, C.A.; Talamonti, M.S.; et al. Overexpression of 5-lipoxygenase in colon polyps and cancer and the effect of 5-lox inhibitors in vitro and in a murine model. *Clin. Cancer Res.* **2008**, *14*, 6525–6530. [CrossRef] [PubMed]

35. Hennig, R.; Grippo, P.; Ding, X.Z.; Rao, S.M.; Buchler, M.W.; Friess, H.; Talamonti, M.S.; Bell, R.H.; Adrian, T.E. 5-lipoxygenase, a marker for early pancreatic intraepithelial neoplastic lesions. *Cancer Res.* **2005**, *65*, 6011–6016. [CrossRef] [PubMed]

36. Hennig, R.; Ding, X.Z.; Tong, W.G.; Witt, R.C.; Jovanovic, B.D.; Adrian, T.E. Effect of LY293111 in combination with gemcitabine in colonic cancer. *Cancer Lett.* **2004**, *210*, 41–46. [CrossRef] [PubMed]

37. Mao, F.; Xu, M.; Zuo, X.; Yu, J.; Xu, W.; Moussalli, M.J.; Elias, E.; Li, H.S.; Watowich, S.S.; Shureiqi, I. 15-lipoxygenase-1 suppression of colitis-associated colon cancer through inhibition of the IL-6/stat3 signaling pathway. *FASEB J.* **2015**, *29*, 2359–2370. [CrossRef] [PubMed]

38. Mao, F.; Wang, M.; Wang, J.; Xu, W.R. The role of 15-LOX-1 in colitis and colitis-associated colorectal cancer. *Inflamm. Res.* **2015**, *64*, 661–669. [CrossRef] [PubMed]

39. Cooper, H.S.; Murthy, S.N.; Shah, R.S.; Sedergran, D.J. Clinicopathologic study of dextran sulfate sodium experimental murine colitis. *Lab. Investig.* **1993**, *69*, 238–249. [PubMed]

40. Livak, K.J.; Schmittgen, T.D. Analysis of relative gene expression data using real-time quantitative PCR and the 2(-Delta Delta C(T)) method. *Methods* **2001**, *25*, 402–408. [CrossRef] [PubMed]

41. Pervin, M.; Hasnat, M.A.; Lim, J.H.; Lee, Y.M.; Kim, E.O.; Um, B.H.; Lim, B.O. Preventive and therapeutic effects of blueberry (vaccinium corymbosum) extract against dss-induced ulcerative colitis by regulation of antioxidant and inflammatory mediators. *J. Nutr. Biochem.* **2016**, *28*, 103–113. [CrossRef] [PubMed]

42. Urushima, H.; Nishimura, J.; Mizushima, T.; Hayashi, N.; Maeda, K.; Ito, T. Perilla frutescens extract ameliorates dss-induced colitis by suppressing proinflammatory cytokines and inducing anti-inflammatory cytokines. *Am. J. Physiol. Gastrointest. Liver Physiol.* **2015**, *308*, G32–G41. [CrossRef] [PubMed]

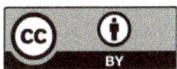

marine drugs

MDPI

Article

Correlation between Fatty Acid Profile and Anti-Inflammatory Activity in Common Australian Seafood by-Products

Tarek B. Ahmad [1,2,†], David Rudd [1,3], Michael Kotiw [2], Lei Liu [4] and Kirsten Benkendorff [1,*,†]

[1] Marine Ecology Research Centre, Southern Cross University, Lismore 2480, Australia; Tarek.Ahmad@usq.edu.au (T.B.A.); david.rudd@monash.edu (D.R.)
[2] Division of Research & Innovation, University of Southern Queensland, Toowoomba 4350, Australia; Michael.Kotiw@usq.edu.au
[3] Monash Institute of Pharmaceutical Sciences, Monash University, Parkville 3052, Australia
[4] Southern Cross Plant Science, Southern Cross University, Lismore 2480, Australia; Ben.liu@scu.edu.au
* Correspondence: kirsten.benkendorff@scu.edu.au; Tel.: +61-2-6620-3755
† These authors contributed equally to the manuscript.

Received: 29 January 2019; Accepted: 2 March 2019; Published: 6 March 2019

Abstract: Marine organisms are a rich source of biologically active lipids with anti-inflammatory activities. These lipids may be enriched in visceral organs that are waste products from common seafood. Gas chromatography-mass spectrometry and fatty acid methyl ester (FAME) analyses were performed to compare the fatty acid compositions of lipid extracts from some common seafood organisms, including octopus (*Octopus tetricus*), squid (*Sepioteuthis australis*), Australian sardine (*Sardinops sagax*), salmon (*Salmo salar*) and school prawns (*Penaeus plebejus*). The lipid extracts were tested for anti-inflammatory activity by assessing their inhibition of nitric oxide (NO) and tumor necrosis factor alpha (TNFα) production in lipopolysaccharide (LPS)-stimulated RAW 264.7 mouse cells. The lipid extract from both the flesh and waste tissue all contained high amounts of polyunsaturated fatty acids (PUFAs) and significantly inhibited NO and TNFα production. Lipid extracts from the cephalopod mollusks *S. australis* and *O. tetricus* demonstrated the highest total PUFA content, the highest level of omega 3 (ω-3) PUFAs, and the highest anti-inflammatory activity. However, multivariate analysis indicates the complex mixture of saturated, monounsaturated, and polyunsaturated fatty acids may all influence the anti-inflammatory activity of marine lipid extracts. This study confirms that discarded parts of commonly consumed seafood species provide promising sources for the development of new potential anti-inflammatory nutraceuticals.

Keywords: seafood waste; polyunsaturated fatty acid; NO inhibition; fish oil; marine nutraceuticals

1. Introduction

Acute and chronic inflammation is the basis of many serious diseases including asthma, cardiovascular diseases, and rheumatoid arthritis [1]. The stimulation of macrophages during the inflammatory response gives rise to overproduction of several pro-inflammatory mediators, including nitric oxide (NO) via inducible nitric oxide synthase (iNOS) [2]. NO overproduction can lead to tissue damage through cytokine-mediated processes. This molecule can also cause vasodilation, edema, and cytotoxicity [3,4]. Macrophage stimulation also leads to the overproduction of many cytokines including TNFα and interleukins (IL). These pro-inflammatory cytokines have many roles, including the recruitment and activation of more macrophages, effects on the endothelial cells in the blood vessels, as well as playing a role in the perception of pain generated from inflammation [5]. Cytokines such as TNFα are powerful pro-inflammatory mediators during infection, trauma, or surgery, which can trigger short- and long-term effects on the peripheral and central nervous system, leading to exacerbated pain processed by directly affecting specific receptors on sensorial neurons [6,7]. Thus, these pro-inflammatory cytokines and NO are reliable markers for screening new anti-inflammatory treatments *in vitro* and *in vivo*.

The conventional management of inflammation relies mainly on the use of steroidal and non-steroidal anti-inflammatory drugs (NSAIDs). Both drug families are well-known for their common and serious side effects [8], especially when associated with long term consumption, such as is often required for the treatment of chronic inflammatory diseases. Consequently, there is a critical need to identify new sources of less harmful treatments, particularly for the management of diseases associated with chronic inflammation. Our increased understanding of the impact of food and diet on health has driven the search for novel natural medicines [9]. A recent study has shown that patients suffering from chronic inflammatory diseases are more likely to seek out natural anti-inflammatory agents with the intention to minimize the side effects associated with long term use of steroid and NSAIDs [8]. Therefore, the development of new safer anti-inflammatory nutraceuticals is of clinical interest and could have a significant impact on the treatment of inflammatory cases. Functional foods and marine extracts provide a relatively untapped source of potential anti-inflammatory agents, but claims need to be evidence-based.

In comparison to saturated fats, dietary polyunsaturated fatty acids (PUFAs) can have a number of positive impacts on health when incorporated into the diet to meet deficiencies from sub-optimal dietary intake. The human body relies on food as a source of long chain PUFAs, as it is unable to synthesize PUFAs larger than 18 carbons [10]. Both omega 3 (ω-3) alpha-linolenic and omega 6 (ω-6) linoleic PUFAs are considered essential for mammals and can only be obtained from the diet. Seafood (fish and shellfish) lipids are the main sources of biologically active ω-3 long chain PUFAs [10,11]. These PUFAs are known to minimize the occurrence and severity of chronic inflammatory conditions [12–15], cancer [16–18], obesity [19,20], and cardiovascular diseases [10,21,22]. Dietary PUFAs have been shown to improve the quality of life for people suffering from chronic inflammatory diseases such as arthritis, asthma, and neuroinflammatory diseases [11]. Long chain ω-3 PUFAs can directly inhibit inflammation by competing with arachidonic acid or indirectly by affecting the transcription factors or nuclear receptors responsible for inflammatory gene expression [23].

Docosahexaenoic acid (C22:6 ω-3) (DHA) and eicosapentaenoic acid (C20:5 ω-3) (EPA) are the most valuable long chain PUFAs and are considered potent anti-inflammatory agents as a result of the amount and type of the eicosanoids they generate, which interfere with intracellular signaling pathways, transcription factors, and gene expression mechanisms [24]. DHA has been shown to reduce the levels of IL-1β and TNFα in LPS-stimulated peripheral blood mononuclear cells (PBMNC) *in vitro* [25]. Furthermore, studies have shown that a number of health problems including increased inflammatory processes [26], poor fetal development, and a higher risk of Alzheimer's diseases are associated with diets low in EPA and DHA PUFAs [27].

Omega 3 PUFAs can be commercially sourced from oily fishes including salmon, sardine, and mackerel [10]. There is some evidence that seafoods from temperate Australian origins contain higher amounts of DHA compared to seafood from the northern hemisphere [28]. Some of the PUFA-rich Australian marine organisms include crustaceans, such as school prawn and tiger prawn, oily fishes such as sardine and salmon, and mollusks, including octopus, squid, shelled gastropods, and bivalves [28]. In Western countries like Australia, there is a significant level of waste from underutilization of parts of seafood, as only the choice flesh is consumed by many people. However, valuable PUFAs might not only occur in the predominantly eaten components of the seafood organisms, but could also be present in the undervalued presumptive waste tissues of fish and shellfish. For example, in fish, lipids are not only stored in the subcutaneous tissue, belly flap, and muscle, but are also high in mesenteric tissue, head, and liver [29]. A number of previous studies have investigated the quality of fatty acids in seafood waste tissues. For example, high levels of ω-3 rich PUFAs were found in lipid extracts from the head (26%), intestine (24%), and liver (23%) from the sardine *Sardinella lemuru* [30], and similarly in the tuna *Euthynnus affinis* (head 28.77%; intestine 27.43%; liver 23.98%) [31]. Significant amounts of the valuable ω-3 EPA and DHA were also found in eye orbital samples of tuna in an Australia-based study [28,32]. Therefore, the byproducts of the seafood industry could be a source of high-quality anti-inflammatory fatty acids.

To date, investigations on the anti-inflammatory activity of fish oil have been insufficiently investigated, and consequently, results remain inconclusive [33]. Nevertheless, there is some clinical evidence to support the benefits of krill oil in the treatment of inflammatory conditions [34,35], suggesting that the specific PUFA composition may be important for anti-inflammatory activity. Many molluscan products and derivatives are used in traditional medicines for the treatment of inflammatory conditions [36], and mollusks are also known to be rich in beneficial PUFAs [37]. Examples of lipid extracts from mollusk with demonstrated *in vivo* and *in vitro* anti-inflammatory activity include the New Zealand green-lipped mussel *Perna canaliculus* [38], *Filopaludina bengalensis* foot [39], Indian green mussel *Perna viridis* [40,41], *Mytilus unguiculatus* (Hard-shelled mussel) [40], and sea hares *Aplysia fasciata* and *Aplysia punctata* [42]. Despite the promising anti-inflammatory activity of lipid extracts from mollusks, the only natural anti-inflammatory nutraceuticals available over-the-counter as anti-inflammatory medications are Lyprinol and Biolane sourced from the lipid extract of the New Zealand green-lipped mussel *Perna canaliculus* [38], and Cadalmin™, the lipid extract from a closely related species of bivalve *Perna viridis* in India [41,43]. The anti-inflammatory activities of lipid extracts from predatory cephalopod mollusks are yet to be tested.

This study aims to investigate the composition of lipid extracts from common Australian seafoods including oily fish, prawns, and cephalopods, with a comparison of the edible flesh and under-utilized by-products. The anti-inflammatory activity of these lipid extracts was compared using *in vitro* assays for NO and TNFα inhibition and the inhibition concentrations (IC_{50}s) were correlated to the fatty acids composition to provide further insight into how the fatty acid compositions of marine lipid extracts influence the anti-inflammatory potential.

2. Results

2.1. Comparison of Fatty Acid Composition from Lipid Extracts of Different Seafood and Waste Products

As expected for oily fish, the highest yield of lipid extract was recovered from the Australian sardine, followed by salmon (>100 mg/g tissue, Figure 1A). Substantially lower quantities were recovered from the cephalopods and prawns (5–40 mg/100 g tissue, Figure 1A). Higher quantities of oil were recovered from the viscera and/or heads of all species in comparison to the flesh. The lipid extracts from the cephalopod mollusks had the highest proportion of PUFAs comprising over 40% of the fatty acid composition (Figure 1B, Table 1). Salmon had the lowest percentage of PUFAs (<25%), but the highest percentage of MUFAs, with over 45% of the total fatty acids (Figure 1B and Table 1). Permutational analysis of variance (PERMANOVA) revealed a significant difference between species in the composition of fatty acid classes (Pseudo F = 16.4, p = 0.001). Pair-wise analysis revealed that the octopus, squid, prawns, and sardines were not significantly different in the relative proportion of fatty acid classes (p > 0.05); however, salmon was significantly different to octopus (p = 0.0091), squid (p = 0.0066) and sardines (p = 0.0017). Specifically, there were significantly less saturated fatty acids and more monounsaturated fatty acids in salmon compared to squid (SFA p = 0.0035, MUFA, p = 0.0054) and sardines (SFA p = 0.001, MUFA = 0.0031). Salmon had significantly less PUFAs than octopus (p = 0.0144), squid (p = 0.0144), and sardines (p = 0.0202). The PUFAs were also significantly lower in prawns compared to octopus (p = 0.0302) and squid (p = 0.0276). The waste products (viscera and heads), did not have a significantly different profile to the more frequently consumed cephalopod flesh or fish fillets, but the prawn heads and viscera had less MUFA, relative to SFA and PUFA, compared to the body flesh (Figure 1B). All extracts had a healthy ω-6/ω-3 ratio of less than or close to 1 (Table 1B), with the ratio as low as 0.1 in sardines and the flesh of octopus. The ratio of saturated to unsaturated fatty acids was also less than 1 for all species.

(A)

(B)

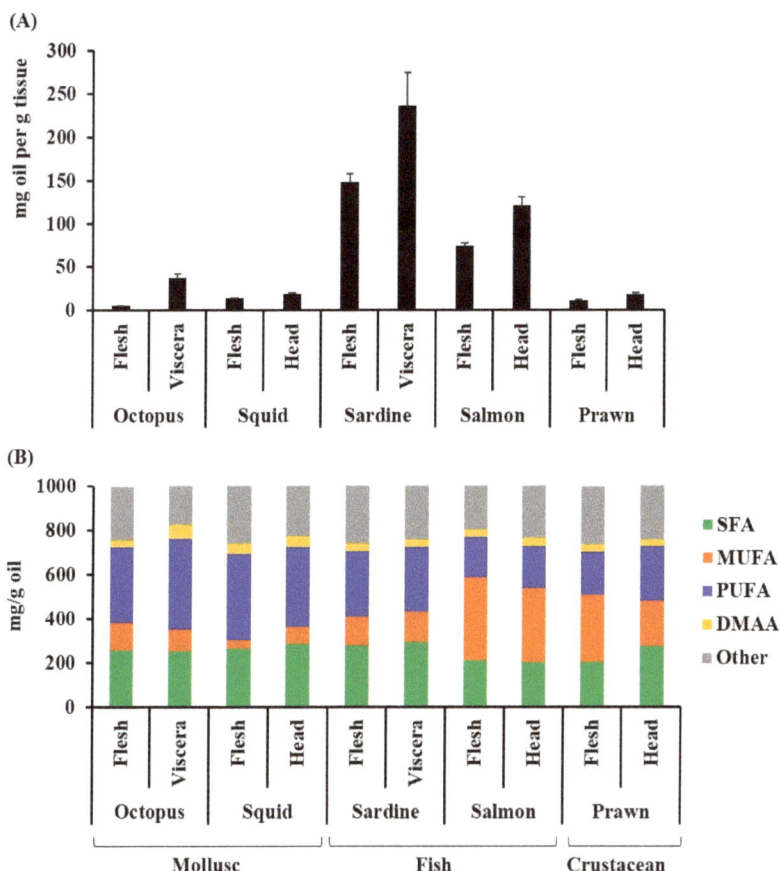

Figure 1. Lipid composition of some common Australian seafood flesh and waste streams: (**A**) The amount of oil extracted from the flesh (mg/g tissue); (**B**) the amount of the main fatty acid classes and other hydrocarbons (dimethyl acetal aldehydes) in the lipid extracts (mg/g oil). The fatty acids were quantified by GC-FID and identified against reference standards with supplementary GC-MS analyses. The samples are: *Octopus tetricus* flesh and viscera, *Sepioteuthis australis* (squid) flesh and head; *Sardinops sagax* (Australian sardine) flesh and viscera, including heads; *Salmo salar* (Atlantic salmon) flesh and head (SH); and *Penaeus plebejus* (Australian school prawn) flesh and head, including viscera.

Multivariate comparison of the overall fatty acid profiles in the oil extracts revealed significant differences between the species (Pseudo-F = 9.59 *p* = 0.0007), but not between the different types of tissue (Pseudo-F = 2.73, *p* > 0.05), and there was no significant interaction between these factors (Pseudo-F = 1.6, *p* > 0.05). Pair-wise tests confirmed that *S. salar* (salmon) has a different fatty acid composition to all species except prawns (*p* < 0.01), which is driven by a higher percentage of oleic, linoleic, and eicosatrienoic acids in the salmon and prawn heads (Figure 2 and Table 1A). The squid contained higher proportions of stearic acid, arachidonic (ARA), and docosahexaenoic acid (DHA), and were significantly different to sardines (*p* = 0.015), which, along with octopus and prawn bodies, have a higher percentage of the SFA arachidic and the ω-3 PUFA, EPA (Figure 2).

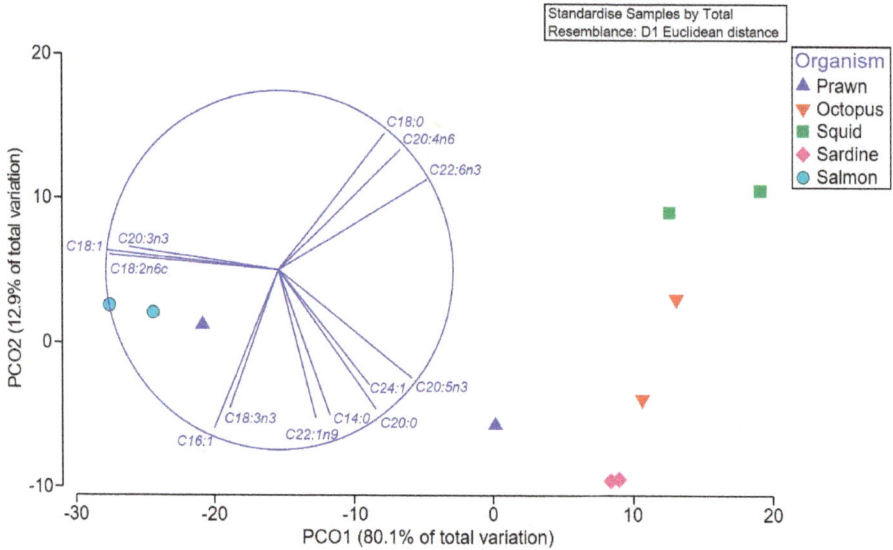

Figure 2. Principal coordinate ordination (PCO) of the fatty acid composition of various Australian seafood species. Vector overlay based on the Pearson correlation (r > 0.8) identifies the main fatty acids contributing to the separation between extracts, with higher levels of the specifically labeled fatty acids occurring in samples in the direction of the vector.

The amounts of EPA, DPA, and DHA per 100g of the seafood tissue were estimated from the yield of oil in the original tissue (Table 1B). Due to high oil yields, the sardines were the best source of these ω-3 PUFAs, with a total amount of over 3500mg/100g tissue in the flesh and over 6000 mg/100 g in the viscera. The viscera of octopus and heads of salmon also had high ω-3 yields with totals of over 1000mg/100g tissue. In all species, the viscera and/or head waste streams produced larger amounts of EPA, DPA, and DHA (Table 1B).

2.2. Cytotoxicity

At 50 µg/mL, none of the seafood extracts caused any reduction in cell viability for either 3T3-ccl-92 fibroblasts or RAW 264.7 macrophages (Table 2).

Table 1. Fatty acid profiles of lipid extracts from the commonly consumed flesh (tentacles, fillet, body) and waste products (viscera, heads) of Australian seafood organisms: (A) µg fatty acid per mg oil extract (estimated from a 2,6-Di-tert-butyl-4-methylpheno (BHT) internal standard and adjusted for molecular mass); (B) percent composition of dimethyl acetal aldehydes and major fatty acid classes in the lipid extract, as well as the estimated quantity of eicosapentanoic (EPA) and docosahexanoic (DHA) per 100g tissue for each seafood.

(A) Fatty Acid	Trivial Name	*Octopus tetricus*		*Sepioteuthis australis*		*Sardinops sagax*		*Salmo salar*		*Penaeus plebejus*	
		Flesh	Viscera	Flesh	Head	Flesh	Viscera & Head	Flesh	Head	Flesh	Head & Viscera
				Saturated Fatty Acids (SFAs)							
C12:0	Lauric	0.7	0	0	0	0.8	0.8	0.8	0.8	0.7	0
C13:0	tridecanoic	0	0	0	0	0.7	0.8	0	0	0	1.6
C14:0	myristic	43.0	20.0	11.3	14.8	57.8	59.7	16.5	20.1	17.8	16.1
C15:0	pentadecanoic	4.1	4.6	4.2	5.9	5.0	6.0	1.6	2.3	5.7	41.0
C16:0	palmitic	146.9	132.0	160.9	176.4	163.1	173.0	142.9	132.2	121.8	112.3
C17:0	heptadecanoic	8.0	14.0	11.1	11.6	65.6	6.9	3.1	4.0	7.4	26.0
C18:0	Stearic	43.7	69.1	69.4	67.2	34.6	37.0	40.1	39.4	39.2	44.5
C20:0	arachidic	3.6	4.1	1.5	1.5	4.5	4.8	0.8	0.8	1.5	3.2
C21:0	henicosanoic	0.7	0	0.8	0	0.8	0.8	0.8	0.8	3.1	21.4
C22:0	Behenic	2.2	2.5	1.6	2.4	2.4	1.7	0.9	0.8	1.6	3.4
C23:0	tricosanoic	0	0	0	0	0	0	1.0	0.9	0.9	1.9
C24:0	lignoceric	6.2	2.6	1.6	4.2	0.8	0.9	0.9	0.9	0.8	1.7
				Monounsaturated Fatty Acids (MUFAs)							
C14:1	myristoleic	6.2	2.3	0	0	1.5	1.5	1.6	1.5	0.7	2.3
C15:1	pentadecanoic	0.7	1.5	0	0	0.7	0.8	0.8	0.7	0.7	1.5
C16:1	palmitoleic	44.1	22.5	5.6	10.9	59.4	60.7	48.5	42.3	39.8	36.8
C17:1	heptadecanoic	0.7	1.5	0.7	2.2	0.7	1.5	2.3	2.2	7.0	50.6

Table 1. Cont.

(B) Fatty Acid	Trivial Name	Octopus tetricus		Sepioteuthis australis		Sardinops sagax		Salmo salar		Penaeus plebejus	
		Flesh	Viscera	Flesh	Head	Flesh	Viscera & Head	Flesh	Head	Flesh	Head & Viscera
C18:1n9t	elaidic	2.1	3.1	1.4	3.0	0.7	0.8	0.8	0.7	1.5	3.9
C18:1n9c	oleic	42.2	43.7	16.7	55.9	50.3	54.2	301.9	261.7	230.3	93.4
C20:1n9	eicosenoic	19.2	14.4	12.6	0	3.8	3.9	15.6	16.8	16.3	8.0
C22:1n9	erucic	8.2	7.6	1.6	4.0	9.5	9.1	4.3	4.8	5.5	5.0
C24:1n9	nervonic	5.3	6.0	1.6	2.5	4.8	5.0	1.7	2.4	3.2	4.3
Polyunsaturated Fatty Acids (PUFAs)											
C18:2n6c	Linoleic (LA)	12.3	8.5	2.8	0	15.2	0.8	82.8	76.3	67.2	20.8
C18:3n6	γ-linolenic (GLA)	1.4	5.4	0.7	11.2	2.2	2.3	1.6	2.2	2.2	1.5
C18:3n3	α-linolenic (ALA)	10.6	4.7	0.7	2.2	13.9	14.5	10.3	8.9	8.6	3.1
C20:2	eicosadienoic	1.4	5.5	2.2	12.2	1.5	1.6	4.8	7.5	6.6	6.3
C20:3n3	eicosatrienoic	2.2	3.3	2.3	4.8	3.1	3.3	4.2	4.7	5.4	5.0
C20:4n6	arachidonic (ARA)	21.6	56.7	77.1	63.2	11.4	12.0	4.8	7.0	10.5	34.0
C20:5n3	eicosapentanoic (EPA)	120.3	107.0	62.5	53.6	123.2	125.6	14.0	19.6	26.2	75.3
C22:2	docosadienoic	1.5	0.9	1.6	0	0.8	0.8	0	0.8	0.8	1.7
C22:5n3	docosapentanoic (DPA)	24.4	22.9	10.1	7.9	18.1	18.0	7.5	12.2	14.4	33.8
C22:6n3	docosahexanoic (DHA)	141.9	192.9	229.8	205.7	105.1	111.0	48.0	50.7	51.9	66.7
Dimethyl Acetal Aldehydes											
dimethyl acetal octadecan-1-al		0	2.5	3.0	2.9	0	0	0	0	0	0
dimethyl acetal nonadecan-1-al		3.3	4	1.4	1.8	3.6	3.7	3.4	3.6	3.9	3.0

Table 1. *Cont.*

	Categories									
SFAs	25.5	24.9	26.2	28.4	27.7	29.2	20.9	20.3	20.0	27.3
MUFAs	12.8	10.3	4.0	7.8	13.1	13.8	37.8	33.3	30.5	20.6
PUFAs	33.7	40.8	39.0	36.1	29.4	29.0	17.9	19.0	19.3	24.8
Total ω-3	29.9	33.1	30.5	27.4	26.3	27.2	8.4	9.6	10.7	18.4
Total ω-6	3.5	17.1	8.6	7.4	2.9	1.5	9.1	8.5	8.0	5.6
Total ω-9	15.0	7.5	3.4	6.5	6.9	7.3	32.4	28.6	25.7	11.5
Total unidentified	24.2	17.6	26.4	23.0	26.1	24.3	20.0	23.8	26.2	24.3
Saturated/unsaturated ratio	0.6	0.5	0.6	0.6	0.7	0.7	0.4	0.4	0.4	0.6
ω-6/ω-3 ratio	0.1	0.2	0.3	0.3	0.1	0.1	1.1	1.0	0.7	0.3
EPA per 100 g tissue	64.2	395.7	88.7	99.3	1845.5	2972.5	104.2	238.5	29.9	138.2
DPA per 100 g tissue	13.1	84.7	14.3	14.6	268.8	426.0	55.8	148.5	16.4	62.0
DHA per 100 g tissue	75.7	713.4	326.0	381.2	1560.7	2627.0	357.2	617.0	59.1	122.4

Table 2. Cytotoxicity and anti-inflammatory activity of the lipid extracts from various tissues of commercial seafood species, as well as two commercially available marine oils, calculated from the average of three repeat assays.

Organism	Extract	3T3 ccl-92 Fibroblasts Viability at 50 µg/mL	RAW 264.7 Macrophages Viability at 50 µg/mL	NO Inhibition IC$_{50}$ (µg/mL)	TNFα Inhibition IC$_{50}$ (µg/mL)
Octopus tetricus (Octopus)	Viscera	100%	100%	64.6	51.0
	Flesh	100%	100%	71.2	71.0
Sepioteuthis australis (Squid)	Head	100%	100%	91.1	67.7
	Flesh	100%	100%	114.2	78.8
Sardinops sagax (Australian Sardine)	Viscera/head	100%	100%	84.6	71.1
	Fillet	100%	100%	66.5	147.7
Salmo salar (Salmon)	Head	100%	100%	97.3	85.8
	Fillet	100%	100%	157.9	157.1
Penaeus plebejus (School Prawn)	Head/viscera	100%	100%	88.0	71.2
	Body	100%	100%	306.4	201.7
Euphausia superba	Krill Oil	100%	100%	337.8	99.8
Perna canaliculus (NZ Green-Lipped Mussel)	Oil (Lyprinol)	100%	100%	No detectable activity	>> max test dose 587.9

2.3. NO Inhibition

Lipid extracts from all Australian seafood organisms demonstrated significant NO inhibition in LPS-stimulated RAW 264.7 cells compared to the solvent positive control, except the lipid extract from school prawn bodies, which only showed weak NO inhibition (Supplementary Figure S1 and Table 2). Lipid extracts from the octopus showed strong NO inhibition with the lowest IC_{50}s of 65 µg/mL. The lipid extracts from the waste by-products showed higher NO inhibition (lower IC_{50}s) than the more commonly consumed flesh for octopus, squid, salmon, and prawns. All of the Australian seafood lipid extracts were active at much lower concentrations than the reference nutraceutical oils, Lyprinol and Deep Sea Krill oil, at the maximum concentration (Table 2). In fact, Lyprinol showed no inhibition of NO in this assay at the maximum solubility.

Multivariate RELATE analysis using a Spearman rank correlation demonstrated a significant relationship between NO inhibition and fatty acid composition (Rho = 0.302, p = 0.0477, 9999 permutations). BEST analysis revealed that a combination of four fatty acids explained the greatest amount of variation in NO inhibiting activity, with a correlation coefficient of 0.428. NO inhibition correlated with lower levels of oleic acid (C18:1) and higher levels of C18:3n-6, C20:2 and C22:2. Univariate correlations to investigate the relationship between IC_{50} for NO and the amount of particular fatty acids in the extracts revealed different trends depending on the fatty acid class (Supplementary Figure S2). Negative relationships (i.e., lower IC_{50} at higher concentrations = stronger activity) were observed for total SFAs (R^2 = 0.4) and PUFA (R^2 = 0.3), as well as ω-3 PUFAs (R^2 = 0.3), EPA (R^2 = 0.4), and to a lesser extent, DHA (R^2 = 0.2). Conversely, MUFAs showed a positive relationship (higher IC_{50}s = weaker activity) (R^2 = 0.3), along with ω-9 FAs (R^2 = 0.3). Surprisingly NO activity increased with higher SFA:UFA ratios (R^2 = 0.4), driven largely by inactive MUFAs, but decreased with higher ω-6:ω-3 ratios (R^2 = 0.3), as expected. There was no relationship between NO inhibitory activity and the amount of ω-6 PUFAs, the ω-3 DPA, or unidentified components in the extracts (Supplementary Figure S2).

2.4. TNF-Alpha Inhibition

Lipid extracts from all the seafood samples demonstrated significant TNFα down-regulatory effects reducing the levels of TNFα in the RAW 264.7 supernatant (Supplementary Figure S3, Table 2). Octopus viscera again showed the lowest IC_{50} (51 µg/mL), whereas the body of prawns had the highest IC_{50} at ~200 µg/mL. The extract from seafood by-products showed greater TNFα inhibition than the edible flesh for all species (Table 2), and this was most noticeable in prawns, with an IC_{50} nearly three times lower in the heads and viscera that are routinely discarded in Australia. The fish viscera and heads were approximately twice as active as the fillets.

There was a significant correlation between NO inhibition and TNFα inhibition (R^2 = 0.631), although the Australian sardine fillet had lower TNFα activity than would have been predicted from the NO inhibition. Multivariate RELATE analysis revealed a marginally significant relationship between TNFα inhibition and fatty acid composition (Rho = 0.269, p = 0.058, 9999 permutations). BEST analysis identified only two fatty acids, with a correlation coefficient of 0.334. TNFα inhibition was weakly correlated with lower levels of linolenic acid (C18:2) and higher levels of stearic acid (C18:0). Univariate correlations investigating the relationship between IC_{50} for TNFα and the amount of particular fatty acids in the extracts (Supplementary Figure S4) revealed similar trends to NO inhibition (Supplementary Figure S2). Decreasing TNFα IC_{50} with higher quantities were observed for total SFAs (R^2 = 0.3) and PUFA (R^2 = 0.4), as well as ω-3 PUFAs (R^2 = 0.4), DHA (R^2 = 0.3), and to a lesser extent, EPA (R^2 = 0.2). MUFAs again showed the reverse trend, along with ω-9 FAs (R^2 = 0.3). TNFα IC_{50} decreased with higher SFA:UFA ratios (R^2 = 0.2), but increased with higher ω-6:ω-3 ratios (R^2 = 0.2). There was again no relationship between TNFα IC_{50} inhibitory activity and the amount of ω-6 PUFAs, the ω-3 DPA, or unidentified components in the extracts (Supplementary Figure S2).

3. Discussion

This study demonstrates the quality and anti-inflammatory activity of lipids extracted from different Australian seafood. Seafood is known to be high in PUFAs, which have been previously associated with anti-inflammatory activity. All of the extracts tested in this study contain a high content of PUFAs, with ω-6/ω-3 ratios less than one. Simopoulos [44] found that lower ratios are desirable for reducing the risk of many chronic diseases, with ratios < 4:1 reducing mortality from chronic disease, and ratios less than 3:1 suppressing inflammation due to arthritis. We found that lower ω-6/ω-3 ratios correlated with higher NO and TNFα inhibitory activity across a range of seafood extracts. Furthermore, Western diets typically contain excessive levels of saturated fats and omega 6 fatty acids, which promote the pathogenesis of many diseases, including inflammatory conditions [44]. Our lipid extracts from Australia seafood all had saturated to unsaturated fatty acid ratios of less than 1, but higher amounts of MUFAs rather than SFAs were related to lower NO and TNFα inhibitory activity. Overall, the entire fatty acid composition appears to influence anti-inflammatory activity *in vitro*. Nevertheless, all of our extracts provided a good source of ω-3 fatty acids and significantly inhibited LPS stimulated NO and TNFα production by macrophages *in vitro*. This indicates the potential to value-add the Australian seafood industry based on high-quality marine oils with anti-inflammatory activities.

Anti-inflammatory fatty acids were not only found in the flesh that is normally consumed in Australian seafood, but are also present in high quantities in unprocessed parts like the head and viscera. In fact, the viscera and heads produced a higher yield of oils and contained higher quantities of commercially important long-chain ω-3 PUFAs EPA, DPA, and DHA with known healthy attributes for seafood consumers. The yields of these ω-3 PUFAs in the under-utilized/non-processed parts were substantially higher than in the edible flesh for most species (e.g., ten times the DHA in octopus viscera compared to flesh; four times the amount of EPA in prawn heads compared to flesh; and nearly double the EPA, DPA, and DHA in salmon heads and sardine viscera/heads compared to the flesh). This data is consistent with previous studies which have demonstrated high-quality fatty acid profiles in the uneaten tissues of mackerel tuna fish *Euthynnus affinis*, ray-finned fish *Sardinella lemuruand*, and Alaska pink salmon *Oncorhynchus gorbuscha* [30,31,45]. Overall the yields of EPA and DHA are similar to the range previously reported for mollusks, fish, and crustaceans (e.g., Reference [46]), although the Australian sardine is particularly notable for containing over 1000mg/100g tissue of both EPA and DHA in both the flesh and viscera. Australian seafood waste streams could therefore be used to generate a sustainable source of high-value marine lipids if they can be rapidly processed in a centralized facility to prevent oxidation and degradation.

All the lipid extracts from Australian seafood tested in this study showed significant inhibition of NO and TNFα, except those from the body of school prawns. As a neurotransmitter, NO is a potent inflammatory mediator, as well as playing a role in wound healing and maintaining blood pressure [47]. However, there are many diseases associated with the overproduction of NO, including liver cirrhosis, rheumatoid arthritis, infection, autoimmune diseases, and diabetes [48]. Similarly, TNFα is an important pro-inflammatory mediator that can lead to damaging effects, including neuropathic pain, when over-expressed [49]. Inflammation and neuropathic pain are complex problems involving many mediators and coupled signaling pathways which reduce the effectiveness of single compounds for drug development [49]. Natural extracts that contain a mixture of potential inhibitors of inducible NO Synthase (iNOS), TNFα expression, and other inflammatory pathway modulators might be effective for controlling chronic inflammation. For example, studies on the NZ Green-lipped mussel extract Lyprinol®, in a rat model for arthritis, have demonstrated that it modulates inflammatory cytokines (TNFα, IL-6, IL-1α, and IL-γ) and decreases the synthesis of some proteins associated with inflammation, whilst increasing malate dehydrogenase synthesis, which is related to glucose metabolism [50]. The effects on regulatory proteins were proposed to reduce energy for MHC-1 activation as a novel mechanism of action with anti-inflammatory efficacy at lower doses than other fish oil preparations. Lyprinol is a patented combination of 50 mg of PCSO-524® (lipid extract from *P. canaliculus*), 100 mg of a proprietary oleic acid blend, and 0.225 mg of vitamin E, so the ω-3 fatty acids in this mussel lipid extract may act synergistically with the anti-oxidant Vitamin E. Similarly, krill oil contains the antioxidant astaxanthin which can prevent lipid peroxidation, thus preserving of the ω-3 fatty acids EPA and DHA, in addition to acting directly on a number of biomarkers [51]. Krill oil has been shown to modulate cytokines, lipidogenesis, lipid peroxide, oxidative enzymes, glucose metabolism, and the endocannabinoid system in a range of animal studies [52]. It is possible that some of the unidentified components in our extracts have anti-oxidant activity and/or immunomodulatory activity that complements or enhances the activity of ω-3 fatty acids. Further *in vivo* studies investigating a range of anti-inflammatory markers and modulators will be required to establish the mechanism of action and novel potential of these Australian seafood lipid extracts.

The anti-inflammatory effects of fish oils and krill oil are typically attributed to long chain ω-3 PUFAs [14,52]. Similarly, we found a correlation between the amount of ω-3 PUFAs in the extracts and the IC_{50}s for both LPS stimulated NO and TNFα inhibition in RAW264.7 macrophages. In particular, the concentrations of both EPA and DHA were found to correlate with higher activity, but with EPA showing a stronger relationship with NO inhibition and DPA explaining more of the variation in TNFα inhibition. Previous studies on pure DHA and EPA have confirmed that these ω-3 PUFAs strongly inhibit NO production (IC_{50} < 25 μM) [53] and inducible NO synthase in LPS stimulated RAW264 macrophages (DHA at 30μM and EPA at 60 μM) [54]. Both EPA and DHA (100 μM) have also been shown to reduce TNFα secretion in LPS stimulated RAW264.7 cells after 24 hr exposure to 100 μM [55], and they significantly inhibit the secretion and transcription of TNFα in LPS stimulated THP-1 macrophages at 25 mM [56]. These studies lend support to the idea that EPA and DHA are contributing to the *in vitro* anti-inflammatory activity in our extracts, however, without further purification and testing against the pure compounds, we cannot conclude that there are no other factors involved. Indeed, higher concentrations of saturated fatty acids were also found to correlate with NO and TNFα inhibition, and our multivariate correlations indicate that the overall composition of fatty acids is important, along with potentially unidentified factors.

In this study, lipid extracts from the two cephalopod mollusks contained the highest proportion of ω-3 PUFAs and were associated with relatively high NO and TNFα inhibition. This supports the use of the flesh from octopus (*Zhang Yu*) and squid (*Qiang Wu Zei*) in traditional Chinese Medicine for inflammatory conditions [36]. Our comprehensive review of the anti-inflammatory, wound healing, and immunomodulatory activity of mollusks [36] found no previous *in vitro* studies on cephalopod extracts, and only a handful of *in vivo* animal models that have tested the ink and melanoprotein of squid [57,58]. Nevertheless, one previous study found that cuttlefish (*Ommastrephes bartrranii*) liver oil significantly reduced formalin and carrageenan-induced paw edema in rats fed 1% cuttlefish liver oil for 45 days [59]. We found that the cephalopods produce a fairly low yield of oil in comparison to oily fish, and consequently, they had lower overall amounts of EPA, DPA, and DHA per mg of tissue. This suggests the cephalopods may not be as good a functional food for dietary intake of ω-3 PUFAs based on the mass obtainable from the wet weight of edible tissue as compared to some other seafood, such as the Australian sardines, which have very high yields of ω-3 PUFAs in their flesh. However, the viscera and heads of octopuses and squids produce a significant waste stream that could be value-added based on their high-quality anti-inflammatory oils. For example, a large proportion of Southern jig squid fishery is sold as processed tubes in Australia, generating approximately 48% viscera as waste from ~1000 t annual harvest [60]. This justifies further investigation into cephalopod lipid extracts for anti-inflammatory applications.

The fatty acid profiles of the cephalopod and sardine lipid extracts are dominated by ω-3 PUFAs, whereas the salmon and prawns contain relatively high MUFA and ω-9 PUFAs. The high NO activity of sardine and cephalopod extracts reflects their richness in ω-3 fatty acids, especially DPA, DHA, and EPA, which are arguably the healthiest PUFAs [12,23,61]. The main ingredients of the well-known anti-inflammatory nutraceutical Lyprinol® and Biolane®, lipid extracts from the New

Zealand green-lipped mussel (GMLE) *Perna canaliculus*, are long chain ω-3 PUFA. The percent of the ω-3 PUFA in GMLE is about 37.1% of the total fatty acids [40]. A similar proportion of ω-3 PUFAs was found in the cephalopod mollusk extracts in this study. Interestingly, however, the different levels of ω-3 fatty acids in the various seafood extracts were not found to correlate directly with either NO or TNFα inhibitory concentrations in this study. Rather, lower levels of the MUFA oleic acid and higher levels of the ω-6 acids gamma-linolenic (C18:3), eicosadienoic (C20:2) and docosadienoic (C22:2) correlated with higher NO activity, whereas lower levels of linolenic (C18:2) and higher levels of the SFA stearic acid (C18:0) explained more of the variation in TNFα inhibitory concentrations. This implies that the overall composition of fatty acids in seafood oils could influence the anti-inflammatory activity, with particular fatty acids having either beneficial or antagonistic effects. This may help explain the variable outcomes from clinical trials on the use of fish oils for some inflammatory conditions [62,63].

The minimal anti-inflammatory activity detected in our prawn flesh extract was similar to that observed for a commercial krill oil in the same assays. The fatty acid composition of our prawn extracts was similar to that previously reported for a commercial krill oil (10% ω-3 PUFAs, 14% ω-6 PUFAs and 35% MUFAs), which was found to significantly modulate inflammation and lipid metabolism in mice transgenic for TNFα [33]. Antarctic krill oil has also been shown to inhibit LPS-induced iNOS in a rodent model [64] and to protect against rheumatoid arthritis in mouse models, but without effects on serum cytokines [35]. Further research on Penaeid extracts is therefore justified despite the relatively low *in vitro* activity. In particular, the waste streams from aquacultured prawns can be sustainably produced in comparison to wild harvested krill, although their fatty acid compositions could be impacted by an artificial diet [65].

Lyprinol®, the anti-inflammatory nutraceutical composed of lipid extracts from the Green-lipped mussel *Perna canaliculus,* was also used as a reference drug but did not show detectable inhibition of NO and TNFα in our *in vitro* assays. Green-lipped mussel extracts have been previously found to suppress iNOS expression and inhibit NO production in LPS-induced RAW264.7 cells by regulating nuclear factor kappa B [66], as well as inhibiting TNFα in LPS-stimulated human THP-1 monocytes [67]. Therefore, the lack of activity in both the commercial marine oils we tested is likely due to their relative insolubility in ethanol as a result of product formulation. Furthermore, *in vitro* assays do not always provide a good predictor of *in vivo* activity. Nevertheless, given the wealth of evidence relating to the beneficial effects of ω-3 PUFAs in clinical trials, the preliminary *in vitro* anti-inflammatory activity observed here, along with the beneficial fatty acid composition of Australian seafood extracts, justifies further research to value-add the industry by developing a sustainable supply of high-quality fish oil.

4. Materials and Methods

4.1. Chemicals and Reagents

Escherichia coli LPS (O128:B12, Sigma-Aldrich, Castle Hill, Australia), sulfanilic acid, N-(1-Naphthyl) ethylenediamine (NED), 85% orthophosphoric acid sodium nitrite ($NaNO_2$), and HPLC grade solvents were obtained from Sigma Aldrich (St. Louis, MO, USA). The mouse TNFα ELISA kit was purchased from BD biosciences (Sparks, MD, USA). Penicillin–streptomycin solution, Dulbecco's Modified Eagle's Medium (DMEM), fetal bovine serum (FBS), sodium pyruvate, and L-glutamine were from Life Technology Australia (Mulgrave, VIC, Australia). The two cell lines, RAW264.7 mouse macrophages and 3T3 Swiss albino (ATCC® CCL92™) cell lines, were purchased from the American Type Culture Collection (ATCC®, Manassas, VA, USA).

4.2. Sample Collection

Fresh seafood used in this study including octopus (*Octopus tetricus* n = 3), Australian sardine (*Sardinops sagax* n = 4), salmon (*Salmo salar* n = 3), school prawn (*Penaeus plebejus*, n = 12), and squid (*Sepioteuthis australis* n = 3) were purchased fresh from Ballina seafood co-op., Ballina, Australia. Salmon and squid viscera are processed during harvesting to prevent degradation and fouling of the prime edible flesh; however, the heads of these organisms are still available as a waste stream. All other species were obtained whole and the typically consumed flesh was separated from the waste streams, including internal organs (viscera) and heads. Lyprinol (BLACKMORES®, Alexandria, Australia) and Krill oil (Swisse, Collingwood Melbourne, Australia) were purchased from a local pharmacy.

4.3. Lipid Extraction

Extracts from the cephalopods, *O. tetricus* and *S. australis*, included the tentacles and mantle tissue (edible flesh) and body viscera, comprised of the gastrointestinal tract and other internal organs for *O. tetricus* and just the heads for *S. australis*. Extracts from the fish included flesh fillets and viscera, including heads from *S. sagax*, and just the head from *S. salar*. The head with viscera (waste) and body (edible flesh) were also extracted from the school prawn *Penaeus plebejus*. Lipids were extracted as above using a solvent to tissue ratio of 19 mL final volume for every 1 g tissue.

The solvent homogenates were vacuum filtered through Whatman paper (No. 1) into separating funnels. Saturated NaCl solution (6.2 M) was added to the solvent phase to a final ratio of 8:4:3 (Chloroform: methanol: NaCl solution). The organic phases were collected and the solvent evaporated on a rotary evaporator (Rotavapor® R-114; BÜCHI Labortechnik AG, Flawil, Switzerland). Extracted lipids were transferred into glass vials, dried under a stream of nitrogen gas, weighed on an analytical balance to calculate yield per g tissue, and then covered and stored in minimal hexane at $-80\ ^{\circ}$C until required.

4.4. Fatty Acid Methyl Ester (FAME) Analysis

Subsamples of 200 µL of foot and viscera lipid extracts from all species were placed in 10 mL pyrex glass vials for derivitization. NaCl in methanol solution (0.5 M, 1.5 mL) was added under nitrogen gas, capped and shaken for 10 secs. Samples were then heated at 100°C for 10 min in a dry block and cooled. Two mL of 14% Boron trifluoride in methanol was added and bubbled with nitrogen gas for 8 s, then placed in a 100 °C dry block for 30 min. After cooling, 1 mL of hexane containing 1 µg 2,6-Di-tert-butyl-4-methylphenol (BHT) was added, and samples were shaken for 30 s. Saturated NaCl solution (5 mL) was added and the samples were shaken to create an upper lipid layer, which was collected and stored at $-80\ ^{\circ}$C for FAMEs and GC-MS analysis.

FAMEs were analyzed using a GC (Agilent 6890N, Santa Clara, CA, USA) coupled to an Agilent 6890 flame ionization detector (FID) using a BPX 70 capillary column (70% cyanopropyl polysilphenylene-siloxane, 50 m length, 0.22 mm internal diameter and 0.25 µm thickness). The FID was operated at 260 °C and the split injector was maintained at 230 °C. High-purity helium was used as the carrier gas and maintained with a linear flux of 1 mL/min. The GC oven was held at 100 °C for 5 min and then raised to 240 °C at a rate of 5 °C/min. 1 µL of each subsample extract was injected with a split ratio of 200:1 and a column flow of 1 mL/min.

FAMEs were identified by peak retention time and elution order and compared against a reference FAMEs standard test mix (SUPELCO 37-Component FAME Mix CRM47885, Bellefonte, PA, USA) and a marine test mix PUFA No.1 (Marine Source, Analytical Standards, Sigma-Aldrich, Castle Hill, Australia). Some samples were further analyzed using an Agilent gas chromatography-mass spectrometer (GC-MS) with an Agilent 5973 Mass Selective Detector to confirm the identity of the fatty acids. The mass spectra were recorded at 70 eV ionization voltage over the mass range of 35–550 amu. To facilitate the identification of DPA, which was not in the test mix, a soft ionization MS technique at 40 eV ionization voltage was employed to ionize the lipid molecules in the *D. orbita* samples without causing extensive fragmentation. The spectrum was compared on MS databases (WILEY 275 online and NIST98, Gaithersburg, MD, USA), along with retention times and elution order from extensive literature searches including the American Oil Chemists' Society. The relative composition of each identified fatty acid was calculated by peak integration from the GC [68]. The concentration of each fatty acid was estimated using BHT as an internal standard. In each sample, the area under the curve for each fatty acid was calibrated against the peak area for BHT and adjusted for molecular weight, then scaled for the concentration on 1mg per g extract. For the ω-3 PUFAs EPA, DHA, and DPA, we also calculated the yield per 100 g of tissue by adjusting for the amount of crude lipid extract obtained per g of tissue that was extracted.

4.5. Cell Lines and Cell Culture

The Murine RAW264.7 macrophages and 3T3 fibroblast cell lines were obtained from American Type Cell Culture (ATCC). Both cell lines were maintained in 10% FBS supplemented DMEM, 100 µg/L streptomycin, and 100 IU/mL penicillin at 37 °C and 5% CO_2 atmosphere. Cells were passaged every 48–72 h [69].

4.6. Lipid Extract Preparation

Lipid extracts were dried under nitrogen gas flow before being weighed and dissolved in HPLC-grade 100% ethanol. The stock solutions of the lipid extracts were diluted in color-free DMEM before being added to the cell culture, and the final concentration of ethanol in all experiments was around 0.35%. Stock solutions of the lipid extracts were prepared fresh on the day of the experiment prior to addition to the cell culture. The solubility of all extracts in the cell cultures was confirmed under an inverted microscope (200 and 400×). Each sample was tested in triplicate and each experiment was repeated independently at least three times on different days.

4.7. Cytotoxicity Assay

Toxicity of the lipid extracts used in this study was assessed using a crystal violet cytotoxicity assay as previously described by Feoktistova, et al. [70] using both the RAW 264.7 macrophages and 3T3 ccl-92 fibroblasts cell lines. Briefly, cells were seeded at a density of 2×10^4 cells/well in a 96-well plate and then incubated for 18–24 h. Lipid extracts were added then and incubated for 24 h before the media was aspirated and the cells washed twice in a gentle stream of water. Water was removed by tapping the plate on a pile of paper towel followed by addition of 50 µL of 0.5% crystal violet staining solution and incubated for 20 min at room temperature. The plate was then washed 4 times with water and air dried for 2 h. Finally, 200 µL of methanol was added to each well and incubated for 20 min at room temperature on a rocker. The optical density was then measured at 570 nm using Anthos Zenyth 200rt plate reader (Anthos Labtec Instruments, Heerhugowaard, Netherlands). Chlorambucil in a gradient concentration was used as a positive control.

4.8. NO Inhibition Assay

The production of NO by LPS stimulated RAW 264.7 macrophages was measured in the cell culture supernatant using the Greiss reaction method as previously described by Ahmad et al. [64]. In brief, RAW 264.7 macrophages were seeded at a density of 10^6 cell/mL and incubated overnight. The following day, cells were incubated with different concentrations of the extracts 50, 25, 12.5, 6.25, or 3.125 µg/mL 1 h prior to LPS stimulation. Twenty-four h after LPS stimulation, the supernatant was collected, and an equal volume of supernatant and Greiss' reagent was mixed in a 96 well plate and incubated in dark for 10–15 min. Absorbance was read at 550 nm using an Anthos Zenyth 200rt plate reader (Anthos Labtec Instruments, Heerhugowaard, Netherlands). Sodium nitrite was used as a standard in this assay, and all assays were repeated in triplicate. The commercially available marine nutraceuticals Lyprinol (BLACKMORES®, Sydney, Australia) and Deep Sea Krill oil (Swisse, Collingwood, Australia) were used as reference anti-inflammatory nutraceuticals at the same test concentrations. Dexamethasone at 2.5 µM concentration was used as a reference drug. All assays were repeated three times.

4.9. TNF Alpha Inhibition Assay

The levels of TNFα produced by LPS stimulated RAW 264.7 macrophages in the cell culture supernatant were measured using a mouse TNFα ELISA kit (R&D Systems, Minneapolis, MN, USA) and performed as per the manufacturer's instructions. All extracts were tested in five different concentrations 50 µg/mL, 25 µg/mL, 12.5 µg/mL, 6.25 µg/mL, and 3.125 µg/mL. Dexamethasone was used as a reference anti-inflammatory drug, and untreated, stimulated cells (LPS + ethanol) were used as a positive control. Absorbance was read at 450 nm using an Anthos Zenyth 200rt plate reader (Anthos Labtec Instruments, Heerhugowaard, Netherlands). The commercially available marine nutraceuticals Lyprinol® (BLACKMORES®, Alexandria, Australia) and Deep Sea Krill oil (Swisse, Collingwood Melbourne, Australia) were used as reference anti-inflammatory nutraceuticals. The assays were repeated in triplicate.

4.10. Statistical Analysis

PRIMER v 7 + PERMANOVA software (version 7, Primer-e, Albany, New Zealand) was used to explore the multivariate differences in lipid profiles, and univariate analyses were used to test differences in specific lipid classes and anti-inflammatory activity between the various seafood extracts. Separate Euclidean distance similarity matrices were created for the fatty acid percent composition, the composition of fatty acid classes, and the totals for each fatty acid class (SFA, MUFA, PUFA and ω-3, ω-6, n-9, ω-3:ω-6 and DMAAs), as well as the IC_{50} for NO inhibition and TNFα inhibition. Principle Coordinate Ordination plots were generated on the fatty acid composition with vector overlay based on Pearson's correlation with a cut-off at r > 0.8 to identify which fatty acids contributed most to the separation between samples.

To assess the relationship between fatty acid composition and NO inhibition or TNFα inhibition, relate analyses were undertaken on PRIMER V7 using Spearman rank correlation and 9999 permutations. This was followed by a BIOENV stepwise model on the Euclidean distance similarity matrix to identify which set of fatty acids explained the most variability for each of the anti-inflammatory markers.

5. Conclusions

In conclusion, lipid extracts from Australian marine seafood were found to contain a high ratio of unsaturated: saturated fatty acids and significant anti-inflammatory activity. The inhibition of NO and TNFα in LPS stimulated macrophages was correlated with higher levels of SFAs and PUFA, and in particular the ω-3 PUFAs EPA and DHA, as well as with lower levels of MUFAs, thus indicating that the overall composition of marine lipid extracts can influence the anti-inflammatory activity. High valued marine oils rich in healthy ω-3 PUFAs were not only demonstrated in the edible parts of seafood, but the under-utilized components of these organisms showed similar if not higher proportions of PUFAs and anti-inflammatory activity. In particular, the byproducts from cephalopod mollusks appear to have good anti-inflammatory activity, with potential for the development of another high-quality marine oil for nutraceutical applications. Further *in vitro* and *in vivo* studies are required to optimize and develop the seafood waste stream as used for natural anti-inflammatory treatments.

Supplementary Materials: The following are available online at http://www.mdpi.com/1660-3397/17/3/155/s1, Figure S1: The NO inhibitory activity of lipid extracts from different seafood organisms; (A) *Penaeus plebejus* (Australian school prawn), body flesh and head, including viscera; (B) *Sardinops sagax* (Australian sardine) flesh and viscera, including heads; (C) *Salmo salar* (Atlantic salmon) flesh and heads; (D) *Sepioteuthis australis*; (E) *Octopus tetricus* * $p < 0.05$, ** $p < 0.01$, *** $p < 0.001$, **** $p < 0.0001$ versus the LPS + Solvent control. Figure S2: Correlations between NO inhibitory activity (IC_{50}) of lipid extracts and the amount of certain fatty acid classes or ratios in different seafood organisms. Figure S3: The TNFα inhibitory activity of lipid extracts from different seafood organisms; (A) *Penaeus plebejus* (Australian school prawn), body flesh and head, including viscera; (B) *Sardinops sagax* (Australian sardine) flesh and viscera, including heads; (C) *Salmo salar* (Atlantic salmon) flesh and heads; (D) *Sepioteuthis australis*; (E) *Octopus tetricus* * $p < 0.05$, ** $p < 0.01$, *** $p < 0.001$, **** $p < 0.0001$ versus the LPS + Solvent control. Figure S4: Correlations between the TNFα inhibitory activity (IC_{50}) of lipid extracts and the amount of certain fatty acid classes or ratios in different seafood organisms.

Author Contributions: This study was conceptualized by D.R., T.B.A., and K.B. T.B.A. undertook all the anti-inflammatory testing, and D.R. undertook the lipid extractions and fatty acid analyses. K.B. performed the statistical analysis. K.B. and M.K. contributed resources and K.B., M.K., and L.L. supervised the project. The original draft manuscript was written by T.B.A., and K.B., D.R., L.L., and M.K. reviewed and edited the manuscript. K.B. and D.R. revised the manuscript to address feedback from reviewers.

Funding: This research received no external funding.

Acknowledgments: We appreciate postgraduate research support from the School of Environment, Science and Engineering and Marine Ecology Research Centre, Southern Cross University and the use of facilities in the Analytical Research Laboratory in Southern Cross Plant Science.

Conflicts of Interest: The authors declare no conflict of interest.

References

1. Guo, L.Y.; Hung, T.M.; Bae, K.H.; Shin, E.M.; Zhou, H.Y.; Hong, Y.N.; Kang, S.S.; Kim, H.P.; Kim, Y.S. Anti-inflammatory effects of schisandrin isolated from the fruit of *Schisandra chinensis* Baill. *Eur. J. Pharm.* **2008**, *591*, 293–299. [CrossRef] [PubMed]

2. MacMicking, J.; Xie, Q.W.; Nathan, C. Nitric oxide and macrophage function. *Annu. Rev. Immunol.* **1997**, *15*, 323–350. [CrossRef] [PubMed]

3. Abramson, S.B.; Amin, A.R.; Clancy, R.M.; Attur, M. The role of nitric oxide in tissue destruction. *Best Pract. Res. Clin. Rheumatol.* **2001**, *15*, 831–845. [CrossRef] [PubMed]

4. Evans, C.H. Nitric oxide: What role does it play in inflammation and tissue destruction? *Agents Actions Suppl.* **1995**, *47*, 107–116. [PubMed]

5. Zhang, J.M.; An, J. Cytokines, inflammation, and pain. *Int. Anesthesiol. Clin.* **2007**, *45*, 27–37. [CrossRef] [PubMed]

6. De Oliveira, C.M.; Sakata, R.K.; Issy, A.M.; Gerola, L.R.; Salomao, R. Cytokines and pain. *Rev. Bras. Anestesiol.* **2011**, *61*, 255–265. [CrossRef]

7. Miller, R.E.; Miller, R.J.; Malfait, A.M. Osteoarthritis joint pain: The cytokine connection. *Cytokine* **2014**, *70*, 185–193. [CrossRef] [PubMed]

8. Saltzman, E.T.; Thomsen, M.; Hall, S.; Vitetta, L. *Perna canaliculus* and the intestinal microbiome. *Mar. Drugs* **2017**, *15*, 207. [CrossRef] [PubMed]

9. Biesalski, H.K.; Dragsted, L.O.; Elmadfa, I.; Grossklaus, R.; Muller, M.; Schrenk, D.; Walter, P.; Weber, P. Bioactive compounds: Definition and assessment of activity. *Nutrition* **2009**, *25*, 1202–1205. [CrossRef] [PubMed]

10. Hamed, I.; Ozogul, F.; Ozogul, Y.; Regenstein, J.M. Marine bioactive compounds and their health benefits: A review. *Comp. Rev. Food Sci. Fod Saf.* **2015**, *14*, 446–465. [CrossRef]

11. Lordan, S.; Ross, R.P.; Stanton, C. Marine bioactives as functional food ingredients: Potential to reduce the incidence of chronic diseases. *Mar. Drugs* **2011**, *9*, 1056–1100. [CrossRef] [PubMed]

12. Calder, P.C. Polyunsaturated fatty acids and inflammatory processes: New twists in an old tale. *Biochimie* **2009**, *91*, 791–795. [CrossRef] [PubMed]

13. Calder, P.C.; Grimble, R.F. Polyunsaturated fatty acids, inflammation and immunity. *Eur. J. Clin. Nutr.* **2002**, *56* (Suppl. 3), S14–S19. [CrossRef]

14. Wall, R.; Ross, R.P.; Fitzgerald, G.F.; Stanton, C. Fatty acids from fish: The anti-inflammatory potential of long-chain omega-3 fatty acids. *Nutr. Rev.* **2010**, *68*, 280–289. [CrossRef] [PubMed]

15. Moreillon, J.; Bowden, R.; Shelmadine, B. *Fish Oil and c-Reactive Protein. Bioactive Food as Dietary Interventions for Arthritis and Related Inflammatory Diseases*; Academic Press: San Diego, CA, USA, 2012; pp. 393–405.

16. Zheng, J.S.; Hu, X.J.; Zhao, Y.M.; Yang, J.; Li, D. Intake of fish and marine n-3 polyunsaturated fatty acids and risk of breast cancer: Meta-analysis of data from 21 independent prospective cohort studies. *Br. Med. J.* **2013**, *346*, f3706. [CrossRef] [PubMed]

17. Yam, D.; Peled, A.; Shinitzky, M. Suppression of tumor growth and metastasis by dietary fish oil combined with vitamins E and C and cisplatin. *Cancer Chemother. Pharmacol.* **2001**, *47*, 34–40. [CrossRef] [PubMed]

18. Hardman, W.E.; Avula, C.P.; Fernandes, G.; Cameron, I.L. Three percent dietary fish oil concentrate increased efficacy of doxorubicin against mda-mb 231 breast cancer xenografts. *Clin. Cancer Res.* **2001**, *7*, 2041–2049. [PubMed]

19. Li, J.J.; Huang, C.J.; Xie, D. Anti-obesity effects of conjugated linoleic acid, docosahexaenoic acid, and eicosapentaenoic acid. *Mol. Nutr. Food Res.* **2008**, *52*, 631–645. [CrossRef] [PubMed]

20. Arai, T.; Kim, H.J.; Chiba, H.; Matsumoto, A. Anti-obesity effect of fish oil and fish oil-fenofibrate combination in female kk mice. *J. Atheroscler. Thromb.* **2009**, *16*, 674–683. [CrossRef] [PubMed]

21. Chan, E.; Cho, L. What can we expect from omega-3 fatty acids? *Cleve Clin. J. Med.* **2009**, *76*, 245–251. [CrossRef] [PubMed]

22. Juturu, V. Omega-3 fatty acids and the cardiometabolic syndrome. *J. Cardiometab. Syndr.* **2008**, *3*, 244–253. [CrossRef] [PubMed]

23. Calder, P.C. N-3 polyunsaturated fatty acids, inflammation, and inflammatory diseases. *Am. J. Clin. Nutr.* **2006**, *83*, 1505S–1519S. [CrossRef] [PubMed]

24. Simopoulos, A.P. Omega-3 fatty acids in inflammation and autoimmune diseases. *J. Am. Coll. Nutr.* **2002**, *21*, 495–505. [CrossRef] [PubMed]

25. Kelley, D.S.; Taylor, P.C.; Nelson, G.J.; Schmidt, P.C.; Ferretti, A.; Erickson, K.L.; Yu, R.; Chandra, R.K.; Mackey, B.E. Docosahexaenoic acid ingestion inhibits natural killer cell activity and production of inflammatory mediators in young healthy men. *Lipids* **1999**, *34*, 317–324. [CrossRef] [PubMed]

26. Kelley, D.S.; Siegel, D.; Fedor, D.M.; Adkins, Y.; Mackey, B.E. Dha supplementation decreases serum c-reactive protein and other markers of inflammation in hypertriglyceridemic men. *J. Nutr.* **2009**, *139*, 495–501. [CrossRef] [PubMed]

27. Leaf, D.A.; Hatcher, L. The effect of lean fish consumption on triglyceride levels. *Phys. Sports Med.* **2009**, *37*, 37–43. [CrossRef] [PubMed]

28. Nichols, P.D.; Elliott, N.G.; Mooney, B.D.; Scientific, C. *Nutritional Value of Australian Seafood II: Factors Affecting Oil Composition of Edible Species*; Division of Marine Research, Commonwealth Scientific and Industrial Research Organization (CSIRO): Hobart, TAS, Australia, 1998.

29. Ackman, R. Seafood lipids. In *Seafoods: Chemistry, Processing Technology and Quality*; Springer: New York City, NY, USA, 1994; pp. 34–48. [CrossRef]

30. Khoddami, A.; Ariffin, A.; Bakar, J.; Ghazali, H. Fatty acid profile of the oil extracted from fish waste (head, intestine and liver)(*Sardinella lemuru*). *World Appl. Sci. J.* **2009**, *7*, 127–131.

31. Khoddami, A.; Ariffin, A.; Bakar, J.; Ghazali, H. Quality and fatty acid profile of the oil extracted from fish waste (head, intestine and liver)(*Euthynnus affinis*). *Afr. J. Biotechnol.* **2012**, *11*, 1683–1689. [CrossRef]

32. Nichols, P.D.; Mooney, B.D.; Elliott, N.G. Value-adding to australian marine oils. In *Developments in Food Science*; Sakaguchi, M., Ed.; Elsevier: Amsterdam, The Netherlands, 2004; Volume 42, pp. 115–130.

33. Vigerust, N.F.; Bjorndal, B.; Bohov, P.; Brattelid, T.; Svardal, A.; Berge, R.K. Krill oil versus fish oil in modulation of inflammation and lipid metabolism in mice transgenic for TNF-alpha. *Eur. J. Nutr.* **2013**, *52*, 1315–1325. [CrossRef] [PubMed]

34. Deutsch, L. Evaluation of the effect of neptune krill oil on chronic inflammation and arthritic symptoms. *J. Am. Coll. Nutr.* **2007**, *26*, 39–48. [CrossRef] [PubMed]

35. Ierna, M.; Kerr, A.; Scales, H.; Berge, K.; Griinari, M. Supplementation of diet with krill oil protects against experimental rheumatoid arthritis. *BMC Musculoskelet. Disord.* **2010**, *11*, 136. [CrossRef] [PubMed]

36. Ahmad, T.B.; Liu, L.; Kotiw, M.; Benkendorff, K. Review of anti-inflammatory, immune-modulatory and wound healing properties of molluscs. *J. Ethnopharmacol.* **2018**, *210*, 156–178. [CrossRef] [PubMed]

37. Giri, A.; Ohshima, T. Bioactive marine peptides: Nutraceutical value and novel approaches. *Adv. Food Nutr. Res.* **2012**, *65*, 73–105. [PubMed]

38. Cobb, C.S.; Ernst, E. Systematic review of a marine nutriceutical supplement in clinical trials for arthritis: The effectiveness of the new zealand green-lipped mussel *Perna canaliculus*. *Clin. Rheumatol.* **2006**, *25*, 275–284. [CrossRef] [PubMed]

39. Bhattacharya, S.; Chakraborty, M.; Bose, M.; Mukherjee, D.; Roychoudhury, A.; Dhar, P.; Mishra, R. Indian freshwater edible snail *bellamya bengalensis* lipid extract prevents t cell mediated hypersensitivity and inhibits lps induced macrophage activation. *J. Ethnopharmacol.* **2014**, *157*, 320–329. [CrossRef] [PubMed]

40. Li, G.; Fu, Y.; Zheng, J.; Li, D. Anti-inflammatory activity and mechanism of a lipid extract from hard-shelled mussel (*Mytilus coruscus*) on chronic arthritis in rats. *Mar. Drugs* **2014**, *12*, 568–588. [CrossRef] [PubMed]

41. Chakraborty, K. Green mussel extract (GME) goes commercial first nutraceutical produced by an ICAR institute. *Cmfri Newsl* **2012**, *135*, 5–6.

42. Pereira, R.B.; Taveira, M.; Valentao, P.; Sousa, C.; Andrade, P.B. Fatty acids from edible sea hares: Anti-inflammatory capacity in lps-stimulated raw 264.7 cells involves inos modulation. *RSC Adv.* **2015**, *5*, 8981–8987. [CrossRef]

43. Chakraborty, K.; Vijayagopal, P.; Vijayan, K.K.; Syda Rao, G.; Joseph, J.; Chakkalakal, S.J. A Product Containing Anti-Inflammatory Principles from Green Mussel *Perna viridis* L. And a Process Thereof. Indian Patent IP 2066/CHE/2010, 22 March 2013.

44. Simopoulos, A.P. The importance if the ratio of omega-6/omega-3 essential fatty acids. *Biomed. Pharmacother.* **2002**, *56*, 365–379. [CrossRef]

45. Oliveira, A.C.M.; Bechtel, P.J. Lipid composition of alaska pink salmon (*Oncorhynchus gorbuscha*) and Alaska Walleye pollock (*Theragra chalcogramma*) byproducts. *J. Aquat. Food Prod. Technol.* **2005**, *14*, 73–91. [CrossRef]

46. Mohanty, B.P.; Ganguly, S.; Mahanty, A.; Sankar, T.V.; Ananda, R.; Chakraborty, K.; Sridhar, N. DHA and EPA content and fatty acid profile of 39 food fishes from India. *Biomed Res. Int.* **2016**, *2016*, 4027437. [CrossRef] [PubMed]

47. Korhonen, R.; Lahti, A.; Kankaanranta, H.; Moilanen, E. Nitric oxide production and signaling in inflammation. *Curr. Drug Targets Inflamm. Allergy* **2005**, *4*, 471–479. [CrossRef] [PubMed]

48. Lechner, M.; Lirk, P.; Rieder, J. In Inducible nitric oxide synthase (iNOS) in tumor biology: The two sides of the same coin. *Semin. Cancer Biol.* **2005**, *15*, 277–289. [CrossRef] [PubMed]

49. Leung, L.; Cahill, C. Tnf-α and neuropathic pain—A review. *J. Neuroinflammation* **2010**, *7*, 27. [CrossRef] [PubMed]

50. Halpern, G. Novel anti-inflammatory mechanism of action of lyprinol in the aia rat model. *Prog. Nutr.* **2008**, *10*, 146–152.

51. Ambati, R.R.; Moi, P.S.; Ravi, S.; Aswathanarayana, R.G. Astaxanthin: Sources, extraction, stability, biological activities and its commercial applications—A review. *Mar Drugs* **2014**, *12*, 128–152. [CrossRef] [PubMed]

52. Burri, L.; Johnsen, L. Krill products: An overview of animal studies. *Nutrients* **2015**, *7*, 3300–3321. [PubMed]

53. Ohata, T.; Fukuda, K.; Takahashi, M.; Sugimura, T.; Wakabayashi, K. Suppression of nitric oxide production in lipopolysaccharide-stimulated macrophage cells by omega 3 polyunsaturated fatty acids. *Jpn. J. Cancer Res.* **1997**, *88*, 234–237. [CrossRef] [PubMed]

54. Komatsu, W.; Ishihara, K.; Murata, M.; Saito, H.; Shinohara, K. Docosahaenoic acid suppresses nitric oxide production and inducible nitric oxide synthase expression in interferon-γ plus lipopolysaccharide-stimulated murine macrophages by inhibiting the oxidative stress. *Free Radic. Biol. Med.* **2002**, *34*, 1006–1016. [CrossRef]

55. Honda, K.L.; Lamon-Fava, S.; Matthan, N.R.; Wu, D.; Lichtenstein, A.H. EPA and DHA Exposure Alters the Inflammatory Response but not the Surface Expression of Toll-like Receptor 4 in Macrophages. *Lipids* **2015**, *50*, 121–129. [CrossRef] [PubMed]

56. Mullen, A.; Loscher, C.E.; Roche, H.M. Anti-inflammatory effects of EPA and DHA are dependent upon time and dose-response elements associated with LPS stimulation in THP-1-derived macrophages. *J. Nutr. Biochem.* **2010**, *21*, 444–450. [CrossRef] [PubMed]

57. Soliman Mimura, T.; Itoh, S.; Tsujikawa, K.; Nakajima, H.; Satake, M.; Kohama, Y.; Okabe, M. Studies on biological activities of melanin from marine animals. V. Antiinflammatory activity of low-molecular-weight melanoprotein from squid (Fr. Sm ii). *Chem. Pharm. Bull.* **1987**, *35*, 1144–1150. [CrossRef]

58. Soliman, A.; Fahmy, S. *in vitro* antioxidant, analgesic and cytotoxic activities of *Sepia officinalis* ink and *Coelatura aegyptiaca* extracts. *Afr. J. Pharm. Pharmacol.* **2013**, *7*, 1512–1522.

59. Joseph, S.; George, M.; Nair, J.; Senan, V.; Pillai, D.; Sherief, P. Effect of feeding cuttlefish liver oil on immune function, inflammatory response and platelet aggregation in rats. *Curr. Sci.* **2005**, *88*, 507–510.

60. Emery, T.; Curtotti, R. Chapter 13: Southern squid jig Fishery. In *Fishery Status Reports*; Australian Bureau Agricultural and Resource Economics and Sciences: Canberra, Australia, 2018. Available online: http://www.agriculture.gov.au/abares/research-topics/fisheries/fishery-status/southern-squid-jig-fishery (accessed on 8 February 2019).

61. Calder, P.C. Omega-3 polyunsaturated fatty acids and inflammatory processes: Nutrition or pharmacology? *Br. J. Clin. Pharmacol.* **2013**, *75*, 645–662. [CrossRef] [PubMed]

62. Turner, D.; Chan, P.; Steinhart, A.; SZlotkin, S.; Griffiths, A. Maintenance of remission in inflammatory bowel disease using omega-3 fatty acids (fish oil): A systematic review and meta-analyses. *Inflamm. Bowel Dis.* **2010**, *17*, 336–345. [CrossRef] [PubMed]

63. Woods, R.; Thien, F.; Abramson, M. Dietary marine fatty acids (fish oil) for asthma in adults and children. *Cochranes Database Syst. Rev.* **2002**, *2002*, CD001283.

64. Choi, J.; Jang, J.; Son, D.; Im, H.-K.; Kim, J.; Patk, J.; Choi, W.; Han, S.; Hong, J. Antarctic krill oil diet protects against lipopolysaccharide-inducde oxidative stress, neuroinflammation and cognitive impairment. *Int. J. Mol. Sci.* **2017**, *18*, 2554. [CrossRef] [PubMed]

65. Strobel, C.; Jahreis, G.; Kuhnt, K. Survey of n-3 and n-6 polyunsaturated fatty acids in fish and fish products. *Lipids Health Dis.* **2012**, *11*, 144. [CrossRef] [PubMed]

66. Chen, J.; Cheng, B.; Cho, S.; Lee, H. Green lipped mussel oil complex suppresses lipopolysaccharide stimulated inflammation via regulating nuclear factor kb and mitogen activated kinases signalling in RAW 264.7 murine macrophages. *Food Sci. Biotech.* **2017**, *26*, 815–822. [CrossRef] [PubMed]

67. Lawson, B.R.; Belkowski, S.M.; Whitesides, J.F.; Davis, P.; Lawson, J.W. Immunomodulation of murine collagen-induced arthritis by *N,N*-dimethylglycine and a preparation of *Perna canaliculus*. *BMC Comp. Alt. Med.* **2007**, *7*, 20. [CrossRef] [PubMed]

68. Valles-Regino, R.; Tate, R.; Kelaher, B.; Savins, D.; Dowell, A.; Benkendorff, K. Ocean warming and CO_2-induced acidification impact the lipid content of a marine predatory gastropod. *Mar. Drugs* **2015**, *13*, 6019–6037. [CrossRef] [PubMed]

69. Ahmad, T.B.; Rudd, D.; Smith, J.; Kotiw, M.; Mouatt, P.; Seymour, L.M.; Liu, L.; Benkendorff, K. Anti-inflammatory activity and structure-activity relationships of brominated indoles from a marine mollusc. *Mar. Drugs* **2017**, *15*, 133. [CrossRef] [PubMed]

70. Feoktistova, M.; Geserick, P.; Leverkus, M. Crystal violet assay for determining viability of cultured cells. *Cold Spring Harb. Protoc.* **2016**, *2016*, pdb prot087379. [CrossRef]

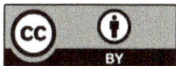

marine drugs

MDPI

Article

Hirsutanol A Attenuates Lipopolysaccharide-Mediated Matrix Metalloproteinase 9 Expression and Cytokines Production and Improves Endotoxemia-Induced Acute Sickness Behavior and Acute Lung Injury

Jing-Shiun Jan [1,2], Chih-Hao Yang [1,2], Mong-Heng Wang [3], Fan-Li Lin [1,2], Jing-Lun Yen [1,2], Irene Hsieh [1,2], Maksim Khotimchenko [4], Tzong-Huei Lee [5,†] and George Hsiao [1,2,6,*,†]

[1]   Graduate Institute of Medical Sciences, College of Medicine, Taipei Medical University, Taipei 110, Taiwan; d119101004@tmu.edu.tw (J.-S.J.); chyang@tmu.edu.tw (C.-H.Y.); fllin@tmu.edu.tw (F.-L.L.); m120102039@tmu.edu.tw (J.-L.Y.); m120105021@tmu.edu.tw (I.H.)

[2]   Department of Pharmacology, School of Medicine, College of Medicine, Taipei Medical University, Taipei 110, Taiwan

[3]   Department of Physiology, Augusta University, Augusta, GA 30912, USA; mwang@augusta.edu

[4]   School of Biomedicine, Far Eastern Federal University, 690091 Vladivostok, Russia; khotimchenko.my@dvfu.ru

[5]   Institute of Fisheries Science, National Taiwan University, Taipei 106, Taiwan; thlee1@ntu.edu.tw

[6]   Ph.D. Program in Biotechnology Research and Development, College of Pharmacy, Taipei Medical University, Taipei 110, Taiwan

*   Correspondence: geohsiao@tmu.edu.tw; Tel./Fax: +886-2-2737-4622

†   These authors contributed equally to this work.

Received: 27 May 2019; Accepted: 14 June 2019; Published: 17 June 2019

Abstract: Activated human monocytes/macrophages, which increase the levels of matrix metalloproteinases (MMPs) and pro-inflammatory cytokines, are the essential mechanisms for the progression of sepsis. In the present study, we determined the functions and mechanisms of hirsutanolA (HA), which is isolated from the red alga-derived marine fungus *Chondrostereum* sp. NTOU4196, on the production of pro-inflammatory mediators produced from lipopolysaccharide (LPS)-treated THP-1 cells. Our results showed that HA suppressed LPS-triggered MMP-9-mediated gelatinolysis and expression of protein and mRNA in a concentration-dependent manner without effects on TIMP-1 activity. Also, HA significantly attenuated the levels of TNF-α, IL-6, and IL-1β from LPS-treated THP-1 cells. Moreover, HA significantly inhibited LPS-mediated STAT3 (Tyr705) phosphorylation, IκBα degradation and ERK1/2 activation in THP-1 cells.   In an LPS-induced endotoxemia mouse model, studies indicated that HA pretreatment improved endotoxemia-induced acute sickness behavior, including acute motor deficits and anxiety-like behavior. HA also attenuated LPS-induced phospho-STAT3 and pro-MMP-9 activity in the hippocampus. Notably, HA reduced pathologic lung injury features, including interstitial tissue edema, infiltration of inflammatory cells and alveolar collapse. Likewise, HA suppressed the induction of phospho-STAT3 and pro-MMP-9 in lung tissues. In conclusion, our results provide pharmacological evidence that HA could be a useful agent for treating inflammatory diseases, including sepsis.

Keywords: signal transducer and activator of transcription 3 (STAT3); matrix metalloproteinases-9 (MMP-9); interleukin (IL); lipopolysaccharide (LPS); acute sickness behavior; acute lung injury (ALI)

1. Introduction

Sepsis is defined as an abnormal host response to infection, which triggers inflammation throughout the body and causes life-threatening organ dysfunction [1]. Sepsis and septic shock are significant public health concerns, affecting millions of people around the world with high mortality and poor diagnosis [1–3]. Notably, in-hospital mortality of sepsis has declined in the last two decades because of established evidence-based managements, which improve the outcome of the critically ill patient [2,4,5]. Nevertheless, deterioration of health after sepsis is still common, including physical disability and cognition impairment [3]. Because of the high mortality rate and serious complications, it is critical to develop new and novel approaches to the treatment of sepsis.

The innate immune system is the first line of defense against microorganism, but the uncontrolled inflammatory response can lead to tissue damage [6,7]. Tissue-resident leukocytes recognize the molecules released from pathogens and dead host cells via a pattern recognition receptor activating downstream transcription factors, especially NF-κB and AP-1, leading to the production of inflammatory mediators. These inflammatory mediators then initiate localized transmigration of leukocytes to the infection site to destroy pathogens [7]. The positive feedback loop between cytokines and immune cells leads to an auto-amplifying phenomenon and cytokine storm, eventually resulting in injuries to multiple organs during sepsis [7–9]. The emblematic pro-inflammatory cytokines, including tumor necrosis factor (TNF)-α, interleukin (IL)-1β and IL-6 are major products generated by monocyte/macrophages and neutrophils. These pro-inflammatory cytokines play a critical role in pathophysiologic processes of sepsis associated-organ injuries and -cognition impairment, as described previously [9,10]. Therefore, pro-inflammatory cytokines are considered as the therapeutic targets for the treatment of sepsis or as diagnostic biomarkers of sepsis [11,12].

Matrix metalloproteinases (MMPs) are zinc- and calcium-dependent endopeptidases; these enzymes involve in biological processes including tissue remodeling and angiogenesis via degrading the extracellular matrix [13]. Also, MMPs can regulate non-matrix substrates in pathological processes. For example, MMP-9 has been shown to cleave and activate pro-inflammatory cytokines, and degrade the complement of tight junction protein [14]. Therefore, several reports [13,15–17] have shown that MMP-9 plays an essential role in the pathogenesis of inflammation diseases, such as multiple sclerosis, arthritis, ischemic stroke, and sepsis. Leukocytes-mediated MMP-9 production and secretion could be induced by inflammatory response, in particular endotoxemia, CD11b^{high} GR-1^{high} neutrophils are the main producers of MMP-9 [18,19]. The serum levels of MMP-9 are elevated in patients with both sepsis and septic animal models [13,20]. The MMP-deficient mice have low lethality in a lipopolysaccharide (LPS)-induced endotoxemia model [21]. In addition, synthetic inhibitor Regasepin1-inhibiting neutrophil MMP-9 and MMP-8 protects mice against endotoxin shock [22]. Further, MMP-9 blockade attenuated blood-brain-barrier dysfunction in a cecal ligation and puncture rat model of sepsis [23]. Thus, MMP-9 inhibition could provide a therapeutic strategy of sepsis.

Hirsutanol A (HA), a hirsutane-type sesquiterpene, which is isolated from marine fungus *Chondrostereum* sp. NTOU4196, attenuates NO production in LPS-activated murine BV-2 microglial cells as described previously [24]. This report [24] supports the notion that HA could be a potential anti-inflammatory agent. In this study, we determined the inhibitory effect and mechanism of HA on production of MMP-9 and pro-inflammatory cytokine (TNF-α, IL-1β, and IL-6) from LPS-treated human monocytic THP-1 cells. In an LPS-induced endotoxemia mouse model, we further evaluated the protective effect of HA on endotoxemia-induced acute sickness behavior and acute lung injury (ALI).

2. Results

2.1. HA Inhibited MMP-9-Mediated Gelatinolysis Induced by LPS

To determine whether HA modulated the production of MMP-9, MMP-2, or TIMP-1 from LPS-activated monocytes, THP-1 cells were pretreated with HA (2, 5, and 10 μM) for 15 min, followed by the addition of LPS (50 ng/mL) within 24 h. Zymography showed that LPS (50 ng/mL) significantly enhanced extracellular MMP-9-mediated gelatinolysis by up to 3.06 ± 0.12-fold, and pretreatment with HA (2, 5, and 10 μM) strongly inhibited MMP-9-mediated gelatinolysis in a concentration-dependent manner by 2.88 ± 0.37-, 2.56 ± 0.25-, 1.97 ± 0.49-, and 1.37 ± 0.48-fold compared with that under the normal condition, respectively (Figure 1A). In addition, the pretreatment of HA (10 μM) had no effect on monocytic extracellular MMP-9 gelatinolysis in the absence of LPS (Figure S1). Systematic TIMP-1 protein levels are increased during endotoxemia [18]. Similarly, as shown in Figure 1B, THP-1 cells constitutively releasing TIMP-1 was enhanced by LPS stimulation. The pretreatment of HA did not upregulate the TIMP-1 production of THP-1. In contrast, HA (10 μM) attenuated TIMP-1 enhanced by LPS challenge. Furthermore, to confirm whether HA suppressed extracellular MMP-9 gelatinolysis by down-regulating MMP-9 expression, intracellular MMP-9 protein expression was evaluated by immunoblotting. As shown in Figure 1C, compared with the resting condition, THP-1 cells treated with LPS for 24 h strongly induced up-regulation of MMP-9 protein expression by up to 3.71 ± 1.18-fold compared with that under the normal condition. Pretreatment with HA at different concentrations for 15 min followed by the addition of LPS (50 ng/mL) within 24 h decreased MMP-9 expression to 2.55 ± 0.98-, 1.70 ± 0.67-, and 1.04 ± 0.14-fold, respectively, in a concentration-dependent manner. Similarly, LPS (50 ng/mL) significantly increased the expression of MMP-9 mRNA in THP-1 cells by up to 25.42 ± 8.53-fold compared with normal conditions, and pretreated with HA (5 and 10 μM) significantly suppressed LPS-mediated MMP-9 mRNA expression down to 9.26 ± 7.17- and 8.62 ± 6.84-fold, respectively (Figure 1D). These results suggested that HA down-regulated MMP-9-mediated gelatinolysis occurred at both transcriptional and protein expression levels.

A

B

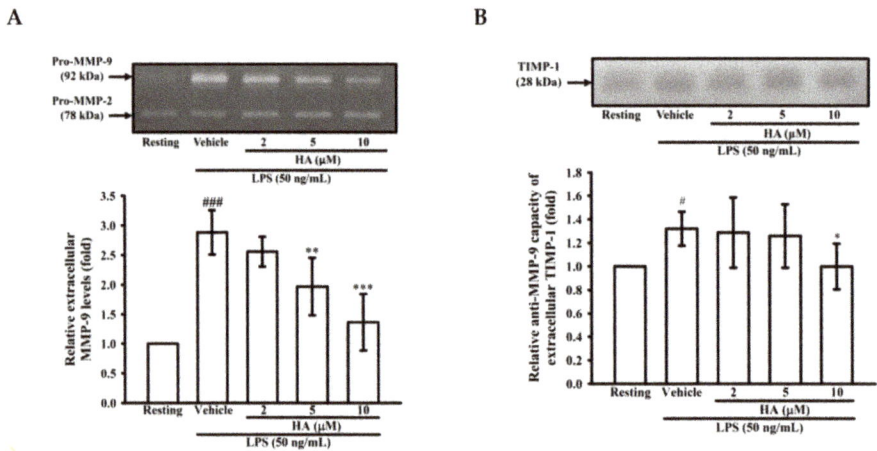

Figure 1. *Cont.*

C   D

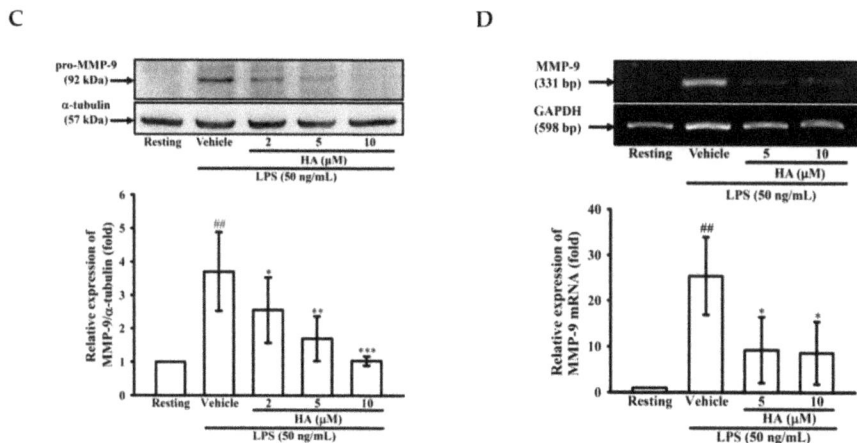

Figure 1. Effect of HA on MMP-9-mediated gelatinolysis and expression induced by LPS. THP-1 cells (5×10^5 cells/0.5 mL) were dispensed onto 24-well plates and treated with LPS (50 ng/mL) for 24 h. Cells were treated with the indicated concentrations of HA (2, 5 and 10 μM) or vehicle for 15 min before treatment with a stimulant. Cell-free supernatants were then assayed for MMPs and TIMP-1 activity by gelatin zymography (**A**) and reverse zymography (**B**). THP-1 cells (10^6 cells/mL) were dispensed onto 6-well plates and were treated with LPS (50 ng/mL) for 24 h (**C**) or 8 h (**D**) at the indicated concentrations of HA or vehicle for 15 min before treatment with LPS. Cell lysates were obtained and analyzed for MMP-9 protein expression by Western blotting or for MMP-9 mRNA expression by RT-PCR. Data represent means ± S.D. from three independent experiments. [#] $p < 0.05$, [##] $p < 0.01$ and [###] $p < 0.001$ as compared with the resting, [*] $p < 0.05$, [**] $p < 0.01$ and [***] $p < 0.001$ as compared with the vehicle.

2.2. HA Attenuated Pro-Inflammatory Cytokines Production Induced by LPS

To determine whether HA down-regulated the level of the pro-inflammatory cytokines TNF-α, IL-6, and IL-1β production by activated monocytes, THP-1 cells were pretreated with different concentrations of HA (0.5–10 μM) for 15 min followed by the addition of LPS (50 ng/mL) within 4 h or 24 h. As shown in Figure 2A, compared with the resting condition, THP-1 cells stimulated with LPS for 4 h significantly increased extracellular TNF-α levels by up to 345.8 ± 73.0 pg/10^6 cells, and pretreatment with HA at different concentrations significantly attenuated the extracellular TNF-α production in a concentration-dependent manner to 249.5 ± 33.5, 198.8 ± 29.1, 94.5 ± 7.1, and 21.0 ± 5.1 pg/10^6 cells, respectively. Likewise, LPS significantly increased extracellular IL-6 levels by up to 303.0 ± 182.5 pg/10^6 cells. Pretreatment with different concentrations of HA significantly suppressed the extracellular IL-6 levels in a concentration-dependent manner to 101.0 ± 54.2, 8.5 ± 6.8, and 6.2 ± 9.5 pg/10^6 cells, respectively (Figure 2B). Also, as shown in Figure 2C, LPS markedly enhancing extracellular IL-1β production to 32.3 ± 17.0 pg/10^6 cells, and pretreatment with HA at different concentrations significantly decreased the extracellular IL-1β levels in a concentration-dependent manner to 23.8 ± 10.6, 18.6 ± 8.4, and 9.5 ± 5.5 pg/10^6 cells, respectively (Figure 2C). In addition, the pretreatment of HA (5 μM) did not induce pro-inflammatory cytokines production of THP-1 without LPS challenge (Figure S2). Notably, HA (2, 5, and 10 μM) and the combination of LPS and HA (10 μM) did not have a significant cytotoxic effect against THP-1 cells based on MTT assay, respectively (Figures 2D and S3).

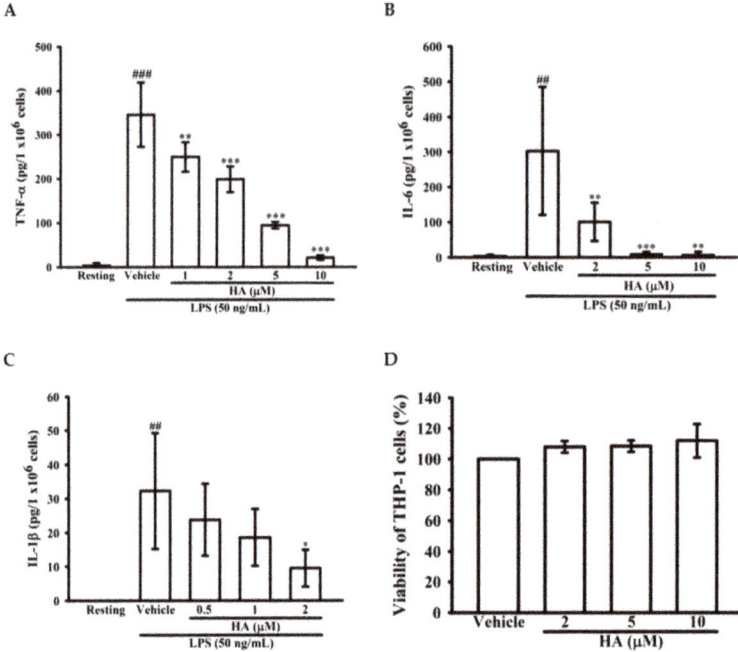

Figure 2. Effect of HA on pro-inflammatory cytokines production induced by LPS in THP-1 cells without cellular toxicity. THP-1 cells (5 × 10⁵ cells/0.5 mL) were dispensed onto 24-well plates and were treated with the indicated concentrations of HA or vehicle for 15 min followed by treatment with LPS (50 ng/mL) for 4 h (**A**) and 24 h (**B,C**). Cell-free supernatants were then assayed for the level of TNF-α (**A**), IL-6 (**B**) and IL-1β (**C**) by ELISA. (**D**) THP-1 cells treated with the indicated concentrations of HA or vehicle for 24 h. Cell viability was quantified by the ability of mitochondria to reduce the tetrazolium dye MTT in viable cells. Data represent means ± S.D. from three independent experiments. ## $p < 0.01$ and ### $p < 0.001$ as compared with the resting; * $p < 0.05$, ** $p < 0.01$ and *** $p < 0.001$ as compared with the vehicle.

2.3. HA Suppressed IκB-α Degradation and the Phosphorylation Level of STAT3 and ERK1/2 Induced by LPS

While the JAK2-STAT3 pathway is essential to regulate the immune response, it is considered to be involved in an "early" inflammatory response during sepsis [25]. To examine the effects of HA on LPS-mediated STAT3 activation, the phosphorylation levels of STAT3 (Tyr705) were determined by western blotting. THP-1 cells stimulated with LPS for 24 h significantly induced the level of phosphorylated-STAT3 (Tyr705) by up to 3.65 ± 0.29-fold, and pretreatment of HA (2, 5, and 10 μM) significantly attenuated LPS-mediated activation of STAT3 (Tyr705) down to 2.27 ± 0.60-, 1.39 ± 0.48-, and 1.08 ± 0.16-fold, respectively (Figure 3A). On the other hand, MMP-9 expression was regulated by various transcription factors, such as NF-κB, AP-1, and SP-1 [26]. Therefore, the effect of HA on the LPS-induced activation of MAPKs (p38, ERK), degradation of the inhibitor of kappa B alpha (IκBα) and the phosphorylation level of IκB kinase alpha/beta (IKKα/β) was determined by western blotting. To examine whether HA regulates the IKKα/IκBα/NF-κB cascade, THP-1 cells were pretreated with HA (2, 5, and 10 μM) or parthenolide (PTL; 10μM, an inhibitor of the NF-κB pathway) for 15 min followed by the addition of LPS (50 ng/mL) within 60 min. As shown in Figure 3B, significant degradation of IκBα was observed in THP-1 stimulated with LPS (50 ng/mL) for 60 min, and the pretreatment with different concentrations of HA significantly prevented the degradation of IκBα in a concentration-dependent manner by 0.55 ± 0.13-, 0.74 ± 0.13-, and 0.95 ± 0.10-fold, respectively. Similarly, LPS significantly enhanced the level of phosphorylated IKKα by up to 4.60 ± 0.72-fold, and pretreatment with HA (5 and

10 μM) attenuated the IKKα phosphorylation down to 3.79 ± 0.27-, and 3.14 ± 0.16-foldcompared with basal levels of the normal condition, respectively (Figure S4). To investigate whether HA regulates the activation of ERK or p38 MAPK, THP-1 cells were pretreated with HA (2, 5, and 10 μM), PD (PD98059, a MEK MAPK inhibitor; 20 μM), or SB (SB203580, a p38 MAPK inhibitor; 10 μM) for 15 min followed by the stimulation of LPS within 30 min. As shown in Figure 3C, the phosphorylation levels of ERK was strongly induced by LPS to 1.80 ± 0.46-fold compared with the resting condition, while the pretreatment with HA at different concentrations significantly inhibited LPS-stimulated ERK phosphorylation in a concentration-dependent manner by 1.39 ± 0.16-, 1.14 ± 0.03-, and 1.08 ± 0.21-fold, respectively. Notably, LPS significantly enhanced the phosphorylation levels of p38 by up to 1.68 ± 0.12-fold, and pretreatment with SB (10 μM) attenuated the p38 phosphorylation down to 0.44 ± 0.13-fold compared with the resting condition. However, unlike SB, pretreatment with HA at different concentrations did not affect p38 activation (Figure 3D). On the other hand, the pretreatment of HA (10 μM) did not induce phosphorylation of STAT3 and degradation of IκBα in THP-1 without LPS challenge (Figure S5). These results suggested that HA attenuated MMP-9 expression through regulating IKKα/IκBα/NF-κB- and ERK-associated signaling in THP-1 cells during LPS treatment.

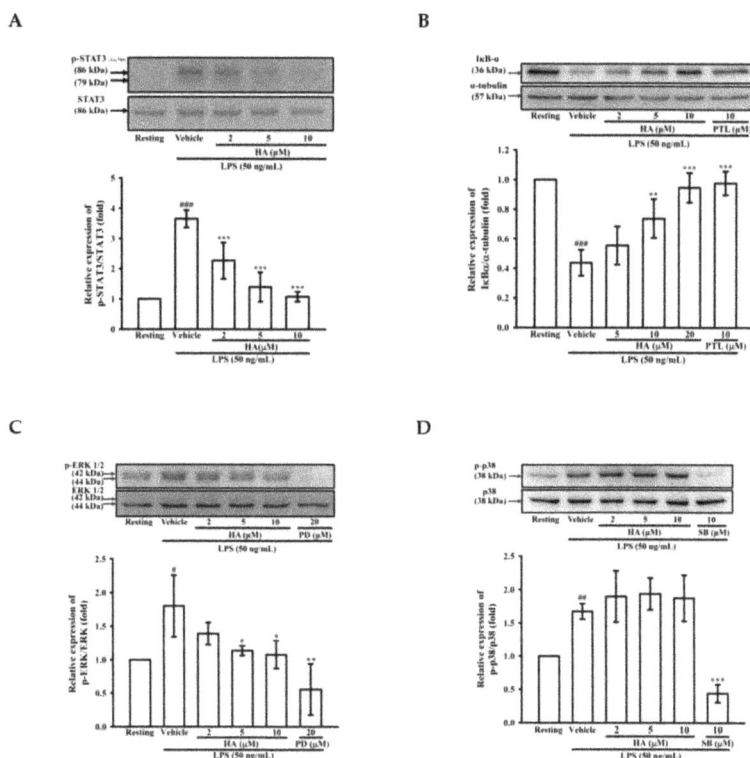

Figure 3. Effect of HA on STAT3, MAPK and NF-κB activation induced by LPS in THP-1 cells. THP-1 cells (10^6 cells/mL) were dispensed onto 6-well plates and were treated with the indicated concentrations of HA (2, 5 and 10 μM), parthenolide (PTL, 10 μM), PD98059 (PD, 20 μM), SB203580 (SB, 10 μM) or vehicle followed by treatment of LPS (50 ng/mL) for 24 h (**A**), 60 min (**B**), and 30 min (**C,D**), respectively. Cell lysates were obtained and analyzed for IκBα degradation and the level of phosphorylated-STAT3, ERK and p38 MAPK by Western blotting. Data represent means ± S.D. from three independent experiments. [#] $p < 0.05$, [##] $p < 0.01$ and [###] $p < 0.001$ as compared with the resting; [*] $p < 0.05$, [**] $p < 0.01$ and [***] $p < 0.001$ as compared with the vehicle.

2.4. The Activation of JAK2-STAT3 Cascade Was Associated with LPS-Mediated MMP-9 Production

To determine the effects of JAK2-STAT3 inhibition on MMP-9 production, THP-1 cells were pretreated with AG490 (a JAK2 inhibitor; 5, 10, 20, and 40 μM) or HA (5, and 10μM) for 15 min followed by the addition of LPS (50 ng/mL) for 24 h. As described in zymography, compared with the LPS-stimulating condition, the pretreatment of AG490 (20, 40 μM) significantly lessened extracellular MMP-9-mediated gelatinolysis down to 1.71 ± 0.41-, and 0.92 ± 0.15-fold, respectively (Figure 4A). Interestingly, at the same concentration, HA was more potent than AG490 on attenuating MMP-9-mediated gelatinolysis induced by LPS. The ERK1/2 inhibition suppress LPS-mediated STAT3 (Tyr705) activation and AP-1 expression in THP-1 cells [27]. Also, the inhibition of JAK2-STAT3 cascade lessens NF-κB phosphorylation in LPS-stimulated THP-1 cells [25]. As shown in Figure 3, HA pretreatment both down-regulated ERK1/2 phosphorylation and prevented IκBα degradation in LPS-challenged THP-1 cells. To investigate the difference between MEK inhibition and HA pretreatment on LPS-mediated STA3 (Tyr705) phosphorylation and whether HA regulated STAT3 activation in LPS-challenged-monocytes, THP-1 cells were pretreated with HA (10 μM) or PD (10 μM) for 15 min followed by the addition of LPS within 3 h or 5 h. As shown in Figure 4B, THP-1 cells stimulated with LPS for 5 h significantly induced STAT3 (Tyr 705) phosphorylation by up to 5.03 ± 0.50-fold, and pretreatment with HA (10 μM) significantly inhibited the phosphorylation levels to 1.44 ± 0.41-fold (Figure 4B). At the same concentration, HA was more potent than PD to inhibit STAT3 phosphorylation. To compare the difference between the effect of HA and JAK2-inhibitor on LPS-mediated IκBα/NF-κB cascade, THP-1 cells were pretreated with HA (10 μM) or AG490 (20 μM) for 15 min followed by the addition of LPS for 60 min. As indicated in Figure 4C, HA (10 μM) and AG490 (20 μM) caused similar efficacy on the inhibition of extracellular MMP-9 activity. At the same condition as stated above, HA was more effective than JAK inhibitor for preventing LPS-induced IκBα degradation in THP-1 cells. Taken together, these results suggested that HA regulated the functions of various signal molecules, including ERK1/2, NF-κB, and STAT3 to regulate the production of MMP-9 and pro-inflammatory cytokines.

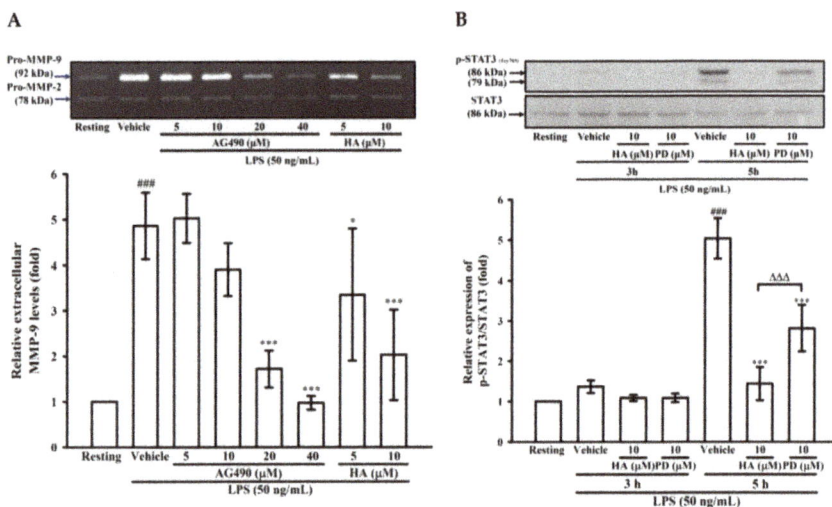

Figure 4. *Cont.*

C

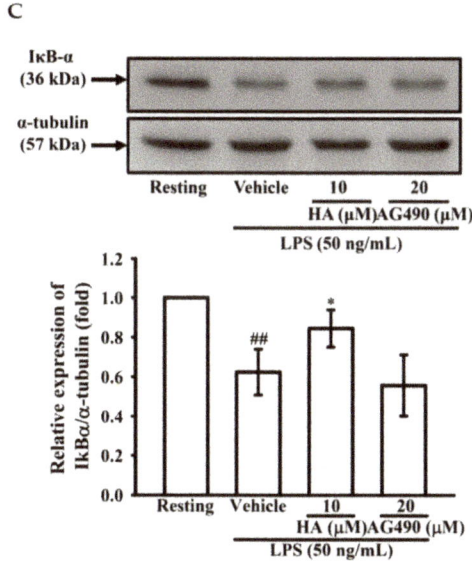

Figure 4. Effect of JAK2-STAT3 cascade inhibition on LPS-mediated MMP-9 expression. THP-1 cells $(5 \times 10^5$ cells/0.5 mL) were dispensed onto 24-well plates and treated with LPS (50 ng/mL) for 24 h. Cells were treated with the indicated concentrations of AG490 (5, 10, 20, and 40 μM), HA (5 and 10 μM) or vehicle for 15 min before treatment with LPS. Cell-free supernatants were then assayed for MMPs activity by gelatin zymography (**A**). THP-1 cells (10^6 cells/mL) were dispensed onto 6-well plates and were treated with LPS (50 ng/mL) for 3 h, 5h (**B**) and 60 min (**C**) at the indicated concentrations of HA, PD (10 μM), AG490 (10 μM) or vehicle for 15 min before treatment with LPS. Cell lysates were obtained and analyzed for STAT3 (Tyr705) phosphorylation and IκBα degradation by Western blotting. Data represent means ± S.D. from three to four independent experiments, respectively. $^{##}$ $p < 0.01$ and $^{###}$ $p < 0.001$ as compared with the resting; * $p < 0.05$ and *** $p < 0.001$ as compared with the vehicle; $^{\Delta\Delta\Delta}$ $p < 0.001$ as compared with the group pretreated with HA pre-treatment.

2.5. HA Decreased LPS-Mediated Acute Sickness Behavior

Body weight loss, acute motor deficits, and anxiety-like behavior are typical sickness behaviors that are mediated by systemic immune responses [28]. As indicated in Figure 5A, the 5-min period of OFT after LPS-injection for 2 h and 24 h, respectively, were presented using heat-maps. The total distance traveled by LPS-challenged mice was dramatically reduced by 57% compared to control mice (Saline-2073.0 ± 224.9 vs. LPS-888.9 ± 625.5, $p < 0.001$). HA (30 mg/kg) pretreatment significantly prevented LPS-induced acute locomotor deficits compared to the LPS-challenged group at 2 h (Figure 5C, $p < 0.05$). As shown in Figure 5D, the LPS-injected mice group spent significantly less time in the open area than the control group ($p < 0.001$). HA pretreatment significantly lessened the LPS-induced reduction in the time spent in the open area ($p < 0.001$). One day after LPS injection, HA pretreatment still significantly improved the reduction of the time spent in the open area and the total distance traveled induced by LPS-injection ($p < 0.05$, Figure 5E,F). Also, pretreatment reduced body weight loss and body temperature abnormalities mediated by LPS at 24 h compared with the LPS-challenged group (Figure S6A,B). As shown in Figure 6 A, the 5-min period of the EZM tests were tracked as a Heat-map at one day after the LPS injection. As shown in Figure 6B, the percentage of entries in the open quadrants was significantly lower in the LPS-challenged group than in the control group ($p < 0.01$). HA-pretreatment significantly lessened the decline of time spent in the open quadrants compared to the behaviors observed in the LPS challenge group ($p < 0.05$). A slight decrease in the percentage of entries in the open quadrants was observed in the LPS challenge group compared to the control group, but no significant differences were observed among the 3 groups ($p > 0.05$, Figure 6C). To further determine whether HA pretreatment regulated STAT3 activation and pro-MMP-9 expression in the hippocampus during endotoxemia-mediated acute sickness behavior and anxiety-like behavior, the expression levels of phosphorylated STAT3 (Tyr705) and pro-MMP-9 expression were evaluated by immunoblotting and gelatin zymography, respectively. Compared with the control group, LPS significantly increased the expression levels of STAT3 phosphorylated on Tyr705 in the hippocampus to 2.55 ± 0.90 fold. The increase in phosphorylated STAT3 protein levels was reduced by HA pretreatment to 50% as compared with the LPS-challenged group (LPS-2.55 ± 0.90-fold vs. HA-1.29 ± 0.37 fold, $p < 0.01$) (Figure 6D). Additionally, zymography showed that sample of hippocampus post-LPS challenged significantly enhanced MMP-9-mediated gelatinolysis by up to 1.44 ± 0.17-fold, and pretreatment with HA significantly attenuated MMP-9-mediated gelatinolysis by 28% as compared with the LPS-challenged group (LPS-1.44 ± 0.17-fold vs. HA 1.03 ± 0.09, $p < 0.01$) (Figure 6E). Furthermore, LPS injection significantly increased the number of CD68[+] phagocytes in the CA3 hippocampal region compared with the control group. Compared with the septic group, the pretreatment of HA reduced the infiltration of CD68[+] phagocytes (Figure S7).

A

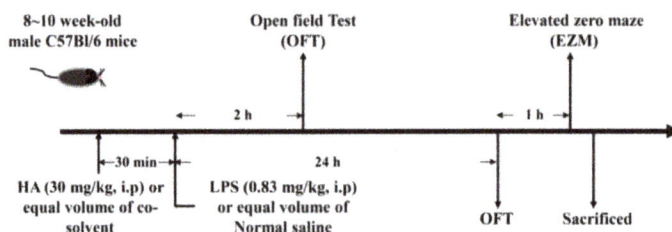

B

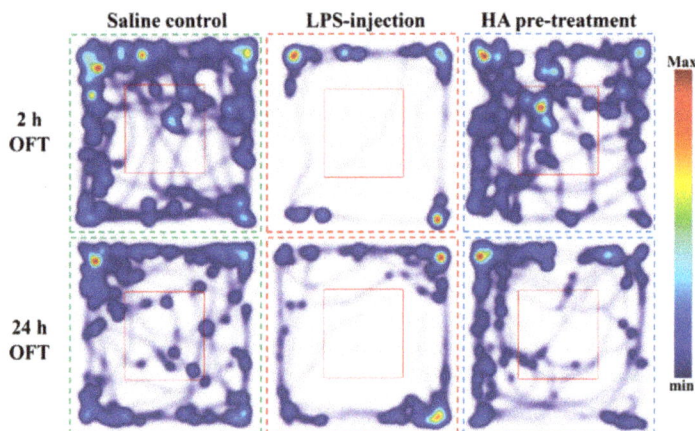

Figure 5. *Cont.*

C

D

E

F

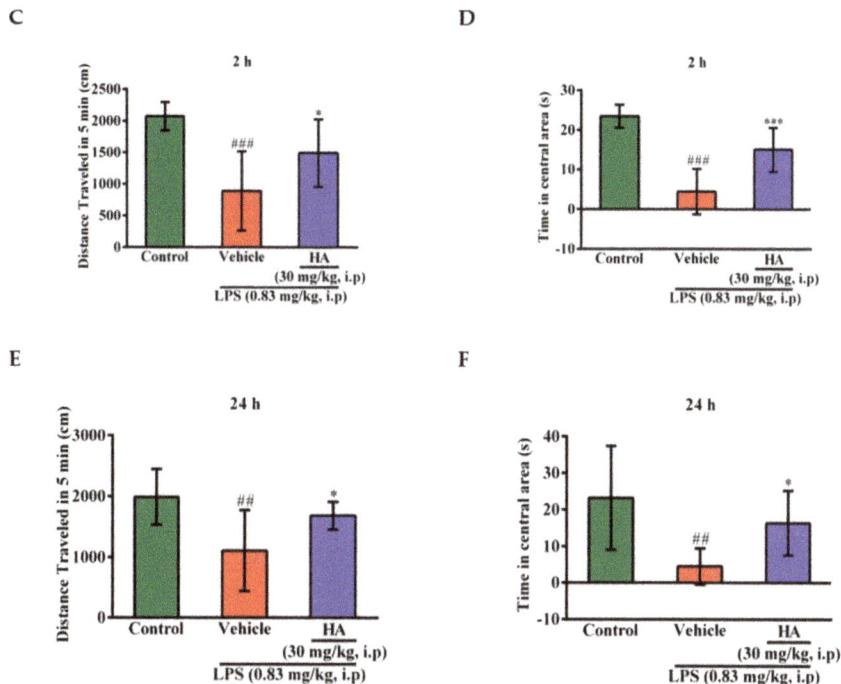

Figure 5. Effect of HA on sickness behavior in the open field test following a systemic LPS challenge. (**A**) Experimental timeline and design. (**B**) Heat-map represented the tracks of mice in the different groups in OFT, red = more time, blue = less time. (**C**) Total distance traveled 5 min in the different groups administrated with sterile saline or LPS (0.83 mg/kg, i.p) for 2 h. (**D**) Percentage of time spent in 5 min in the open area in the different groups for 2 h. (**E**) Total distance traveled 5 min in the different groups challenged with sterile saline or LPS (0.83 mg/kg, i.p) for 24 h. (**F**) Percentage of time spent in 5 min in the central area in the different groups for 24 h. Data represent group means ± S.D., $n = 7$ mice/group. [##] $p < 0.01$ and [###] $p < 0.001$ as compared with the saline control group (Control); * $p < 0.05$ and *** $p < 0.001$ as compared with the co-solvent group (vehicle).

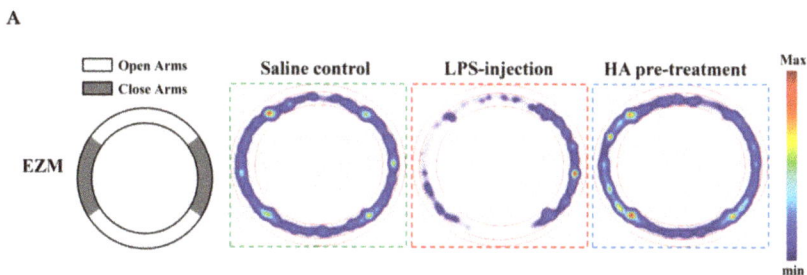

A

Figure 6. *Cont.*

B

C

D

E

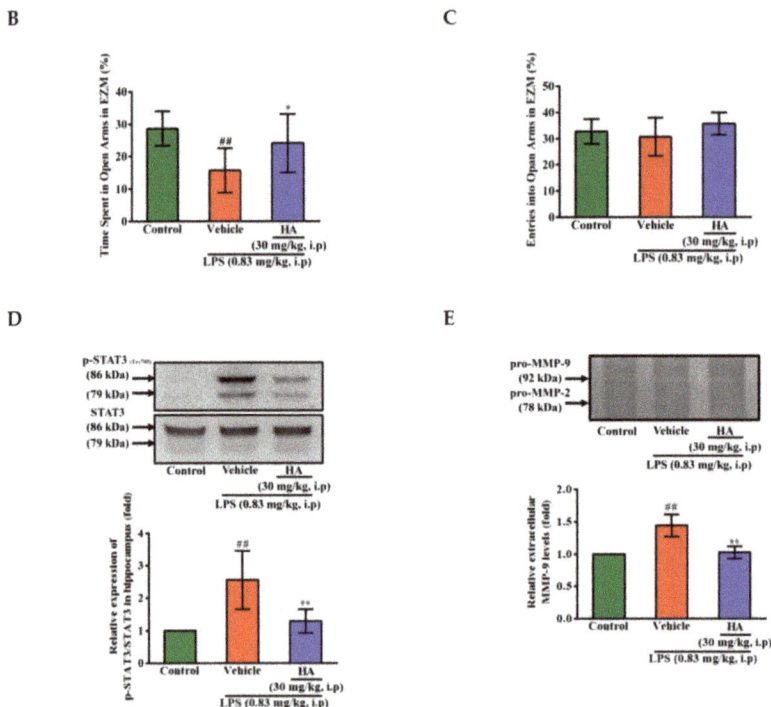

Figure 6. Effect of HA on anxiety-like behavior in the elevated zero maze test, and the expression of phospho-STAT3 and MMP-9 in the hippocampus following systemic LPS challenge. (**A**) The structure diagram of EZM was described as the left panel. Heat-map illustrated the tracks of mice in the different groups in EZM test, red = more time, blue = less time. (**B**) Percentage of time spent in 5 min in the open arms (gray) in the different groups administrated with sterile saline or LPS (0.83 mg/kg, i.p) for 25 h. (**C**) Percentage of entries into the open arms in 5 min in the different groups for 25 h. Mice were sacrificed after behavior tests, and then hippocampus was collected immediately. Homogenates of the hippocampus were obtained and analyzed for the phosphorylation of STAT3 by Western blotting (**D**, $n = 5$), and assayed for MMPs activity by gelatin zymography (**E**, $n = 3$). Data represent group means ± S.D., $n = 3$ to 7 mice/group. $^{##}$ $p < 0.01$ as compared with the saline control group (Control); * $p < 0.05$ and ** $p < 0.01$ as compared with the co-solvent group (vehicle).

2.6. HA Improved Pulmonary Histological Changes during Endotoxemia

Pulmonary edema caused by Gram-negative bacterial infection is the primary manifestation of organ failure and the most common cause of sepsis-related death [29]. It has been reported [30] that STAT3 blocker inhibits the LPS-mediated inflammatory response in mice with acute lung injuries (ALI). One day after intraperitoneal injection of LPS (0.83 mg/kg), histology image analysis was done to assess the effect of HA pretreatment on endotoxemia-mediated lung injury. As shown in Figure 7A, LPS induced pathologic lung injury, including interstitial tissue edema, infiltration of inflammatory cells, and alveolar collapse, which were reduced in the HA-pretreated group compared to the LPS-challenged group. Furthermore, LPS significantly augmented the expression levels of phosphorylated STAT3 (Tyr705) in lung tissue compared to the control group, and HA pretreatment reversed the upregulation of STAT3 phosphorylation induced by LPS (Figure 7B). On the other hand, one day after LPS was challenged, the protein levels of MMP-9 were significantly increased, and pretreatment with HA significantly attenuated the MMP-9 expression induced by LPS of the lung tissues (Figure 7C). Notably, BALF collected from mice injected at one day after LPS treatment also showed an increase in the MMP-9-mediated gelatinolysis by 1.65 ± 0.25 fold compared to control mice. The pretreatment of HA significantly reduced MMP-9 activity in BALF collected from the HA group compared with the LPS-challenged group (LPS-1.65 ± 0.25-fold vs. HA-1.04 ± 0.36 fold, $p < 0.05$) (Figure 7D).

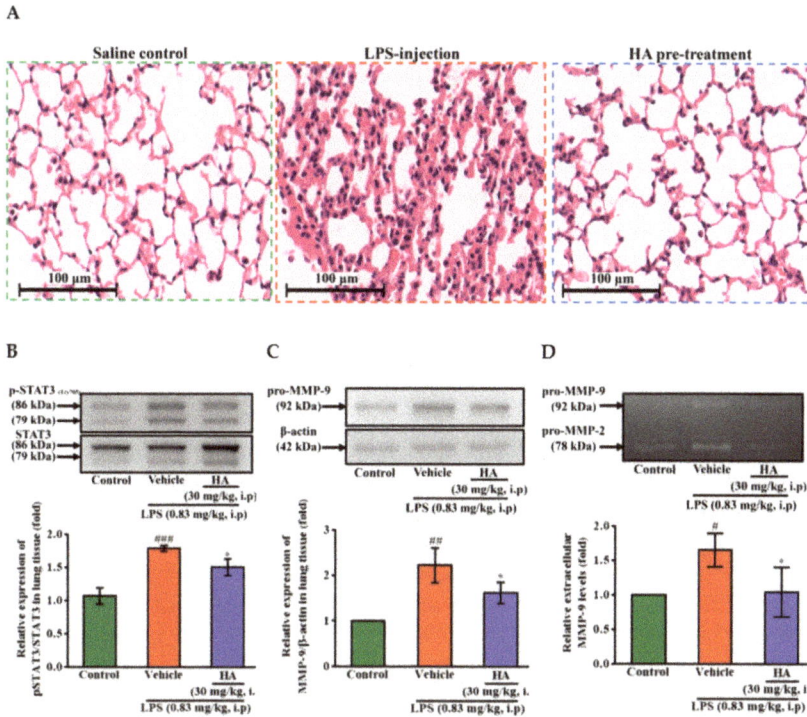

Figure 7. Effect of HA on LPS-mediated histopathological changes and the production of phospho-STAT3 and MMP-9 in lung tissues and BALF. Mice in the different groups administrated with sterile saline or LPS (0.83 mg/kg, i.p) which were sacrificed after behavior tests, and then BALF and lung tissues were collected immediately for following experiments. (**A**) Representative hematoxylin and eosin (H&E)-stained sections of right lung lobes at 400 × original magnification showed exaggerated acute inflammatory infiltration, alveoli destruction and interstitial edema in LPS group (scale bar = 100 μm). Homogenates of the left lung lobes were obtained and analyzed for the expression of phospho-STAT3 (**B**) and pro-MMP-9 (**C**, $n = 3$) by Western blotting, and assayed for MMPs activity in BALF by gelatin zymography (**D**, $n = 3$). Data represent group means ± S.D., $n = 3$ to 7 mice/group. # $p < 0.05$, ## $p < 0.01$ and ### $p < 0.001$ as compared with the saline control group (Control); * $p < 0.05$ as compared with the co-solvent group (vehicle).

3. Discussion

The course of sepsis is often accompanied by many serious complications, such as acute lung injury or sepsis-associated encephalomyelitis, which causes high mortality and poor prognosis [7–9]. Systemic inflammatory response during sepsis promotes the abnormal activation of immune cells such as monocyte, which plays a crucial role in organ damage. The infiltration of monocytes causes organ damage, which are associated with the elevation of MMPs and cytokines. MMPs degrade the extracellular matrix leading to abnormal leakage of endothelial tight junctions, which is responsible for the development of edema and organ dysfunction [31–34]. It had been reported that MMP-9 blockade attenuates the cellular transmigration of monocytes induced by LPS [35]. MMP-2 and MMP-9 blocker could reverse the increase of permeability of the blood-brain barrier and improve acute cognitive alteration associated with sepsis [23]. LPS activates TLR4 downstream signaling including ERK, p38, and NF-κB pathway to upregulate the production of MMP-9 and pro-inflammatory cytokines [26,36]. In the present study, HA pretreatment inhibited LPS-induced ERK1/2 phosphorylation and IκB degradation without cytotoxicity. Notably, HA significantly attenuated LPS-induced MMP-9 mRNA and protein expression and suppressed LPS-mediated extracellular TNF-α, IL-1β, and IL-6 levels. Taken together, these results suggested that HA downregulated THP-1 cells expressing MMP-9 and pro-inflammatory cytokines. These results support our hypothesis that HA improved monocyte-mediated lung injury and anxiety-like behavior during endotoxemia.

In the present study, we showed that HA pretreatment significantly inhibited STAT3 tyrosine phosphorylation in THP-1 cells during LPS stimulation for 24 h. Variety of different stimuli including LPS and pro-inflammatory cytokines activate JAK-STAT3 signaling which exhibits crosstalk between different pathways and involves in the up-regulation of pro-inflammatory mediators, such as IL-6 [25,27,37]. JAK2-STAT3 cascade is activated after 30 min of LPS stimulation, whereas JAK2 blockade strongly inhibits LPS-induced STAT3 (tyr705) phosphorylation [25], and JAK2 also modulates the phosphorylation of the IκBα in neurons [38]. Our study showed that AG490 significantly suppressed both LPS-mediated IκBα degradation and MMP-9 production, indicating that JAK2 was also involved in the regulation of MMP-9 expression during LPS stimulation. Interestingly, the effects of HA on attenuating LPS-induced IκBα degradation and MMP-9 production were more potent than JAK2 inhibitor AG490. Contrary to other studies, we found significant STAT3 tyrosine phosphorylation after LPS challenged THP-1 cells were given LPS for 3 h. Inhibition of ERK-AP-1 pathway downregulate LPS-induced phosphorylation of STAT3 [27]. Similarly, in the present study, pretreatment with MEK inhibitor PD98059 significantly prevented LPS-induced ERK1/2 phosphorylation in THP-1 cells. But, at the same concentration, HA pretreatment was more potent than MEK inhibitors to suppress LPS-mediated STAT3 phosphorylation. These results suggested that HA might suppress phosphorylation of STAT3 via regulating upstream signal molecules, such as JAK2 and Myd88. However, the detailed mechanisms of HA regulating STAT3 activation need further investigation in future studies.

During central nervous system (CNS) inflammation, infiltrated immune cells released chemokines and cytokines that recruited and activated more leukocytes into inflamed site resulting complex long-term immune responses and accumulation of neurotoxic products [39,40]. It has been reported that circulating IL-6 and TNF-α levels were significantly linked to patients with the severity of anxiety, depression and cognitive impairment [10,41]. Similarly, elevated systemic pro-inflammatory cytokines levels were associated with sickness behavior, including locomotor activity deficiency, anxiety- and depressive-like behavior in systemic LPS-challenged mice [42–46]. LPS-induced acute-sickness behavior, including anxiety- and depressive-like behavior was prevented by attenuating among TNF-α, IL-1β, and IL-6 levels of brain and plasma of mice [46,47]. In the present study, intraperitoneal administration of LPS-induced significant locomotor deficits, body weight loss, and anxiety-like behavior, while pretreatment with HA was effective in preventing acute sickness behavior caused by LPS. Additionally, the hippocampus in mice sacrificed after 24 h of behavioral testing showed that pretreatment with HA reduced the level of MMP-9 induced by LPS. It had been indicated that inhibition of MMP-9 and MMP-2 levels could effectively reduce the level of inflammatory cytokines in the brain and improve cognitive impairment caused by sepsis [23]. CCR2+/CD68+ activated microglia/macrophages were increased following LPS challenge in the hippocampus [48]. Similarly, LPS challenge induced CD68+ inflammatory cell recruitment in the CA3 hippocampal region, and HA pretreatment prevented the infiltration of CD68+ microglia/macrophages in the hippocampus induced by LPS injection. However, whether HA could regulate the elevation of pro-inflammatory cytokine levels in the hippocampus and serum in the acute phase (2 h) remains to be confirmed.

During endotoxemia, high levels of TNF-α and IL-6 could activate JAK2-STAT3 cascade in CNS [23,37]. STAT3 was associated with the expression of serotonin reuptake transporter (SERT) known to affect food intake and body weight [49]. The blockade of STAT3 activation in the hippocampus and in the hypothalamus attenuated depression-like behavior and anorexia in mice suffered neuroinflammation, respectively [50,51]. In the present study, intraperitoneal administration of LPS did significantly induce increase STAT3 phosphorylation in the hippocampus, whereas pretreatment with HA significantly lessened the level of phosphorylated STAT3 in the hippocampus, which may help further explain that HA could improve the body weight loss and sickness behavior caused by LPS. However, whether HA could regulate the performance of SERT or serotonin in the hippocampus still needs further verification. On the other hand, STAT3 rapidly activates in the lungs during LPS-induced systemic inflammation, and STAT3 activation occurs before significant lung injury [30,52]. Blockade of STAT3 activity could attenuate LPS-mediated inflammatory cell infiltration and damage in the lung [30]. Our results demonstrated that HA obviously attenuated lung injury features accompanied by suppression of LPS-induced STAT3 activation and MMP-9 production in lung tissues or BALF. These results provided evidence that HA reduced LPS-mediated upregulation of pro-inflammatory mediators and increased vascular permeability.

Although hirsutanol A was reported to be effective on anti-tumor growth in vivo [53], we found HA attenuated the activation of monocyte and microglia [24]. The disruption of blood-brain barrier (BBB) was induced by LPS-associated leukocyte activation. Inhibition of pro-inflammatory TLR4 activation represents an impairment of BBB dysfunction and neuroinflammation [54]. The lung inflammation and injuries are also implicated with monocyte activation [55]. According to these findings, we supposed HA regulated monocyte- and microglia-mediated injuries in brain and lung during inflammatory cascade. However, this study still has some potential limitations. CD11b^{high} GR-1^{high} neutrophils are not only the main source of MMP-9, but also the recruitment of neutrophils play important roles in MMP-9-associated tissue damages during endotoxemia [18]. HA may also block the recruitment of neutrophils, thereby preventing MMP-9-induced lung injuries. However, it is necessary to further investigate the effects of HA on neutrophils during endotoxemia. In addition, according to our findings, HA pre-treatment attenuated STAT-3 phosphorylation induced by LPS challenge. However, we had not directly assessed HA regulates the expression of MMP-9 in hippocampus and lung tissue through regulating STAT3. Clinical sepsis treatment is often administered after the onset of the disease; although HA treatment improves several symptoms induced by endotoxemia in in vivo model, it is still different from the actual clinical situation. In further study, the detail molecular mechanism of HA interacted with STAT3 and the suitability for septic preclinical studies should be determined.

4. Materials and Methods

4.1. Materials

Hirsutanol A (HA), was obtained from Professor Tzong-Huei Lee [24]. Anti-mouse immunoglobulin (Ig) G-conjugated horseradish peroxidase (HRP) complexes (cat. No NA934) and anti-rabbit IgG-conjugated HRP complexes (cat. No NA931) were purchased from Amersham Biosciences (Sunnyvale, CA, USA). Anti-rat IgG-conjugated CF^{TM}488A (cat. No #20014) were purchased from Biotium (Fremont, CA, USA). The rabbit polyclonal antibody (pAb) specific for human native 92-kDa MMP-9 (cat. No AB19016) was purchased from MilliporeSigma (St. Louis, MO, USA). The mouse mAb specific for α-tubulin (cat. No MS-581-P1) was purchased from LabVision/NeoMarkers (Fremont, CA, USA). The rabbit mAb specific for STAT3 (cat. No 12640S), phospho-STAT3 (Tyr705; cat. No 9145S), IκB-α (cat. No 4812S), and p-IKKα/β (Ser176/Ser177) (cat. No 2697S) were purchased from Cell Signaling (Danvers, MA, USA). The rabbit pAb specific for phospho-ERK (Thr202/Tyr204) (cat. No 9101S) and phospho-p38 MAPK (Thr180/Tyr182; cat. No 9211S) were purchased from Cell Signaling (Danvers, MA, USA). The mouse mAb specific for ERK (cat. No 9107S) was purchased from Cell Signaling (Danvers, MA, USA). The rabbit pAb specific for p38 MAPK (cat. No GTX110720), β-actin (cat. No GTX109239) and IKKα (cat. No GTX132964) were purchased from GeneTex (Irvine, CA, USA). Thiazolyl blue tetrazolium bromide (MTT; cat. No M5655-1G), 4-(2-hydroxyethyl)-1-piperazineethanesulphonic acid

(HEPES; cat. No H4034-1KG), sodium dodecyl sulfate (SDS; cat. No L3771-500G), phenylmethylsulfonyl fluoride (PMSF; cat. No P-7626), leupeptin (cat. No L2023-5MG), aprotinin (cat. No A1153-5MG), sodium fluoride, sodium orthovanadate (cat. No S6508-10G), sodium pyrophosphate (cat. NO S6422-100G), diethyl pyrocarbonate (DEPC; cat. No 159220-5G), lipopolysaccharide (LPS; cat. No L3880-100mg), parthenolide (PTL; cat. No P0667-5MG), SB203580 (SB; cat. No S8307-1MG), PD98059 (PD; cat. No P215-1MG), AG490 (cat. No 658401-5MGCN) and bovine serum albumin (BSA; cat. No A7906-100G) were purchased from MilliporeSigma (St. Louis, MO, USA). All other chemicals used in this study were of reagent grade.

4.2. Cell Cultivation

THP-1 cells (human acute monocytic leukemia line) were obtained from American Type Culture Collection (Manassas, VA, USA). Cells (passage 6 to passage 30) were maintained in RPMI 1640 medium supplemented with 10% heat-inactivated fetal bovine serum (FBS). HEPES (18 mM), NaHCO$_3$ (23.57 mM), L-glutamine (3.65 mM), penicillin (90 units/mL) and streptomycin (90 µg/mL) (cat. NO 10378-016, PSQ, GIBCO^{TM}, Thermo Fisher Scientific; Waltham, MA, USA). Cells were sub-cultured regularly twice a week (1.2×10^6 cells/ml in 75T flask), as previously described [56].

4.3. Gelatin and Reverse Zymography

THP-1 cells (5×10^5 cells/0.5 mL), seeding into 24-well plate in RPMI 1640 medium containing 0.5% FBS were pretreated with or without HA for 15 min and were subsequently stimulated with LPS (50 ng/mL) for 24 h, followed by the collection of the supernatants. The extracellular MMPs levels were evaluated by MMP-mediated gelatinolysis via gelatin zymography. TIMP-1 activity was determined via reverse zymography, as previously described [56,57].

4.4. Cellular Viability Assay

THP-1 cells (5×10^5 cells/0.5 mL) were seeded into 24-well plate in RPMI 1640 medium containing 0.5% FBS, then incubated in 24-well plates with indicated concentrations of HA at 37 °C for 24 h. The cytotoxic effects of HA on the viability of THP-1 cells were determined by the MTT colorimetric assay, as previously described [56].

4.5. Western Blot Analyses

THP-1 cells (1.0×10^6 cells/mL) were seeded into 6-well plate in RPMI 1640/FBS (0.5%) medium were pretreated with or without indicated concentrations of HA for 15 min, followed by stimulation of LPS (50 ng/mL) for the indicated time. Cells were harvested and lysed as previously described [56]. The samples separated by SDS-PAGE and were blotted onto PVDF or nitrocellulose membranes (cat. NO RPN303F and RPN303D, Hybond™, Amersham™, GE Healthcare, Chicago, IL, USA). The blots were probed with the indicated antibodies and then were visualized by using the enhanced chemiluminescence (cat. NO 32106, Pierce™, Thermo Fisher Scientific; Waltham, MA, USA) and exposure to UVP GelDoc-It2 310 Imaging System (Labrepco; Horsham, PA, USA). The images were cropped, formatted, and adjusted for brightness in Adobe Illustrator. The respective fold was analyzed as previously described [56].

4.6. Reverse Transcription Polymerase Chain Reaction (RT-PCR) Analysis

THP-1 cells (1.0×10^6 cells/mL) were seeded into 6-well plate in RPMI 1640/FBS (0.5%) medium were pretreated with or without indicated concentrations of HA for 15 min, followed by stimulation of LPS (50 ng/mL) for 8 h. Total RNA was isolated from THP-1 cells using TRIsure™ (cat. NO BIO-38033, Bioline, Trento, Italy) following the manufacturer's instructions, and 1 µg of total RNA was reverse transcribed into cDNA using a commercial kit (cat. NO 10928-042, Super Script On-Step RT-PCR system, GIBCO^{TM}, Thermo Fisher Scientific; Waltham, MA, USA). The nucleotide sequences of the primers used for amplification were as follows: for MMP-9, sense 5′-CGTGG AGAGT CGAAA TCTCT G-3′ and antisense 5′-CCAAA CTGGA TGACG ATGTC T-3′; for GAPDH, sense 5′-CCACC CATGG CAAAT TCCAT GGCA-3′ and antisense 5′-TCTAG ACGGC AGGTG CAAAT CACC-3′. PCR was performed using the following conditions: 28 cycles of a 15 s denaturation step at 94 °C, a 30 s annealing step at 54 °C, and a 60 s extension step at 72 °C for MMP-9; followed by 25 cycles of a 15 s denaturation step at 94 °C, a 30 s annealing step at 67 °C, and a 60 s extension step at 72 °C for GAPDH. The respective amplified PCR products were analyzed as previously described [56].

4.7. Measurement of Cytokine Levels by the Enzyme-Linked Immunosorbent Assay (ELISA)

THP-1 cells (5×10^5 cells/0.5 mL) were seeded into 24-well plate in RPMI 1640 medium (cat. NO 31800-022, GIBCO^{TM}, Thermo Fisher Scientific; Waltham, MA, USA) containing 0.5% FBS, then pretreated with or without HA for 15 min and were subsequently stimulated with LPS (50 ng/mL) for the indicated time, and followed by collection of the supernatants. The extracellular levels of TNF-α, IL-6, and IL-1β produced by THP-1 cells were determined using the ELISA Ready-SET-Go! kit (cat. NO #88-7346-88 TNF-α, #88-7066-2 IL-6, and #88-7010-88 IL-1β, eBioscience; San Diego, CA, USA). The quantitative levels of the cytokines were analyzed as previously described [58].

4.8. LPS-Induced Endotoxemia In Vivo and Drug Treatment

Male C57BL/6 mice (8–10 weeks, 25–28 g) were purchased from bioLASCO, Taiwan Co., Ltd (Taipei, Taiwan). The Institutional Animal Care and Use Committee (IACUC) of Taipei Medical University approved the animal experiments in this study (LAC-2015-0195). To develop mouse endotoxemia models, LPS (E. coli LPS, serotype 0127:B8) was dissolved in pyrogen-free sterile saline (0.9% *w/v* NaCl) at a concentration of 0.5 mg/mL and intraperitoneally injected at the dose of 0.83 mg/kg of body weight [45]. C57BL/6 mice were assigned to receive a volume of 1.66 mL/kg LPS or an equal amount of normal saline via intraperitoneal injection. For evaluating the effects of HA on the endotoxemia-mediated sickness behavior, anxiety-like behavior and lung inflammation, HA was dissolved in co-solvent as cremophor EL (cat. NO C5135-500G, MilliporeSigma, St. Louis, MO, USA)/ethanol (1:1) and was diluted (1:10) with pyrogen-free sterile saline (0.9% *w/v* NaCl), and intraperitoneally administered 30 min before LPS-injection at 30 mg/kg of body weight. Animals were randomized into three experimental groups (*n* = 7) for behavioral and biochemical assessment. The group III (HA group) were intraperitoneally administrated with HA, and the group I (Saline control group) group II were injected with an equal volume of vehicle (co-solvent) before LPS injection. After 30 min, the group I challenged with Saline, group II and group III challenged with LPS (0.83 mg/kg, i.p.), respectively. LPS-mediated behavior impairments were assessed by OFT and EPM 2/24 h and 25 h, respectively, post-LPS or saline challenge. Animals were continuously monitored for 26 h. At the end of the above behavioral test, the mice were sacrificed and the target organs were harvested.

4.9. Behavioral Testing

The Open Field Test (OFT)—The OFT was performed in an opaque white plastic box (46.5 × 50.5 × 50.5 cm) and illuminated from overhead (an average of 30 lux). The central zone was defined as the 23.25 × 25.25 cm interior portion of the box. Mice were gently and individually placed in the center of the apparatus and allowed to explore for 5 min. The test period was recorded by a video camera located above the center of the apparatus. Between trials, the box was cleaned with 75% ethanol. Exploratory locomotor activity (eLMA) was used to reflect acute sickness behavior and was measured as the total distance traveled by each mouse in the box. The anxiety-like phenotype of an individual mouse's behavior was assessed by measuring the percentage of time spent in the central or peripheral area of the box [45]. All of the variables were analyzed using Ethovision XT 11 tracking software (Noldus, Leesburg, VA, USA).

The Elevated Zero Maze test (EZM test)—The maze was constructed of opaque white plastic in a circular track 5 cm wide, 68 cm in diameter, elevated 51 cm from the floor, and illuminated from overhead (average 30 lux). The maze was divided into four quadrants of equal length with two opposing open quadrants and two opposing closed quadrants with white plastic walls 12 cm in height. Mice were gently placed in the center in the center of a closed quadrant. An overhead video camera recorded the location of the mice in a 5 min test period. The anxiety-like behavior was assessed by measuring the percent time and entries in the open quadrants. The maze was cleaned with 75% ethanol between mice. All of the variables were analyzed using Ethovision XT 11 tracking software (Noldus, Leesburg, VA, USA).

4.10. Bronchoalveolar Lavage Fluid (BALF) and Lung Tissues Collection

At the end of the above behavioral test, the mice were sacrificed by an excess of anesthetic. The chest was opened, a 20 Gauge blunt needle was inserted, and 0.8 mL of ice-cold sterile PBS was dropped into the lungs through a tracheal incision. The recovered BALF was centrifuged at $500 \times g$ for 10 min, the protein levels of the cell-free supernatant were quantified and used to evaluate the pro-MMP-9 concentration by gelatin zymography [59]. The lung tissues were harvested immediately after collection of BALF. Right lobes of the lung were fixed in 4% formalin and paraffin embedded and stained with hematoxylin and eosin (HE). Whole digital images were obtained using virtual microscopy (Aperio CS2 Leica Microsystems, Wetzlar, Germany). Tagged Image File Format (TIFF) images extracted using image processing software (ImageScope, ver. 9.1.19.1567, Leica Microsystems). Left lobes of lung were immediately frozen in liquid nitrogen, and 50 mg samples of frozen lung tissue were subsequently homogenized with 2 mL Precellys homogenization tube containing three 1.4-mm and three 2.8-mm ceramic beads (Bertin Technologies, Rockville, Maryland) with 7 volumes (7 mL/g tissue) of homogenization buffer which containing 1× protease inhibitor (cat. NO 11 873, 580 001, Roche, Mannheim, Germany). The samples were homogenized (Minilys®; Bertin Technologies, Rockville, Maryland) twice at 5000 rpm for 30 s and then centrifuged at $5000 \times g$ for 5 min at 4 °C. The collected supernatant was incubated at 4 °C for 30 min, then centrifuged at $12,000 \times g$ for 20 min and then stored at −80 ° C before additional experiments.

4.11. Hippocampus Tissues Collection

The hippocampus tissue was harvested immediately after the lung tissues were preserved. The hippocampus was quickly removed on an ice-cold metal plate, and was transferred into a 2 mL Precellys homogenization tube containing three 1.4-mm ceramic beads (Bertin Technologies, Rockville, MD, USA) with a homogenization buffer (7 mL/g tissue) which containing 1× protease inhibitor (cat. NO 11 873, 580 001, Roche, Mannheim, Germany). The samples were homogenized (Minilys®; Bertin Technologies, Rockville, MD, USA) twice at 5000 rpm for 15 s and then centrifuged at $5000 \times g$ for 5 min at 4 °C. The collected supernatant was incubated at 4 °C for 30 min, then centrifuged at $12,000 \times g$ for 20 min and then stored at −80 °C before additional experiments.

4.12. Statistical Analyses

The experimental results are represented as the means ± S.D. for the number of observations. Analysis of experiments was performed using one-way analysis of variance (ANOVA) followed by a multiple comparison test (Student–Newman–Keuls test) via SigmaStat v3.5 software (SYSTAT Software, San Jose, CA, USA). $p < 0.05$ was considered to indicate statistical significance.

5. Conclusions

These results indicated that HA strongly attenuated MMP-9, TNF-α, and IL-6 via regulating the TLR4 downstream signaling pathways, including ERK-1/2, NF-κB, and STAT3. Our findings demonstrated that the novel fungal sesquiterpene HA could provide new opportunities for the development of different strategies on pro-inflammatory cytokines- and MMP-9-associated diseases, such as endotoxemia.

Supplementary Materials: Supplementary Materials are available at http://www.mdpi.com/1660-3397/17/6/360/s1. Supplementary Method-Immunohistochemistry. Figure S1. Effect of HA on monocytic MMP-9-mediated gelatinolysis; Figure S2. Effect of HA on the pro-inflammatory cytokines production of THP-1 cells; Figure S3. Effect of the combination of LPS and HA on the cell viability of THP-1 cells; Figure S4. Effect of HA on LPS-mediated phosphorylation of IKKα in THP-1 cells; Figure S5. Effect of HA on the STAT3 and NF-κB cascade in THP-1 cells; Figure S6. Effect of HA on LPS-induced body weight loss and hypothermia; Figure S7. Effect of HA the numbers of CD68⁺ inflammatory cells in the hippocampus following systemic LPS challenge.

Author Contributions: Conceptualization, J.-S.J., C.-H.Y., M.-H.W., T.-H.L. and G.H.; methodology, J.-S.J.; software, J.-S.J. and M.K.; validation, J.-S.J., F,-L.L., J.-L.Y. and I.H.; formal analysis, J.-S.J.; investigation, J.-S.J.; resources, C.-H.Y.,T.-H.L. and G.H.; writing—original draft preparation, J.-S.J.; writing—review and editing, C.-H.Y., M.-H.W, M.K. and G.H.; visualization, J.-S.J.

Funding: This research was supported by the Ministry of Science and Technology, Taiwan (MOST 105-2320-B-038-041 and MOST 107-2320-B-038-025-MY3).

Conflicts of Interest: The authors declare no conflict of interest.

References

1. Singer, M.; Deutschman, C.S.; Seymour, C.W.; Shankar-Hari, M.; Annane, D.; Bauer, M.; Bellomo, R.; Bernard, G.R.; Chiche, J.D.; Coopersmith, C.M.; et al. The Third International Consensus Definitions for Sepsis and Septic Shock (Sepsis-3). *JAMA* **2016**, *315*, 801–810. [CrossRef] [PubMed]

2. Rhodes, A.; Evans, L.E.; Alhazzani, W.; Levy, M.M.; Antonelli, M.; Ferrer, R.; Kumar, A.; Sevransky, J.E.; Sprung, C.L.; Nunnally, M.E.; et al. Surviving Sepsis Campaign: International Guidelines for Management of Sepsis and Septic Shock: 2016. *Intensive Care Med.* **2017**, *43*, 304–377. [CrossRef] [PubMed]

3. Prescott, H.C.; Angus, D.C. Enhancing Recovery From Sepsis: A Review. *JAMA* **2018**, *319*, 62–75. [CrossRef]

4. Kaukonen, K.M.; Bailey, M.; Suzuki, S.; Pilcher, D.; Bellomo, R. Mortality related to severe sepsis and septic shock among critically ill patients in Australia and New Zealand, 2000–2012. *JAMA* **2014**, *311*, 1308–1316. [CrossRef] [PubMed]

5. Marik, P.E. Surviving sepsis: Going beyond the guidelines. *Ann. Intensive Care* **2011**, *1*, 17. [CrossRef] [PubMed]

6. Kantari, C.; Pederzoli-Ribeil, M.; Witko-Sarsat, V. The role of neutrophils and monocytes in innate immunity. *Contrib. Microbiol.* **2008**, *15*, 118–146. [PubMed]

7. Medzhitov, R. Origin and physiological roles of inflammation. *Nature* **2008**, *454*, 428–435. [CrossRef]

8. Su, X.; Matthay, M.A.; Malik, A.B. Requisite role of the cholinergic α7 nicotinic acetylcholine receptor pathway in suppressing Gram-negative sepsis-induced acute lung inflammatory injury. *J. Immunol.* **2010**, *184*, 401–410. [CrossRef]

9. Schulte, W.; Bernhagen, J.; Bucala, R. Cytokines in sepsis: Potent immunoregulators and potential therapeutic targets—An updated view. *Mediat. Inflamm.* **2013**, *2013*, 165974. [CrossRef]

10. Calsavara, A.J.C.; Costa, P.A.; Nobre, V.; Teixeira, A.L. Factors Associated With Short and Long Term Cognitive Changes in Patients With Sepsis. *Sci. Rep.* **2018**, *8*, 4509. [CrossRef]

11. Ma, L.; Zhang, H.; Yin, Y.L.; Guo, W.Z.; Ma, Y.Q.; Wang, Y.B.; Shu, C.; Dong, L.Q. Role of interleukin-6 to differentiate sepsis from non-infectious systemic inflammatory response syndrome. *Cytokine* **2016**, *88*, 126–135. [CrossRef] [PubMed]

12. Lv, S.; Han, M.; Yi, R.; Kwon, S.; Dai, C.; Wang, R. Anti-TNF-α therapy for patients with sepsis: A systematic meta-analysis. *Int. J. Clin. Pract.* **2014**, *68*, 520–528. [CrossRef] [PubMed]

13. Vandenbroucke, R.E.; Libert, C. Is there new hope for therapeutic matrix metalloproteinase inhibition? *Nat. Rev. Drug Discov.* **2014**, *13*, 904–927. [CrossRef] [PubMed]

14. Nissinen, L.; Kahari, V.M. Matrix metalloproteinases in inflammation. *Biochim. Biophys. Acta* **2014**, *1840*, 2571–2580. [CrossRef] [PubMed]

15. Xue, M.; McKelvey, K.; Shen, K.; Minhas, N.; March, L.; Park, S.Y.; Jackson, C.J. Endogenous MMP-9 and not MMP-2 promotes rheumatoid synovial fibroblast survival, inflammation and cartilage degradation. *Rheumatology* **2014**, *53*, 2270–2279. [CrossRef] [PubMed]

16. Sellebjerg, F.; Bornsen, L.; Ammitzboll, C.; Nielsen, J.E.; Vinther-Jensen, T.; Hjermind, L.E.; von Essen, M.; Ratzer, R.L.; Soelberg Sorensen, P.; Romme Christensen, J. Defining active progressive multiple sclerosis. *Mult. Scler.* **2017**, *23*, 1727–1735. [CrossRef]

17. Chaturvedi, M.; Kaczmarek, L. Mmp-9 inhibition: A therapeutic strategy in ischemic stroke. *Mol. Neurobiol.* **2014**, *49*, 563–573. [CrossRef]

18. Vandooren, J.; Swinnen, W.; Ugarte-Berzal, E.; Boon, L.; Dorst, D.; Martens, E.; Opdenakker, G. Endotoxemia shifts neutrophils with TIMP-free gelatinase B/MMP-9 from bone marrow to the periphery and induces systematic upregulation of TIMP-1. *Haematologica* **2017**, *102*, 1671–1682. [CrossRef]

19. Soumyarani, V.S.; Jayakumari, N. Oxidatively modified high density lipoprotein promotes inflammatory response in human monocytes-macrophages by enhanced production of ROS, TNF-α, MMP-9, and MMP-2. *Mol. Cell. Biochem.* **2012**, *366*, 277–285. [CrossRef]

20. Lauhio, A.; Hastbacka, J.; Pettila, V.; Tervahartiala, T.; Karlsson, S.; Varpula, T.; Varpula, M.; Ruokonen, E.; Sorsa, T.; Kolho, E. Serum MMP-8, -9 and TIMP-1 in sepsis: High serum levels of MMP-8 and TIMP-1 are associated with fatal outcome in a multicentre, prospective cohort study. Hypothetical impact of tetracyclines. *Pharmacol. Res.* **2011**, *64*, 590–594. [CrossRef]

21. Dubois, B.; Starckx, S.; Pagenstecher, A.; Oord, J.; Arnold, B.; Opdenakker, G. Gelatinase B deficiency protects against endotoxin shock. *Eur. J. Immunol.* **2002**, *32*, 2163–2171. [CrossRef]

22. Hu, J.; Van den Steen, P.E.; Dillen, C.; Opdenakker, G. Targeting neutrophil collagenase/matrix metalloproteinase-8 and gelatinase B/matrix metalloproteinase-9 with a peptidomimetic inhibitor protects against endotoxin shock. *Biochem. Pharmacol.* **2005**, *70*, 535–544. [CrossRef] [PubMed]

23. Dal-Pizzol, F.; Rojas, H.A.; dos Santos, E.M.; Vuolo, F.; Constantino, L.; Feier, G.; Pasquali, M.; Comim, C.M.; Petronilho, F.; Gelain, D.P.; et al. Matrix metalloproteinase-2 and metalloproteinase-9 activities are associated with blood-brain barrier dysfunction in an animal model of severe sepsis. *Mol. Neurobiol.* **2013**, *48*, 62–70. [CrossRef] [PubMed]

24. Hsiao, G.; Chi, W.C.; Pang, K.L.; Chen, J.J.; Kuo, Y.H.; Wang, Y.K.; Cha, H.J.; Chou, S.C.; Lee, T.H. Hirsutane-Type Sesquiterpenes with Inhibitory Activity of Microglial Nitric Oxide Production from the Red Alga-Derived Fungus *Chondrostereum* sp. NTOU4196. *J. Nat. Prod.* **2017**, *80*, 1615–1622. [CrossRef] [PubMed]

25. Pena, G.; Cai, B.; Deitch, E.A.; Ulloa, L. JAK2 inhibition prevents innate immune responses and rescues animals from sepsis. *J. Mol. Med.* **2010**, *88*, 851–859. [CrossRef] [PubMed]

26. Sato, H.; Seiki, M. Regulatory mechanism of 92 kDa type IV collagenase gene expression which is associated with invasiveness of tumor cells. *Oncogene* **1993**, *8*, 395–405. [PubMed]

27. Yang, L.; Guo, H.; Li, Y.; Meng, X.; Yan, L.; Dan, Z.; Wu, S.; Zhou, H.; Peng, L.; Xie, Q.; et al. Oleoylethanolamide exerts anti-inflammatory effects on LPS-induced THP-1 cells by enhancing PPARα signaling and inhibiting the NF-κB and ERK1/2/AP-1/STAT3 pathways. *Sci. Rep.* **2016**, *6*, 34611. [CrossRef]

28. Szentirmai, E.; Krueger, J.M. Sickness behaviour after lipopolysaccharide treatment in ghrelin deficient mice. *Brain Behav. Immunity* **2014**, *36*, 200–206. [CrossRef]

29. Gandhirajan, R.K.; Meng, S.; Chandramoorthy, H.C.; Mallilankaraman, K.; Mancarella, S.; Gao, H.; Razmpour, R.; Yang, X.F.; Houser, S.R.; Chen, J.; et al. Blockade of NOX2 and STIM1 signaling limits lipopolysaccharide-induced vascular inflammation. *J. Clin. Investig.* **2013**, *123*, 887–902. [CrossRef]

30. Zhao, J.; Yu, H.; Liu, Y.; Gibson, S.A.; Yan, Z.; Xu, X.; Gaggar, A.; Li, P.K.; Li, C.; Wei, S.; et al. Protective effect of suppressing STAT3 activity in LPS-ind.ced acute lung injury. *Am. J. Physiol. Lung Cell. Mol. Physiol.* **2016**, *311*, L868–L880. [CrossRef]

31. Parks, W.C.; Wilson, C.L.; Lopez-Boado, Y.S. Matrix metalloproteinases as modulators of inflammation and innate immunity. *Nat. Rev. Immunol.* **2004**, *4*, 617–629. [CrossRef] [PubMed]

32. Harrois, A.; Huet, O.; Duranteau, J. Alterations of mitochondrial function in sepsis and critical illness. *Curr. Opin. Anesthesiol.* **2009**, *22*, 143–149. [CrossRef] [PubMed]

33. Wiig, H. Pathophysiology of tissue fluid accumulation in inflammation. *J. Physiol.* **2011**, *589*, 2945–2953. [CrossRef] [PubMed]

34. Calebrant, H.; Sandh, M.; Jansson, I. How the Nurse Anesthetist Decides to Manage Perioperative Fluid Status. *J. Perianesth. Nurs.* **2016**, *31*, 406–414. [CrossRef] [PubMed]

35. Mishra, M.K.; Wang, J.; Silva, C.; Mack, M.; Yong, V.W. Kinetics of proinflammatory monocytes in a model of multiple sclerosis and its perturbation by laquinimod. *Am. J. Pathol.* **2012**, *181*, 642–651. [CrossRef] [PubMed]

36. Akira, S.; Takeda, K. Toll-like receptor signalling. *Nat. Rev. Immunol.* **2004**, *4*, 499–511. [CrossRef]

37. Minogue, A.M.; Barrett, J.P.; Lynch, M.A. LPS-induced release of IL-6 from glia modulates production of IL-1β in a JAK2-dependent manner. *J. Neuroinflamm.* **2012**, *9*, 126. [CrossRef]

38. Digicaylioglu, M.; Lipton, S.A. Erythropoietin-mediated neuroprotection involves cross-talk between Jak2 and NF-κB signalling cascades. *Nature* **2001**, *412*, 641–647. [CrossRef]

39. Gonzalez, H.; Elgueta, D.; Montoya, A.; Pacheco, R. Neuroimmune regulation of microglial activity involved in neuroinflammation and neurodegenerative diseases. *J. Neuroimmunol.* **2014**, *274*, 1–13. [CrossRef]

40. Eyre, H.; Baune, B.T. Neuroplastic changes in depression: A role for the immune system. *Psychoneuroendocrinology* **2012**, *37*, 1397–1416. [CrossRef]

41. Vogelzangs, N.; de Jonge, P.; Smit, J.H.; Bahn, S.; Penninx, B.W. Cytokine production capacity in depression and anxiety. *Transl. Psychiatry* **2016**, *6*, e825. [CrossRef] [PubMed]

42. Hennessy, E.; Gormley, S.; Lopez-Rodriguez, A.B.; Murray, C.; Cunningham, C. Systemic TNF-α produces acute cognitive dysfunction and exaggerated sickness behavior when superimposed upon progressive neurodegeneration. *Brain Behav. Immunity* **2017**, *59*, 233–244. [CrossRef] [PubMed]

43. Mello, B.S.; Monte, A.S.; McIntyre, R.S.; Soczynska, J.K.; Custodio, C.S.; Cordeiro, R.C.; Chaves, J.H.; Vasconcelos, S.M.; Nobre, H.V., Jr.; Florenco de Sousa, F.C.; et al. Effects of doxycycline on depressive-like behavior in mice after lipopolysaccharide (LPS) administration. *J. Psychiatr. Res.* **2013**, *47*, 1521–1529. [CrossRef] [PubMed]

44. Skelly, D.T.; Hennessy, E.; Dansereau, M.A.; Cunningham, C. A systematic analysis of the peripheral and CNS effects of systemic LPS, IL-1β, [corrected] TNF-α and IL-6 challenges in C57BL/6 mice. *PLoS ONE* **2013**, *8*, e69123. [CrossRef]

45. Salazar, A.; Gonzalez-Rivera, B.L.; Redus, L.; Parrott, J.M.; O'Connor, J.C. Indoleamine 2,3-dioxygenase mediates anhedonia and anxiety-like behaviors caused by peripheral lipopolysaccharide immune challenge. *Horm. Behav.* **2012**, *62*, 202–209. [CrossRef] [PubMed]

46. Sulakhiya, K.; Keshavlal, G.P.; Bezbaruah, B.B.; Dwivedi, S.; Gurjar, S.S.; Munde, N.; Jangra, A.; Lahkar, M.; Gogoi, R. Lipopolysaccharide induced anxiety- and depressive-like behaviour in mice are prevented by chronic pre-treatment of esculetin. *Neurosci. Lett.* **2016**, *611*, 106–111. [CrossRef] [PubMed]

47. Swiergiel, A.H.; Dunn, A.J. The roles of IL-1, IL-6, and TNFα in the feeding responses to endotoxin and influenza virus infection in mice. *Brain Behav. Immunity* **1999**, *13*, 252–265. [CrossRef] [PubMed]

48. Cerri, C.; Genovesi, S.; Allegra, M.; Pistillo, F.; Puntener, U.; Guglielmotti, A.; Perry, V.H.; Bozzi, Y.; Caleo, M. The Chemokine CCL2 Mediates the Seizure-enhancing Effects of Systemic Inflammation. *J. Neurosci.* **2016**, *36*, 3777–3788. [CrossRef] [PubMed]

49. Chen, X.; Margolis, K.J.; Gershon, M.D.; Schwartz, G.J.; Sze, J.Y. Reduced serotonin reuptake transporter (SERT) function causes insulin resistance and hepatic steatosis independent of food intake. *PLoS ONE* **2012**, *7*, e32511. [CrossRef] [PubMed]

50. Kong, E.; Sucic, S.; Monje, F.J.; Savalli, G.; Diao, W.; Khan, D.; Ronovsky, M.; Cabatic, M.; Koban, F.; Freissmuth, M.; et al. STAT3 controls IL6-dependent regulation of serotonin transporter function and depression-like behavior. *Sci. Rep.* **2015**, *5*, 9009. [CrossRef]

51. Yamawaki, Y.; Kimura, H.; Hosoi, T.; Ozawa, K. MyD88 plays a key role in LPS-induced Stat3 activation in the hypothalamus. *Am. J. Physiol. Regul. Integr. Comp. Physiol.* **2010**, *298*, R403–R410. [CrossRef] [PubMed]

52. Severgnini, M.; Takahashi, S.; Rozo, L.M.; Homer, R.J.; Kuhn, C.; Jhung, J.W.; Perides, G.; Steer, M.; Hassoun, P.M.; Fanburg, B.L.; et al. Activation of the STAT pathway in acute lung injury. *Am. J. Physiol. Lung Cell. Mol. Physiol.* **2004**, *286*, L1282–L1292. [CrossRef] [PubMed]

53. Yang, F.; Chen, W.D.; Deng, R.; Zhang, H.; Tang, J.; Wu, K.W.; Li, D.D.; Feng, G.K.; Lan, W.J.; Li, H.J.; et al. Hirsutanol A, a novel sesquiterpene compound from fungus *Chondrostereum* sp., induces apoptosis and inhibits tumor growth through mitochondrial-independent ROS production: Hirsutanol A inhibits tumor growth through ROS production. *J. Transl. Med.* **2013**, *11*, 32. [CrossRef] [PubMed]

54. Yang, Y.L.; Cheng, X.; Li, W.H.; Liu, M.; Wang, Y.H.; Du, G.H. Kaempferol Attenuates LPS-Induced Striatum Injury in Mice Involving Anti-Neuroinflammation, Maintaining BBB Integrity, and Down-Regulating the HMGB1/TLR4 Pathway. *Int. J. Mol. Sci.* **2019**, *20*, 491. [CrossRef]

55. Brittan, M.; Barr, L.C.; Anderson, N.; Morris, A.C.; Duffin, R.; Marwick, J.A.; Rossi, F.; Johnson, S.; Dhaliwal, K.; Hirani, N.; et al. Functional characterisation of human pulmonary monocyte-like cells in lipopolysaccharide-mediated acute lung inflammation. *J. Inflamm.* **2014**, *11*, 9. [CrossRef] [PubMed]

56. Chou, Y.C.; Sheu, J.R.; Chung, C.L.; Chen, C.Y.; Lin, F.L.; Hsu, M.J.; Kuo, Y.H.; Hsiao, G. Nuclear-targeted inhibition of NF-κB on MMP-9 production by *N*-2-(4-bromophenyl) ethyl caffeamide in human monocytic cells. *Chem.-Biol. Interact.* **2010**, *184*, 403–412. [CrossRef] [PubMed]

57. Vandooren, J.; Geurts, N.; Martens, E.; Van den Steen, P.E.; Opdenakker, G. Zymography methods for visualizing hydrolytic enzymes. *Nat. Methods* **2013**, *10*, 211–220. [CrossRef]

58. Jan, J.S.; Chou, Y.C.; Cheng, Y.W.; Chen, C.K.; Huang, W.J.; Hsiao, G. The Novel HDAC8 Inhibitor WK2-16 Attenuates Lipopolysaccharide-Activated Matrix Metalloproteinase-9 Expression in Human Monocytic Cells and Improves Hypercytokinemia In Vivo. *Int. J. Mol. Sci.* **2017**, *18*, 1394. [CrossRef] [PubMed]

59. Lee, H.S.; Kang, P.; Kim, K.Y.; Seol, G.H. Foeniculum vulgare Mill. Protects against Lipopolysaccharide-induced Acute Lung Injury in Mice through ERK-dependent NF-κB Activation. *Korean J. Physiol. Pharmacol.* **2015**, *19*, 183–189. [CrossRef]

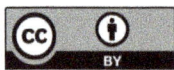

marine drugs

MDPI

Article

Zoanthamine Alkaloids from the Zoantharian *Zoanthus* cf. *pulchellus* and Their Effects in Neuroinflammation

Paul O. Guillen [1,2]**, Sandra Gegunde** [3]**, Karla B. Jaramillo** [1,4]**, Amparo Alfonso** [3]**, Kevin Calabro** [2]**,
Eva Alonso** [3]**, Jenny Rodriguez** [1]**, Luis M. Botana** [3,*] **and Olivier P. Thomas** [2,*]

[1]   ESPOL Escuela Superior Politécnica del Litoral, ESPOL, Centro Nacional de Acuacultura e Investigaciones
      Marinas, Campus Gustavo Galindo km. 30.5 vía Perimetral, P.O. Box 09-01-5863 Guayaquil, Ecuador;
      P.GUILLENMENA1@nuigalway.ie (P.O.G.); K.JARAMILLOAGUILAR1@nuigalway.ie (K.B.J.);
      jenrodri@espol.edu.ec (J.R.)
[2]   Marine Biodiscovery, School of Chemistry and Ryan Institute, National University of Ireland Galway
      (NUI Galway), University Road, H91 TK33 Galway, Ireland; kevin.calabro@nuigalway.ie
[3]   Departamento de Farmacología, Facultad de Veterinaria, Universidade de Santiago de Compostela,
      27002 Lugo, Spain; sandra.gegunde@rai.usc.es (S.G.); amparo.alfonso@usc.es (A.A.);
      eva.alonso@usc.es (E.A.)
[4]   Zoology, School of Natural Sciences and Ryan Institute, National University of Ireland Galway
      (NUI Galway), University Road, H91 TK33 Galway, Ireland
*   Correspondence: luis.botana@usc.es (L.M.B.); olivier.thomas@nuigalway.ie (O.P.T.);
      Tel.: +34-982-82-22-33 (L.M.B.); Tel.: +353-91-493563 (O.P.T.)

Received: 1 July 2018; Accepted: 19 July 2018; Published: 20 July 2018

Abstract: Two new zoanthamine alkaloids, namely 3-acetoxynorzoanthamine (**1**) and 3-acetoxyzoanthamine (**2**), have been isolated from the zoantharian *Zoanthus* cf. *pulchellus* collected off the coast of the Santa Elena Peninsula, Ecuador, together with three known derivatives: zoanthamine, norzoanthamine, and 3-hydroxynorzoanthamine. The chemical structures of **1** and **2** were determined by interpretation of their 1D and 2D NMR data and comparison with literature data. This is the first report of zoanthamine-type alkaloids from *Zoanthus* cf. *pulchellus* collected in the Tropical Eastern Pacific. The neuroinflammatory activity of all the isolated compounds was evaluated in microglia BV-2 cells and high inhibitory effects were observed in reactive oxygen species (ROS) and nitric oxide (NO) generation.

Keywords: zoantharia; Tropical Eastern Pacific; *Zoanthus pulchellus*; zoanthamine; inflammation

---

1. Introduction

Zoanthamines are a bioactive family of marine alkaloids featuring a unique chemical architecture of fused cycles culminating in an unusual azepane ring. They have been isolated essentially from marine zoantharians, particularly from the genus *Zoanthus*. The first alkaloid of this group was isolated in 1984 from an unidentified species of *Zoanthus*, collected off the coast of India by Faulkner et al. [1]. Following this first description, several studies on the chemical diversity of species of the genus *Zoanthus* have led to the discovery of additional zoanthamine-type alkaloids, including zoanthenamine, zoanthenamide [2], norzoanthamine, oxyzoanthamine, norzoanthaminone, cyclozoanthamine, epinorzoanthamine [3], zoanthaminone [4], zoaramine [5], kuroshines [6], epioxyzoanthamine [7], zoanthenol [8], hydroxylated zoanthamines and norzoanthamines [9], and two halogenated zoanthamines [10]. This interesting family of alkaloids has been structurally classified in two different groups based on the presence of a methyl at C-19 (Type I) or its absence (Type II), also called norzoanthamines [10]. Due to the structural complexity of these natural products, the first total synthesis of norzoanthamine was accomplished by Miyashita et al. in 2004 [11], who also synthesized other analogues [12,13]. Other research groups are now addressing this synthetic challenge through alternative approaches [14–16]. Up to date, 38 zoanthamine-type alkaloids have been reported from zoantharian species essentially inhabiting the Central Indo-Pacific and these polycyclic alkaloids seem to be chemical markers of zoantharians from the genus *Zoanthus*. In addition, some members of this family have displayed a wide range of biological activities against P388 murine leukemia cells [3] as well as anti-osteoporosis, anti-inflammatory, and anti-bacterial activity, and have also been found to inhibit human platelet aggregation [9,17]. The most promising therapeutic application is associated with norzoanthamine in the treatment of osteoporosis, as it inhibits interleukin-6, a primary mediator of bone resorption. Furthermore, an interesting study by Tachibana et al. suggested that the principal function of norzoanthamine in *Zoanthus* sp. is collagen strengthening [18].

In our continuous investigation of the bio- and chemodiversity of marine invertebrates present in the understudied Marine Protected Area El Pelado, Santa Elena, Ecuador, located in the Tropical Eastern Pacific [19,20], we came across a massive substrate cover of the intertidal region by undescribed fluorescent green zoantharians. A first taxonomic assessment of these zoantharian species led to the identification of the main species as being closely related to *Zoanthus* cf. *pulchellus*, previously described in the Caribbean [21]. No chemical study of this species has been reported so far, and our first chemical screening by UHPLC-HRMS revealed unknown masses related to the zoanthamine family as major compounds of the extract. In this paper, we describe the isolation and structure elucidation of two new zoanthamine alkaloids, namely 3-acetoxynorzoanthamine (**1**) and 3-acetoxyzoanthamine (**2**) (Figure 1), along with the known zoanthamine [1], norzoanthamine [3], and 3-hydroxynorzoanthamine [8] from the Eastern Pacific zoantharian *Zoanthus* cf. *pulchellus*, as well as their biological activity in cellular pathways related to oxidative stress and neuroinflammation.

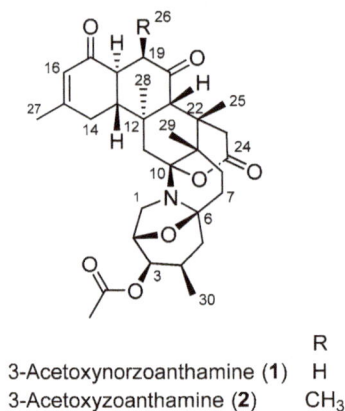

		R
3-Acetoxynorzoanthamine (**1**)		H
3-Acetoxyzoanthamine (**2**)		CH$_3$

Figure 1. Structures of 3-acetoxynorzoanthamine (**1**) and 3-acetoxyzoanthamine (**2**), isolated from *Zoanthus* cf. *pulchellus*.

2. Results

Colonies of the zoantharian *Zoanthus* cf. *pulchellus* were collected by hand in the intertidal coast of San Pedro, Santa Elena, Ecuador. The sample was freeze-dried and extracted with a mixture of solvents $CH_3OH:CH_2Cl_2$ (*v*/*v*; 1:1). The extract was then fractionated through reversed-phase C18 Vacuum Liquid Chromatography (VLC) using a mixture of solvents of decreasing polarity. The aqueous methanolic fractions were analyzed by UPLC-DAD-ELSD, combined, and then subjected to semipreparative RP-HPLC using a C18 column to yield two new zoanthamine-type alkaloids: 3-acetoxynorzoanthamine (**1**) and 3-acetoxyzoanthamine (**2**), along with the known zoanthamine [1], norzoanthamine [18], and 3-hydroxynorzoanthamine [8].

Compound **1** was obtained as a brown amorphous powder and (+)-HRESIMS analyses revealed a major molecular peak at m/z 540.2956 [M + H]$^+$, consistent with the molecular formula $C_{31}H_{41}NO_7$ for the neutral molecule. A preliminary inspection of the ^{1}H and ^{13}C NMR data revealed characteristic signals of the zoanthamine family, as already speculated on the basis of the HRMS data: an olefinic proton at δ_H 5.90 (H-16) along with four methyl singlets at δ_H 0.97 (H-28), 0.99 (H-25), 1.15 (H-29), and 2.00 (H-27), and a methyl doublet at δ_H 0.87 (H-30) together with two ketone signals at δ_C 198.5 (C-17) and δ_C 209.0 (C-20), one ester signal at δ_C 172.3 (C-24), and two olefinic carbons at δ_C 125.6 (C-16) and 160.0 (C-15) (Table 1). The absence of a second doublet of a methyl present in zoanthamines was indicative of a loss of the methyl CH$_3$-26 at C-19; therefore, the compound belonged to the norzoanthamine-type. Unlike most studies on norzoanthamines, in order to make the NMR table more homogeneous, we decided to keep the numbering of the zoanthamines especially for the methyls 27, 28, 29, and 30. Comparing with analogues of this type, we observed the presence of an additional methyl singlet signal at δ_H 2.11 corresponding to an acetyl moiety (Table 1). The presence of the acetyl group on an oxygen at C-3 was evidenced by the deshielding of the signal corresponding to the methine H-3 with δ_H 4.62 and key H-3/C-1' and H$_3$-2'/C-1' HMBC correlations.

Table 1. ^{1}H and ^{13}C NMR data in ppm for compounds **1** and **2** in CDCl$_3$ (500 MHz for ^{1}H NMR and 125 MHz for ^{13}C NMR data).

No.	1 δ_H, mult. (*J* in Hz)	1 δ_C	2 δ_H, mult. (*J* in Hz)	2 δ_C
1	3.24, t (7.0) 3.19, d (7.0)	45.3	3.24, t (7.5) 3.20, d (7.0)	45.5
2	4.58, br d (6.5)	75.6	4.59, d (7.0)	75.7
3	4.62, br t (3.0)	72.5	4.63, t (3.0)	72.6
4	2.44, br sext (5.5)	26.0	2.43, br sext (6.0)	26.1
5	1.92, dd (12.0, 6.0) 1.36, t (12.5)	40.3	1.95, dd (12.5, 6.0) 1.37, t (13.0)	40.4
6	-	90.1	-	90.2
7	1.88, dd (12.5, 4.5) 1.80, dt (12.5, 3.5)	29.8	1.90, dd (12.5, 4.5) 1.80, dt (12.5, 3.5)	29.9
8	1.66, td (13.5, 3.5) 1.57, dt (13.5, 4.0)	23.7	1.67, td (14.0, 3.5) 1.57, dt (14.0, 4.0)	23.8
9	-	40.0	-	40.5
10	-	100.9	-	101.0
11	2.08, d (13.0) 1.94, d (13.0)	41.8	2.11, d (13.0) 1.93, d (13.0)	42.0
12	-	39.9	-	39.8
13	2.20, td (12.0, 4.5)	53.1	2.41, td (12.0, 4.5)	48.1
14	2.26, br s 2.24, br s	32.0	2.24, br s 2.22, br s	30.7
15	-	160.0	-	160.1
16	5.90, s	125.6	5.92, s	127.0
17	-	198.5	-	197.3
18	2.69, td (12.0, 6.5)	46.4	2.66, dd (12.5, 6.5)	48.2
19	2.62, dd (14.5, 6.5) 2.50, dd (14.5, 12.0)	42.4	3.02, dq (7.0, 6.5)	45.9
20	-	209.0	-	212.2

Table 1. *Cont.*

No.	δ_H, mult. (J in Hz)	δ_C	δ_H, mult. (J in Hz)	δ_C
	1		**2**	
21	2.83, s	59.1	3.23, s	53.9
22	-	36.5	-	40.3
23	3.65, d (20.0) 2.36, d (20.0)	35.9	3.68, d (20.0) 2.37, d (20.0)	36.1
24	-	172.3	-	172.4
25	0.99, s	21.1	0.98, s	20.8
26	-	-	1.17, d (7.0)	13.9
27	2.00, s	24.4	2.01, s	24.6
28	0.97, s	18.5	0.99, s	18.5
29	1.15, s	18.4	1.21, s	18.4
30	0.87, d (7.0)	16.3	0.89, d (7.0)	16.4
Ac	-	171.2	-	171.4
	2.11, s	21.1	2.14, s	21.2

We then addressed the question of the relative configurations of the different chiral centers. To the best of our knowledge, this is the first occurrence of an acetoxy group at position C-3 for zoanthamines; however, other analogues oxygenated at this position have already been described. First, 3-hydroxynorzoanthamine was isolated from an undescribed species of *Zoanthus* from the Canary Islands in the Atlantic Ocean [8]. Later, kuroshines C and F as well as 3β-hydroxyzoanthenamide also possess an hydroxyl group at this position [6]. All these four derivatives were shown to have a hydroxyl group on the β-side of the polycyclic compound and this position was deduced from nOes between H-3 and other protons of the azepane ring. In our case, and because both H-3/H-4a and H-3/H-4b coupling constant values were not fully conclusive, we relied on the key H-3/H-1b nOe correlation to place H-3 on the opposite side of the bridged oxygen (α-side). Subsequently, the acetoxy group was located on the β-side like for the other four 3-hydroxylated analogues. The very low coupling constant values of H-3 with H-2 and H-4 were similar to those observed for all 3-hydroxylated compounds and in perfect agreement with this relative configuration. Additionally, a previous study by Uemura et al. assigned the absolute configuration of norzoanthamine as 2*R*, 4*S*, 6*S*, 9*S*, 10*R*, 12*R*, 13*R*, 18*S*, 21*S*, and 22*S* and suggest the same absolute configuration for all norzoanthamine-type alkaloids [22]. In our case, the positive specific rotation obtained for **1** was in accordance with that obtained for 3-hydroxyzoanthamine and therefore confirmed the same absolute configuration [8].

Compound **2** was isolated as an amorphous yellowish powder and the molecular formula $C_{32}H_{43}NO_7$ was deduced from HRESIMS revealing a major peak at m/z 554.3115 [M + H]$^+$; therefore, **2** is an homologue of **1**. A quick inspection of the ^{1}H NMR spectrum evidenced the presence of the acetoxy group at C-3 as in **1**. An additional methyl signal at δ_H 1.17 (d, *J* = 7.0 Hz, H$_3$-26) suggested that **2** is a member of the zoanthamine-type alkaloids. The presence of the methyl at C-19 was confirmed by the key H-19/C-26 and H$_3$-26/C-18/C-19 HMBC correlations. The β-position of the methyl 26 was then inferred from the coupling constant value $J_{H-18/H-19}$ of 6.0 Hz, reminiscent of an axial/equatorial coupling. Because H-18 is placed in an axial position, H-19 should be placed in an equatorial position; therefore, the methyl 26 occupies the corresponding axial β-position at C-19. The β-position of the acetoxy at C-3 was deduced from the same coupling constant values of H-3 as for **1**, and the absolute configuration was supposed to be the same as that of **1**, again because of similar positive specific rotations.

The compounds were tested for biological activity in the BV-2 microglia cell line, a cellular model often used in neuroinflammation studies. The first step was to determine the effect of compounds on cell viability. Five concentrations (from 0.001 to 10 μM) were investigated and after

24 h of incubation no effects on cell viability were observed, which suggested non-toxic compounds. Microglia-mediated inflammation is known to produce reactive oxygen species (ROS) and release nitric oxide (NO), and thus induce oxidative damage [23]. Therefore, zoanthamines were checked as modulators within these processes. BV-2 cells were activated with lipolysaccharide (LPS) to simulate neuroinflammatory conditions. As shown in Figure 2, when cells were pre-treated with the same concentrations of compounds for 1 h and then incubated for 24 h with LPS (500 ng/mL), a significant reduction in ROS production was observed. As expected, the stimulation of BV-2 cells with LPS significantly increased the ROS production, 50% ($p < 0.001$), while the compounds alone did not induce any effect. However, when cells were pre-treated with norzoanthamine and **1**, a dose-dependent inhibitory effect was observed, while 3-hydroxynorzoanthamine, zoanthamine, or **2** were effective at all concentrations tested, with **2** being the most potent ROS inhibitor. From these results, 0.1 and 1 μM were chosen to investigate the effect on NO release (Figure 3). Zoanthamine alkaloids alone did not produce any effect on NO production, while LPS treatment increased it by three times. In the presence of this family of compounds, NO release was significantly inhibited. The anti-inflammatory effect of zoanthamines was previously investigated in neutrophils [10]. From our results in the BV-2 cellular model, zoanthamine and derivatives show effective properties as protective drugs in neuroinflammation processes.

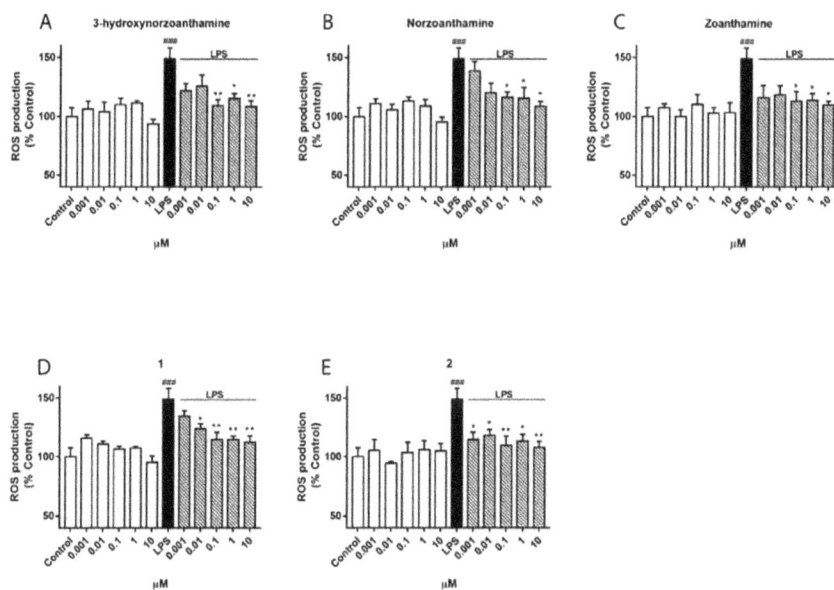

Figure 2. Effect of zoanthamines on intracellular reactive oxygen species (ROS) production in microglia BV-2 cell line. Cells were pre-treated with 3-hydroxynorzoanthamine (**A**); norzoanthamine (**B**); zoanthamine (**C**); **1** (**D**); and **2** (**E**) at different concentrations (0.001, 0.01, 0.1, 1, and 10 μM) 1 h and then stimulated with lipolysaccharide (LPS) (1 μg/mL) for 24 h. ROS production is presented as a percentage of cells control, being the result of mean fluorescence intensity ± SEM of three independent experiments. The values are shown as the difference between cells treated with LPS alone versus cells treated with zoanthamines in presence of LPS by ANOVA followed by *post hoc* Dunnett's test. * $p < 0.05$ and ** $p < 0.01$, and LPS-treated cells versus control cells ### $p < 0.001$.

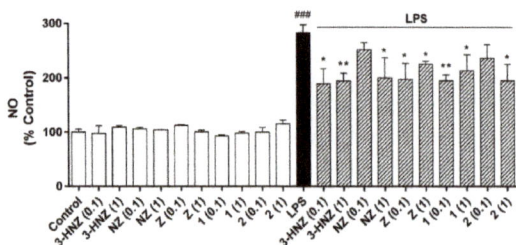

Figure 3. Effect of zoanthamines on nitric oxide (NO) production in BV-2 microglia cell line. Cells were pre-treated with 3-hydroxynorzoanthamine (3-HNZ), norzoanthamine (NZ), zoanthamine (Z), **1**, and **2** (0.1 or 1 μM) for 1 h and then stimulated with lipolysaccharide (LPS) (500 ng/mL) for 24 h. The values are presented in percentage of cells control, being the result of mean ± SEM of a minimum of three independent experiments. The cells treated only with LPS were compared to cells treated with compounds in presence of LPS by ANOVA followed by *post hoc* Dunnett's test. * $p < 0.05$ and ** $p < 0.01$, and LPS-treated cells versus control cells ### $p < 0.001$.

3. Discussion

The isolation of two 3-acetoxy derivatives of zoanthamine and norzoanthamine in *Zoanthus* cf. *pulchellus* strengthens the hypothesis that zoanthamines are markers of the genus *Zoanthus*. However, another species identified as *Zoanthus* cf. *sociatus* was found in the same area and did not present any zoanthamine derivatives [21]. Nevertheless, even if these compounds should not be considered as taxonomic markers of the genus *Zoanthus*, they are clear and characteristic features of some species of *Zoanthus* and could facilitate a more precise classification of this group.

Interestingly, we first ran the NMR analyses of **1** in a different solvent, CD_3OD, and observed clear changes for the signals surrounding the nitrogen atom. Especially, the signals corresponding to H-11 disappeared. This observation reinforced the conclusions on zoanthamine analogues reached by the group of Norte [8]. In a highly polar and protic solvent, the opening of the lactone ring would give rise to an iminium ion at C-11 in equilibrium with its enamine base that can be trapped by exchangeable deuterium atoms provided by the protic deuterated solvent. This behavior signals the high reactivity of this family of compounds at this particular position.

Because these compounds were isolated after a purification step involving acetic acid in the eluent of the HPLC, we wanted to ascertain the presence of these compounds in the collected specimen. For this purpose, we inspected the chemical profiles obtained before any contact with acetic acid and were able to observe the masses corresponding to the new compounds **1** and **2**. These analyses rule out the possibility of a transformation during the purification process.

Finally, the activity observed for all compounds highlights the potential of zoanthamine derivatives as new ROS and NO modulators in neuronal processes, and we will continue our efforts in the study of their mode of action in neuroinflammatory related diseases.

4. Materials and Methods

4.1. General Experimental Procedures

Optical rotation measurements were obtained at the sodium D line (589.3 nm) with a 10-cm cell at 20 °C on a UniPol L1000 polarimeter (Schmidt + Haensch, Berlin, Germany). The UV measurements were obtained on a Cary 300 UV-Visible spectrophotometer (Agilent, Santa-Clara, CA, USA). NMR spectra were recorded on a Inova 500 MHz spectrometer (500 and 125 MHz for ^{1}H and ^{13}C, respectively) (Varian, Palo Alto, CA, USA), and signals were referenced in ppm to the residual solvent signals ($CDCl_3$, at δ_H 7.26 and δ_C 77.16 ppm). HRESIMS data were obtained with a UHPLC-qTOF 6540 mass spectrometer (Agilent, Santa Clara, CA, USA). Purification was carried out on a HPLC equipped with a PU4087 pump (JASCO, Tokyo, Japan) and a UV4070 UV/Vis detector (JASCO, UV, Tokyo, Japan).

4.2. Biological Material

Specimens of *Zoanthus* cf. *pulchellus* were collected by hand on rocks of the shoreline of San Pedro located in the Santa Elena Peninsula, Ecuador. A sample with a voucher 161125SP-01 is stored at CENAIM-ESPOL (San Pedro, Santa Elena, Ecuador). This species has been previously identified using morphological and molecular data [21].

4.3. Extraction and Isolation

The freeze-dried sample of *Z.* cf. *pulchellus* (200 g) was extracted with a mixture of solvents DCM/MeOH (1:1) three times (500 mL) at room temperature. The collected extract was concentrated under reduced pressure to obtain the extract (10 g). The extract was subjected to C18 reversed-phase VLC (LiChroprep® (Merck KGaA, Darmstadt, Germany) RP-18, 40–63 µm, 1:25 ratio for the weight of C18 used, funnel of 10 cm × 10 cm) using a mixture of solvents of decreasing polarity (1) H_2O; (2) H_2O/MeOH (1:1); (3) H_2O/MeOH (1:3); (4) MeOH; (5) MeOH/DCM (3:1); (6) MeOH/DCM (1:1); and (7) DCM using 500 mL of each solvent. The aqueous-methanolic fraction F3 was purified by reversed-phase HPLC (Ultra AQ C18, 10 × 250 mm, 5 µm) using an isocratic method CH_3CN:H_2O:Acetic acid (30:70:0.1) as a mobile phase with a flow rate of 3 mL/min with detection at λ 254 nm for 20 min yielding compound **1** (52.7 mg) and the known compounds norzoanthamine (6.3 mg) [3] and zoanthamine (6.6 mg) [1]. The methanolic fraction F4 was purified by reversed-phase HPLC (Ultra AQ C18, 10 × 250 mm, 5 µm) using the following mobile phases: (A) CH_3CN/Acetic acid 0.1%; (B) H_2O/Acetic acid 0.1%; starting with an isocratic 0–25 min with A 22, B 78; linear gradient for 25–30 min until A 100; then isocratic for 30–60 min at a flow rate of 3 mL/min with UV detection at λ 254 nm to yield compounds **2** (12.3 mg) and the known 3-hydroxynorzoanthamine (2.7 mg) [8].

4.4. 3-Acetoxynorzoanthamine (**1**)

Amorphous yellow powder; $[\alpha]_D^{20}$ +10 (*c* 0.45, CH_3OH); UV (CH_3OH) λ_{max} (log ε) 237 (4.1) nm; ^1H NMR and ^{13}C NMR data see Table 1; HRESIMS (+) *m*/*z* [M + H]$^+$ 540.2956 (calc. for $C_{31}H_{42}NO_7$ 540.2956Δ + 0.0 ppm) (Spectra in the Supplementary Materials).

4.5. 3-Acetoxyzoanthamine (**2**)

Amorphous yellowish powder; $[\alpha]_D^{20}$ + 6.7 (*c* 0.12, CH_3OH); UV (CH_3OH) λ_{max} (log ε) 238 (4.0) nm; ^1H NMR and ^{13}C NMR data see Table 1; HRESIMS (+) *m*/*z* [M + H]$^+$ 554.3115 (calc. for $C_{32}H_{44}NO_7$ 554.3112Δ + 0.5 ppm) (Spectra in the Supplementary Materials).

4.6. Biological Assays

4.6.1. Cell Culture

The microglia BV-2 cell line was obtained from InterLab Cell Line Collection (ICLC) (Genova, Italy), number ATL03001. Cells were maintained in Roswell Park Memorial Institute Medium (RPMI) supplemented with 10% fetal bovine serum (FBS), penicillin (100 U/mL), and 100 µg/mL streptomycin at 37 °C in a humidified atmosphere of 5% CO_2 and 95% air. Cells were dissociated twice a week using 0.05% trypsin/EDTA.

4.6.2. Cell Viability

The 3-(4,5-dimethyl thiazol-2-yl)-2,5-diphenyl tetrazolium bromide (MTT) assay was used to analyzed cell viability as previously described [24]. Briefly, the microglia BV-2 cell line was grown in a 96-well plate at a density of 4 × 10^4 cells per well. Cells were exposed to different compounds concentration (0.001, 0.01, 0.1, 1 and 10 µM) for 24 h. Then, cells were rinsed and incubated with

Mar. Drugs **2018**, 16, 242

MTT (500 µg/mL) diluted in a saline buffer for 1 h at 37 °C. The resulting formazan crystals were dissolved with 5% sodium dodecyl sulfate, (SDS) and the absorbance values were obtained using a spectrophotometer plate reader (595 nm). Saponin was used for cellular death control and its absorbance was substrate from the other data.

4.6.3. Measurement of Intracellular ROS Production

The intracellular ROS levels in microglia activation were performed using $7',2'$-dichlorofluorescein diacetate (DCFH-DA), as previously described [25]. Cells were pre-treated with different compounds concentration (0.001, 0.01, 0.1, 1, and 10 µM) 1 h prior to the stimulation with LPS (500 ng/mL) for 24 h. Afterwards, cells were rinsed twice with saline solution and incubated 1 h at 37 °C with 20 µM DCFH-DA. Then, cells were washed and kept in saline solution for 30 min at 37 °C. Intracellular production of ROS was measured by fluorescence detection of dichlorofluorescein (DCF) as the oxidized product of DCFH-DA on a spectrophotometer plate reader (495 nm excitation and 527 nm emission).

4.6.4. NO Determination

The NO concentration in the culture media was established by measuring nitrite formed by the oxidation of NO, using the Griess reagent kit, according to manufacturer instructions. The detection limit of this method is 1 µM. Briefly, microglia cells were seeded in a 12-well plate at a density of 1×10^6 cells per well and pre-incubated with compounds (0.1 and 1 µM) for 1 h and then stimulated with LPS (500 ng/mL) for 24 h. Thereafter, the following were mixed in a microplate: 150 µL of cells supernatant, 130 µL of deionized water, and 20 µL of Griess Reagent, which was incubated for 30 min at room temperature. The absorbance was measured on a spectrophotometer plate reader at a wavelength of 548 nm.

4.6.5. Statistical Analysis

Results were expressed as mean ± SEM of a minimum of three experiments, repeated twice or three times. Comparisons were performed using Student's *t*-test or one-way ANOVA with Dunnett's *post hoc* analysis. *p* values < 0.05 were considered statistically significant.

Supplementary Materials: The following are available online at http://www.mdpi.com/1660-3397/16/7/242/s1/: HRMS and NMR data for compounds **1** and **2**.

Author Contributions: Methodology and Formal Analysis, P.O.G., S.G., K.B.J., K.C.; Validation, E.A., A.A., K.C.; Writing—Original Draft Preparation, P.O.G.; Writing—Review & Editing, A.A., O.P.T.; Supervision, E.A., O.P.T.; Project Administration, J.R., O.P.T.; Funding Acquisition, J.R., L.M.B., O.P.T.

Funding: The project is originally funded by the Secretaria de Educación Superior, Ciencia, Tecnología e Innovación (SENESCYT) in the framework of the PIC-14-CENAIM-001 Project Caracterización de la Biodiversidad Microbiológica y de Invertebrados de la Reserva Marina "El Pelado" a Escala Taxonómica, Metabolómica y Metagenómica para su Uso en Salud Humana y Animal. Part of this project (Grant-Aid Agreement No. PBA/MB/16/01) is carried out with the support of the Marine Institute and is funded under the Marine Research Programme by the Irish Government. P.O.G. and K.B.J. acknowledge NUI Galway for supporting part of their Ph.D. scholarship. The research leading to the results of the biological assays has received funding from the following FEDER cofunded-grants: Consellería de Cultura, Educación e Ordenación Universitaria, Xunta de Galicia, 2017 GRC GI-1682 (ED431C 2017/01); CDTI and Technological Funds, supported by Ministerio de Economía, Industria y Competitividad, AGL2014-58210-R, AGL2016-78728-R (AEI/FEDER, UE), ISCIII/PI16/01830 and RTC-2016-5507-2, ITC-20161072; European Union POCTEP 0161-Nanoeaters-1-E-1, Interreg AlertoxNet EAPA-317-2016, and H2020 778069-EMERTOX.

Acknowledgments: We acknowledge the support of Cristobal Dominguez (CENAIM-ESPOL, Ecuador) in the collection of the sample and Frederic Sinniger (University of the Ryukyus, Japan) for his help with the taxonomic identification of this species through the training of K.B.J.

Conflicts of Interest: The authors declare no conflict of interest. The funders had no role in the design of the study; in the collection, analyses, or interpretation of data; in the writing of the manuscript; or in the decision to publish the results.

References

1. Rao, C.B.; Anjaneyula, A.S.R.; Sarma, S.S.; Venkatateswarlu, Y.; Chen, M.; Clardy, J.; Rosser, R.; Faulkner, J. Zoanthamine: A novel alkaloid from a marine zoanthid. *J. Am. Chem. Soc.* **1984**, *106*, 7984–7985. [CrossRef]
2. Rao, C.B.; Anjaneyulu, A.S.R.; Sarma, N.S.; Venkateswarlu, Y.; Rosser, R.M.; Faulkner, J. Alkaloids from a marine zoanthid. *J. Org. Chem.* **1985**, *50*, 3757–3760. [CrossRef]
3. Fukuzawa, S.; Hayashi, Y.; Uemura, D.; Nagatsu, A.; Yamada, K.; Ijuin, Y. The isolation and structures of five new alkaloids, norzoanthamine, oxyzoanthamine, norzoanthamine, cyclozoanthamine and epinorzoanthamine. *Heterocycl. Commun.* **1995**, *1*, 207–214. [CrossRef]
4. Atta-ur-Rahman; Alvi, K.A.; Abbas, S.A.; Choudhary, M.I.; Clardy, J. Zoanthaminone, a new alkaloid from a marine zoanthid. *Tetrahedron Lett.* **1989**, *30*, 6825–6828. [CrossRef]
5. Cen-Pacheco, F.; Norte, M.; Fernández, J.J.; Daranas, A.H. Zoaramine, a zoanthamine-like alkaloid with a new skeleton. *Org. Lett.* **2014**, *16*, 2880–2883. [CrossRef] [PubMed]
6. Cheng, Y.-B.; Lo, I.-W.; Shyur, L.-F.; Yang, C.-C.; Hsu, Y.-M.; Su, J.-H.; Lu, M.-C.; Chiou, S.-F.; Lan, C.-C.; Wu, Y.-C.; et al. New alkaloids from Formosan zoanthid *Zoanthus kuroshio*. *Tetrahedron* **2015**, *71*, 8001–8006. [CrossRef]
7. Daranas, A.H.; Fernández, J.J.; Gavin, J.A.; Norte, M. Epioxyzoanthamine, a new zoanthamine-type alkaloid and the unusual deuterium exchange in this series. *Tetrahedron* **1998**, *54*, 7891–7896. [CrossRef]
8. Daranas, A.H.; Fernandez, J.J.; Gavin, J.A.; Norte, M. New alkaloids from a marine zoanthid. *Tetrahedron* **1999**, *55*, 5539–5546. [CrossRef]
9. Behenna, D.C.; Stockdill, J.L.; Stoltz, B.M. The biology and chemistry of the zoanthamine alkaloids. *Angew. Chem. Int. Ed.* **2008**, *47*, 2365–2386. [CrossRef] [PubMed]
10. Hsu, Y.-M.; Chang, F.-R.; Lo, I.W.; Lai, K.-H.; El-Shazly, M.; Wu, T.-Y.; Du, Y.-C.; Hwang, T.-L.; Cheng, Y.-B.; Wu, Y.-C. Zoanthamine-type alkaloids from the zoanthid *Zoanthus kuroshio* collected in Taiwan and their effects on inflammation. *J. Nat. Prod.* **2016**, *79*, 2674–2680. [CrossRef] [PubMed]
11. Miyashita, M.; Sasaki, M.; Hattori, I.; Sakai, M.; Tanino, K. Total synthesis of norzoanthamine. *Science* **2004**, *305*, 495–499. [CrossRef] [PubMed]
12. Takahashi, Y.; Yoshimura, F.; Tanino, K.; Miyashita, M. Total synthesis of zoanthenol. *Angew. Chem. Int. Ed.* **2009**, *48*, 8905–8908. [CrossRef] [PubMed]
13. Yoshimura, F.; Sasaki, M.; Hattori, I.; Komatsu, K.; Sakai, M.; Tanino, K.; Miyashita, M. Synthetic studies of the zoanthamine alkaloids: The total syntheses of norzoanthamine and zoanthamine. *Chem. Eur. J.* **2009**, *15*, 6626–6644. [CrossRef] [PubMed]
14. Yoshimura, F.; Tanino, K.; Miyashita, M. Total synthesis of zoanthamine alkaloids. *Acc. Chem. Res.* **2012**, *45*, 746–755. [CrossRef] [PubMed]
15. Fischer, D.; Nguyen, T.X.; Trzoss, L.; Dakanali, M.; Theodorakis, E.A. Intramolecular cyclization strategies toward the synthesis of zoanthamine alkaloids. *Tetrahedron Lett.* **2011**, *52*, 4920–4923. [CrossRef] [PubMed]
16. Nakajima, T.; Yamashita, D.; Suzuki, K.; Nakazaki, A.; Suzuki, T.; Kobayashi, S. Different modes of cyclization in zoanthamine alkaloid system, bisaminal versus spiroketal formation. *Org. Lett.* **2011**, *13*, 2980–2983. [CrossRef] [PubMed]
17. Villar, R.M.; Gil-Longo, J.; Daranas, A.H.; Souto, M.L.; Fernández, J.J.; Peixinho, S.; Barral, M.A.; Santafé, G.; Rodríguez, J.; Jiménez, C. Evaluation of the effect of several zoanthamine-type alkaloids on the aggregation of human platelets. *Bioorg. Med. Chem.* **2003**, *11*, 2301–2306. [CrossRef]
18. Genji, T.; Fukuzawa, S.; Tachibana, K. Distribution and possible function of the marine alkaloid, norzoanthamine, in the zoanthid *Zoanthus* sp. using MALDI imaging mass spectrometry. *Mar. Biotechnol.* **2010**, 81–87. [CrossRef] [PubMed]
19. Guillen, P.O.; Calabro, K.; Jaramillo, K.B.; Dominguez, C.; Genta-Jouve, G.; Rodriguez, J.; Thomas, O.P. Ecdysonelactones, ecdysteroids from the Tropical Eastern Pacific zoantharian *Antipathozoanthus hickmani*. *Mar. Drugs* **2018**, *16*, 58. [CrossRef] [PubMed]
20. Guillen, P.O.; Jaramillo, K.B.; Genta-Jouve, G.; Sinniger, F.; Rodriguez, J.; Thomas, O.P. Terrazoanthines, 2-aminoimidazole alkaloids from the Tropical Eastern Pacific zoantharian *Terrazoanthus onoi*. *Org. Lett.* **2017**, *19*, 1558–1561. [CrossRef] [PubMed]

21. Jaramillo, K.B.; Reverter, M.; Guillen, P.O.; McCormack, G.; Rodriguez, J.; Sinniger, F.; Thomas, O.P. Assessing the zoantharian diversity of the Tropical Eastern Pacific through an integrative approach. *Sci. Rep.* **2018**, *8*, 7138. [CrossRef] [PubMed]

22. Kuramoto, M.; Hayashi, K.; Fujitani, Y.; Yamaguchi, K.; Tsuji, T.; Yamada, K.; Ijuin, Y.; Uemura, D. Absolute configuration of norzoanthamine, a promising candidate for an osteoporotic drug. *Tetrahedron Lett.* **1997**, *38*, 5683–5686. [CrossRef]

23. Dumont, M.; Beal, M.F. Neuroprotective strategies involving ROS in Alzheimer disease. *Free Radic. Biol. Med.* **2011**, *51*, 1014–1026. [CrossRef] [PubMed]

24. Sanchez, J.A.; Alfonso, A.; Leiros, M.; Alonso, E.; Rateb, M.E.; Jaspars, M.; Houssen, W.E.; Ebel, R.; Tabudravu, J.; Botana, L.M. Identification of *Spongionella* compounds as cyclosporine A mimics. *Pharmacol. Res.* **2016**, *107*, 407–414. [CrossRef] [PubMed]

25. Leiros, M.; Alonso, E.; Rateb, M.E.; Houssen, W.E.; Ebel, R.; Jaspars, M.; Alfonso, A.; Botana, L.M. Gracilins: Spongionella-derived promising compounds for Alzheimer disease. *Neuropharmacology* **2015**, *93*, 285–293. [CrossRef] [PubMed]

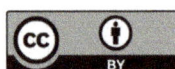

marine drugs

MDPI

Article

Anti-Inflammatory Effects of a *Mytilus coruscus* α-D-Glucan (MP-A) in Activated Macrophage Cells via TLR4/NF-κB/MAPK Pathway Inhibition

Fuyan Liu [1,2,*], Xiaofeng Zhang [3], Yuqiu Li [4], Qixin Chen [1,2], Fei Liu [1,2,*], Xiqiang Zhu [1], Li Mei [1,2], Xinlei Song [2], Xia Liu [1], Zhigang Song [1,2], Jinhua Zhang [1], Wen Zhang [5], Peixue Ling [1,2,*] and Fengshan Wang [2,*]

[1]   Shandong Academy of Pharmaceutical Science, Jinan 250101, China; chenqixin1010@aliyun.com (Q.C.); 15066696818@163.com (X.Z.); huoruhun@163.com (L.M.); ivyliu@yahoo.com (X.L.); zgangsong@163.com (Z.S.); 15098978003@163.com (J.Z.)
[2]   School of Pharmaceutical Sciences, Shandong University, Jinan 250012, China; xinleisongsxl@126.com
[3]   School of Life Sciences, Lanzhou University, Lanzhou 730000, China; xfzhang2014@lzu.edu.cn
[4]   Shandong University of Traditional Chinese Medicine, Jinan 250355, China; xiaoyusd2010@163.com
[5]   School of Pharmacy, Second Military Medical University, Shanghai 200433, China; lfyflying@sohu.com
*   Correspondence: fuyanliu@mail.sdu.edu.cn (Fu.L.); lfshwu@163.com (Fe.L.); lpx@sdfmg.com or lpxsdf@163.com (P.L.); fswang@sdu.edu.cn (F.W.); Tel.: +86-531-8121-3080 (Fe.L.); +86-531-8121-3002 (P.L.); +86-531-8838-2589 (F.W.); Fax: +86-531-8852-4738 (P.L.); +86-531-8838-2548 (F.W.)

Received: 25 July 2017; Accepted: 15 September 2017; Published: 20 September 2017

Abstract: The hard-shelled mussel (*Mytilus coruscus*) has been used as Chinese traditional medicine for thousands of years; however, to date the ingredients responsible for the various beneficial health outcomes attributed to *Mytilus coruscus* are still unclear. An α-D-Glucan, called MP-A, was isolated from *Mytilus coruscus*, and observed to exert anti-inflammatory activity in THP-1 human macrophage cells. Specifically, we showed that MP-A treatment inhibited the production of inflammatory markers, including TNF-α, NO, and PGE2, inducible NOS (iNOS), and cyclooxygenase-2 (COX-2), in LPS-activated THP-1 cells. It was also shown to enhance phagocytosis in the analyzed cells, but to severely inhibit the phosphorylation of mitogen-activated protein kinases (MAPKs) and the nuclear translocation of NF-κB P65. Finally, MP-A was found to exhibit a high binding affinity for the cell surface receptor TLR4, but a low affinity for TLR2 and dectin-1, via surface plasmon resonance (SPR) analysis. The study indicates that MP-A suppresses LPS-induced TNF-α, NO and PEG2 production via TLR4/NF-κB/MAPK pathway inhibition, and suggests that MP-A may be a promising therapeutic candidate for diseases associated with TNF-α, NO, and/or PEG2 overproduction.

Keywords: THP-1 macrophages; anti-inflammatory; TLR4; NF-κB; MAPK; SPR analysis

1. Introduction

The hard-shelled mussel (*Mytilus coruscus*) is one of the main species of marine shellfish inhabiting broad regions of East Asian coastal areas, and has been used as both a food and medicine for thousands of years [1]. Many health benefits have been attributed to its use as a Chinese traditional medicine, including the nourishment of the liver and kidneys, the strengthening of the immune system, and the treatment of various diseases, such as goiter tumors, male impotence, and female menoxenia. In recent years, some biologically active polysaccharides [1], peptides [2,3], and lipid extracts [4] have been isolated from *Mytilus coruscus*, and evaluated to determine their pharmacological efficacy; nevertheless, to date, the ingredients responsible for the various beneficial health outcomes attributed to *Mytilus coruscus* are still unclear.

Polysaccharides isolated from natural sources can affect a variety of biological activities, such as immunity, suggesting their potential use as immunomodulatory agents with broad applications [5,6]. For example, a glycogen polysaccharide extracted from *Perna canaliculus* has been shown to exert anti-inflammatory activities [7], and similarly, a heparin-like substance isolated from the marine clams *Anomalocardia brasiliana*, has been shown to bind anti-thrombin III (ATIII) and to thereby exert a strong anticoagulant effect [8].

Various polysaccharides isolated from the hard-shelled mussel have received increasing attention in recent years. For example, the MP-1 polysaccharide from *Mytilus coruscus* has been demonstrated to exert a protective effect against acute liver injury [1], and the MEP polysaccharide from *Mytihus edulis* Linnaeus has been shown to both significantly ameliorate delayed-type hypersensitivity and phagocytosis, and to improve immune function in mice [9]. In our previous studies, we isolated the MA polysaccharide from *Mytilus coruscus*, and identified it to have anti-hyperlipidemic effects on experimental atherosclerosis in rabbits [10]. In the present study, we isolated a high-molecular-weight α-D-Glucan, named MP-A, from the hard-shelled mussel (*Mytilus coruscus*). We identified MP-A to contain repeating units of D-glucose, and to be structured such that the main chain was connected by α1-4 glucosidic bonds, and that a D-glucose was connected to this chain every twelve monosaccharides by α1-2 glucosidic bonds to form a branch. The molecular weight of MP-A was established to be approximately 1.2×10^3 kDa, and the structure was shown in Figure 1A.

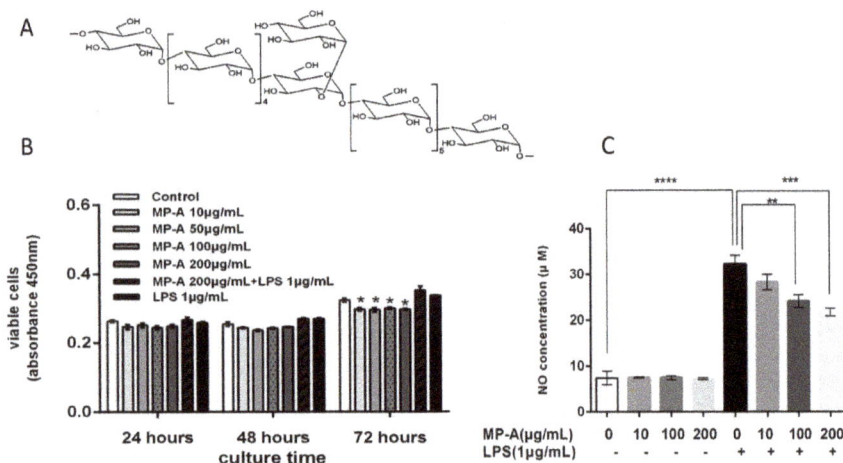

Figure 1. MP-A structure and effects of MP-A on cell viability and nitric oxide (NO) production of THP-1 cells with and without lipopolysaccharide (LPS) treatment. (**A**) MP-A structure; (**B**) Effects of 24, 48, and 72 h of MP-A and/or LPS treatment on THP-1 cell cytotoxicity. * $p < 0.05$ as compared to the control group ($n = 3$); (**C**) Effect of MP-A treatment on NO production in THP-1 cells with or without LPS. NO production was inferred from the level of nitrite formed in the supernatant, as detected using the Griess reagent. The absorbance of treated cells at 540 nm was measured against distilled water using the Griess reagent as a blank, and sodium nitrite as a standard sample. ** $p < 0.01$, *** $p < 0.001$, and **** $p < 0.0001$ compared with 1 μg/mL LPS treatment group ($n = 3$).

Glucans have been previously reported to exhibit significant bioactivity, and in particular, β-Glucans were extensively investigated between 1990 and 2000. These previous studies showed β-Glucans to exert anti-infective and anti-tumorigenic activity via the activation of leukocytes [11–13], and the production of reactive oxygen intermediates, inflammatory mediators such as NO, and TNF-α [11,14,15]. More recently, the α-glucans have begun to attract the attention of various research groups. For example, the α-glucan YCP, which is composed of α-D-(1–4)-linked glucose residues, has been recently revealed to inhibit tumor growth by modulating the innate and adaptive host immune responses to enhance macrophage activity, promote lymphocyte proliferation, and to induce cytokine secretion [16]. Similarly, six homogeneous, low-molecular-weight α-glucans (LMWYCP-1 to LMWYCP-6) have been shown to modulate the activity of toll-like receptors (TLRs), and thus, B lymphocytes [17].

Macrophages play a unique role in the immune system, in that they do not only elicit an innate immune response, but also are effector cells that counteract inflammation and infection. Furthermore, they are also critical to the maintenance of a functional interface between no-adaptive and adaptive immunity, and mediate various other functions, such as antigen processing and presentation to T cells.

THP-1 is a human leukemia monocytic cell line that has been widely used to study monocyte/macrophage function, signaling pathway mechanisms, and drug transport, and is commonly used to investigate the regulation of macrophage activity [18]. Lipopolysaccharide (LPS) is a major component of the outer membrane of gram-negative enteric bacteria [19]. During inflammatory processes, LPS induces the production of pro-inflammatory cytokines and small mediators, such as nitric oxide (NO), and PGE_2 [20]. LPS-stimulated THP-1 macrophages have been shown to express the *MD2*, *CD14*, and *MyD88* genes that are required for LPS signaling in vivo [18]. When macrophages are activated by LPS, the TLR4 signaling pathway is initiated, leading to the phosphorylation of mitogen-activated protein kinase (MAPK), and the activation of the transcription factor nuclear factor-kappa B (NF-κB) [21], and the induction of pro-inflammatory factors including NO, inducible nitric oxide synthase (iNOS), interleukin-1β (IL-1β), interleukin-6 (IL-6), tumor necrosis factor (TNF)-α, and cyclooxygenase-2 (COX-2), etc. The MAPK family of proteins, including extracellular signal regulated kinase (ERK), c-Jun *N*-terminal kinase (JNK), and p38, regulate inflammatory and immune responses, and their respective signaling essential for LPS-induced iNOS and COX-2 expression in macrophages [22,23].

In the present study, LPS-induced THP-1 cells were used as an inflammatory model to investigate the effects of MP-A immunomodulation of THP-1 macrophages. To identify possible cell membrane receptors for MP-A, and putative molecular mechanisms underlying MP-A immunomodulation of THP-1 macrophages, the binding affinity of MP-A for TLR4 and/or TLR2 was assessed using surface plasmon resonance (SPR). To our knowledge, limited publications currently report on the immunomodulatory effects of combined treatment with LPS with MP-A. Thus, in the present study, we investigated the effects of MP-A on LPS-induced pro-inflammatory cytokine secretion by THP-1 cells, and on LPS-induced signal transduction.

2. Materials and Methods

2.1. Reagents and Antibodies

MP-A (purity 97.9% *w/w*) was produced and purified by Shandong Academy of Pharmaceutical Science (Jinan, China), and verified to have an average molecular weight (*Mw*) of 1200 kDa via a size exclusion chromatography multi-angle laser scattering (SEC-MALLS) system (Wyatt Technology Corp, Santa Barbara, CA, USA), the preparation and structural characterization of MP-A has been introduced in other paper. LPS from *Escherichia coli* O55:B5, phorbol-12-myristate-13-acetate (PMA), and FITC-dextran (FD40S) were purchased from Sigma–Aldrich Chemical Co. (St. Louis, MO, USA) and the average MW of Dextran was 40,000 Da. Recombinant human Dectin-1, TLR4, and TLR2 were purchased from R&D Systems (Minneapolis, MN, USA). Fetal bovine serum (FBS), and other cell culture reagents were purchased from Gibco BRL Co. (Grand Island, NY, USA). The Cell Counting Kit-8 (CCK-8) Assay Kit was obtained from Beyotime (Wuhan, China). Penicillin and streptomycin were purchased from HyClone (Logan, UT, USA). ELISA kits for PGE2, and TNF-α were purchased from Biolegend (San Diego, CA, USA). The p-p38, p38, p-JNK1/2, JNK1/2, p-ERK1/2, ERK1/2, p-P65, P65, COX-2, and iNOS antibodies were obtained from Abcam (Cambridge, UK). The β-actin monoclonal antibodies were obtained from Cell Signaling Technology (Beverly, MA,

USA). NF-κB Activation-Nuclear Translocation Assay kits were purchased from Beyotime Institute of Biotechnology (Haimen, China). All of the other chemicals were of analytical grade. The horseradish peroxidase (HRP)-conjugated goat anti-rabbit IgG secondary antibody was purchased from Santa Cruz Biotechnology Inc. (Santa Cruz, CA, USA).

2.2. THP-1 Cell Culture

THP-1, a human leukemia monocytic cell line extensively used to study the modulation of monocytes and macrophages, was purchased from the Shanghai Cell Bank, the Institute of Cell Biology, China Academy of Sciences (Shanghai, China). THP-1 cells in the monocyte state can be differentiated into a macrophage-like phenotype via stimulation with phorbol-12-myristate-13-acetate (PMA) (50 ng/mL, 24 h). The cells were cultivated in RPMI 1640 medium (containing 10% heat-inactivated FBS, and 1% penicillin/streptomycin), at 37 °C in a humidified atmosphere (5% CO_2, 95% air).

2.3. Cell Viability Assay

The viability of THP-1 cells was determined using the Cell Counting Kit-8 (CCK-8) Assay Kit (Beyotime, Wuhan, China). The cells were primed for differentiation with 50 ng/mL PMA for 24 h [24], and then seeded on 96-well plates at a density of 5×10^4 cells/mL, in 100 μL medium, and left to incubate overnight. They were then treated with MP-A (10, 50, 100, or 200 μg/mL dissolved in serum-free medium), and/or LPS (1 μg/mL dissolved in serum-free medium) for 24, 48, or 72 h (37 °C, 5% CO_2). CCK-8 (10 μL) was added to each well 4 h prior to culture termination, and the optical density of each well was measured (450 nm) using a microplate reader (Infinite M200 PRO, TECAN, Männedorf, Switzerland).

2.4. Determination of Phagocytic Uptake of FITC-Labeled Dextran

The cells were primed for differentiation with 50 ng/mL PMA for 24 h [24], and then seeded on 24-well plates at a density of 5×10^4 cells/mL in 1 mL medium and left to incubate overnight. They were then treated with MP-A (10, 100 or 200 μg/mL dissolved in serum-free medium), and/or LPS (1 μg/mL dissolved in serum-free medium) for 24 h. Then THP-1 cells were collected, resuspended, and incubated in 100 μL FITC-labeled dextran (1 mg/mL, 37 °C, 30 min). Cells incubated with FITC-labeled dextran only (4 °C, 30 min) were used as a control and cells incubated without FITC-labeled dextran were used as a blank control. After incubation, ice-cold PBS (2 mL, containing 2% FBS) was added to the cells to inhibit phagocytosis, and they were then washed three times (ice-cold PBS). Cellular uptake of FITC-labeled dextran was analyzed by flow cytometry (BD FACSAria ™ III).

2.5. ELISA for Cytokine Estimation

TNF-α and PGE_2 were measured by using a commercial ELISA kit according to the manufacturers' instructions. THP-1 cells were primed with PMA and seeded in a 96-well plate (density 1×10^6 cells/mL), and cultured overnight. They were then treated first with MP-A (10, 50, 100, or 200 μg/mL, 1 h), and secondly with LPS (1 μg/mL, 6 or 24 h to enable the measurement of TNF-α or PGE_2, respectively. Cell-free supernatants were finally collected and analyzed to measure the levels of both cytokines.

2.6. Nitric Oxide (NO) Production

The total nitrite content in the cell culture supernatant was measured using the Griess reagent. An equal volume of Griess reagent was added to the respective samples, and they were then incubated (30 min, 37 °C). The nitrite concentration was estimated by measuring the absorbance of samples at 545 and 630 nm (wavelength correction) against a sodium nitrite standard using an ELISA plate reader (Infinite M200 PRO, TECAN, Männedorf, Switzerland).

2.7. Western Blot Analyses

THP-1 cells were primed with PMA, seeded in a 100-mm culture dish (density 1×10^6 cells/mL), cultured overnight, and then treated with MP-A (10, 50, 100, or 200 μg/mL) and LPS (1 μg/mL), and the cells were then incubated (37 °C) for 24 h. Cytosolic proteins were isolated using the Cytosol Fractionation Kit, according to the manufacturer's instructions. Total protein was measured by the bicinchoninic acid assay (BCA assay), and proteins were separated by SDS-PAGE and electro-transferred onto a polyvinylidene difluoride (PVDF) membrane. The PVDF membrane blots were blocked (1 h) using 8% non-fat powdered milk in TBST buffer, and then incubated overnight at 4 °C with appropriate primary antibodies against p-p38, p38, p-JNK1/2, JNK1/2, p-ERK1/2, ERK1/2, iNOS, COX-2, P65, and/or p-P65. After three washes (TBST buffer, 5 min), the PVDF membranes were incubated (2 h) with a goat anti-rabbit IgG, or goat anti-mouse IgG second antibody. After a final three washes (TBST buffer, 5 min), specific proteins were detected using an enhanced chemiluminescence kit (ECL, Millipore, Billerica, MA, USA) according to the manufacturer's instructions. β-actin was used as a loading control.

2.8. Detection of NF-κB Activation and Nuclear Translocation

The detection of NF-κB nuclear translocation was carried out following the instruction of the kit (Beyotime Institute of Biotechnology, Haimen, China) [25,26].THP-1 cells were primed with PMA and seeded on glass coverslips in a 24-well plate (density 1×10^6 cells/mL), cultured overnight, and then treated with 200 μg/mL MP-A with or without 1 μg/mL LPS treatments for 2 h. Then, cells grown on coverslips were fixed and blocked, and incubated overnight with the primary antibody against the p65 subunit of NF-κB at 4 °C, then washed in PBS, and incubated with Cy3-labeled secondary antibody for 2 h at room temperature. Finally, the cells were stained with 2 μM 2-(4-amidinophenyl)-6-indolecarbamidine dihydrochloride (DAPI) solution for 5 min. Each step above was followed by washing with ice-cold PBS three times for 5 min each. Then, the activation and nuclear translocation of NF-κB were observed using a laser scanning confocal microscope (LSM 780, Zeiss, Oberkochen, Germany).

2.9. Affinity Assay for MP-A with TLR4, TLR2 and Dectin-1

The affinity of MP-A for recombinant human TLR4, TLR2, and Dectin-1 was examined via SPR, and performed using a BIAcore 3000 (GE Healthcare, Uppsala, Sweden) according to the manufacturer's instructions. Prior to analysis, recombinant human TLR4, TLR2, and Dectin-1 proteins (R&D Systems) were each immobilized on a CM5 sensor chip using an amine coupling kit. The surface of the chip was activated by EDC/NHS, and then TLR4, TLR2, and/or Dectin-1 (25 μg/mL) suspended in 10 mmol/L sodium acetate solution (pH 4.5) was flowed over it. When the ligand density reached the target resonance unit (RU) level, remaining active esters were quenched with a 1 mol/L ethanolamine solution (pH 8.5). (Control flow cells received identical treatment, but no TLR4, TLR2, and/or Dectin-1 protein was added to the 10 mmol/L sodium acetate solution). The resultant sensor chip was stored in 10 mM phosphate-buffered saline as a running buffer, and maintained at 25 °C for all of the experiments. MP-A (dissolved in running buffer at a series of concentrations) was injected into the channels, and resulting signals were detected using the BIAcore program (GE). The sensor chip was regenerated in a 10 mM NaOH solution after each analysis. Affinity constants were calculated using BIA evaluation 4.1 software, by globally fitting the association and dissociation phases of overlay plots to a 1:1 Langmuir binding model.

2.10. Statistical Analyses

Multiple comparisons were statistically assessed using a one-way ANOVA, followed by a Tukey's multiple comparison test. Results were expressed as the mean ± SEM, and a *p*-value of <0.05 was considered to indicate statistical significance.

3. Results

3.1. Effects of MP-A on THP-1 Cell Viability

Treatment of THP-1 cells with up to 200 μg/mL of MP-A over 48 h did not result in any significant cytotoxic effect; however, 72 h of MP-A treatment induced a slight decrease in cell viability (Figure 1B). LPS treatment (1 μg/mL), alone over a 24-h period, was insufficient to cause a significant increase in cell viability, as compared with the negative control ($p > 0.05$). We therefore studied the effects of MP-A on phagocytosis, and on NO and cytokine production, using a 24-h culture model that was unaffected by changes in cell quantity.

3.2. Effect of MP-A on NO Release by THP-1 Cells

LPS stimulation resulted in a significant increase in NO production (nitrite 31.34 ± 1.84 μM) relative to that in of unstimulated controls (nitrite 7.46 ± 1.38 μM) (Figure 1C). MP-A treatment dose-dependently inhibited NO production in LPS-stimulated THP-1 cells, such that approximately 33% inhibition was observed at an MP-A concentration of 200 μg/mL (Figure 1C). In contrast, NO production was not significantly affected by MP-A treatment alone when compared to the negative control group ($p > 0.05$).

3.3. Effect of MP-A on Phagocytic Uptake of FITC-Labeled Dextran by THP-1 Cells

The Phagocytic Uptake of FITC-labeled Dextran by THP-1 cells was analyzed using flow cytometry. The results of this analysis showed that MP-A significantly increased the capacity of cell phagocytic uptake of FITC labeled dextran in a dose-dependent manner at concentrations as low as 10 μg/mL, as compared to controls (e.g., phagocytic uptake of FITC labeled dextran was 1.13 ± 0.06% and 0.73 ± 0.15% in MP-A-treated and control cells, respectively, $p < 0.05$, $n = 3$; Figure 2A–D). LPS treatment also markedly stimulated THP-1 cell phagocytosis (e.g., phagocytic uptake of FITC labeled dextran was 16.73 ± 1.01% and 0.73 ± 0.15% in LPS-treated and control cells, respectively, $p < 0.0001$, $n = 3$; Figure 2A,E), and combined LPS and MP-A treatment further stimulated phagocytosis in a dose-dependent manner (Figure 2F–H).

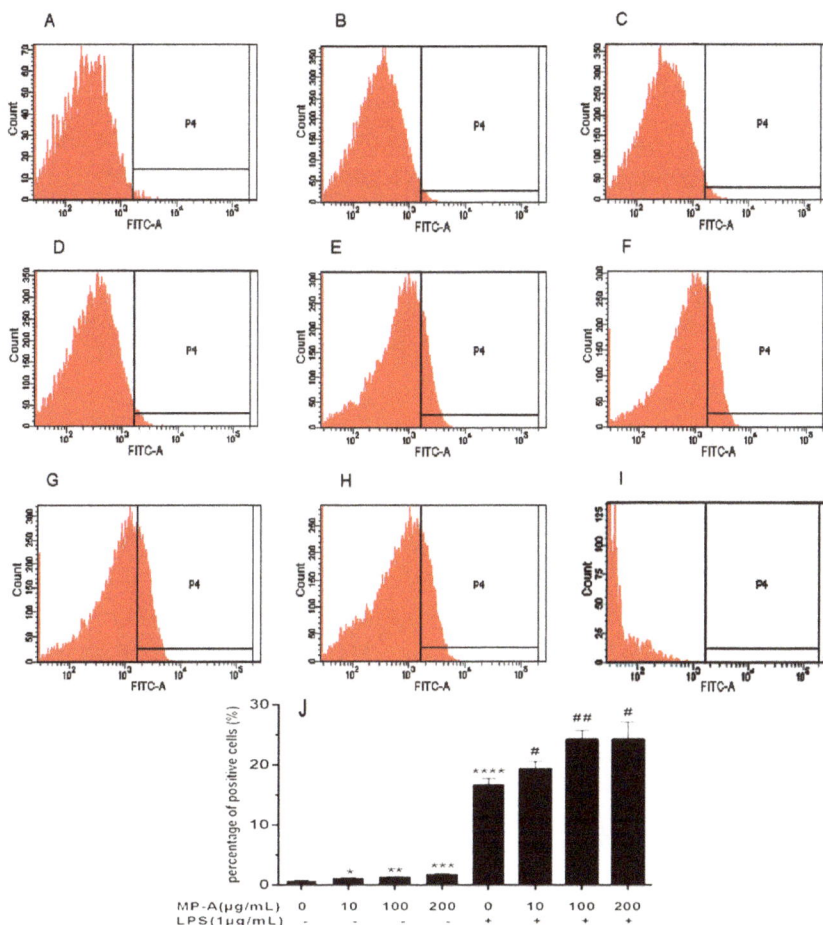

Figure 2. Effect of MP-A on THP-1 cell phagocytosis. (**A–H**) Representative fluorescence activated cell sorter (FACS) plots (three independent experiments), showing phagocytosis of THP-1 cells treated with (**A**) vehicle only (control); (**B**) 10 μg/mL MP-A; (**C**) 100 μg/mL MP-A; (**D**) 200 μg/mL MP-A; (**E**) 1 μg/mL LPS; (**F**) 1 μg/mL LPS + 10 μg/mL MP-A; (**G**) 1 μg/mL LPS + 100 μg/mL MP-A; and (**H**) 1 μg/mL LPS + 200 μg/mL MP-A; (**I**) blank control (**J**) Statistical analysis of results shown in (**A–H**). * $p < 0.05$, ** $p < 0.01$, *** $p < 0.001$, and **** $p < 0.0001$ compared to control (MP-A) group; # $p < 0.05$, and ## $p < 0.01$, when compared to LPS group ($n = 3$).

3.4. MP-A Inhibition of TNF-α and PGE₂ Release by LPS-Stimulated THP-1 Cells

When compared with control cells, LPS treatment significantly increased TNF-α and PGE$_2$ production in THP-1 cells. In contrast, MP-A treatment suppressed TNF-α production such that 60% inhibition was achieved by treating cells with 200 μg/mL MP-A for 6 h. Similarly, 24 h of MP-A treatment (200 μg/mL) resulted in a 35%-inhibition of PGE$_2$ production (Figure 3A,B).

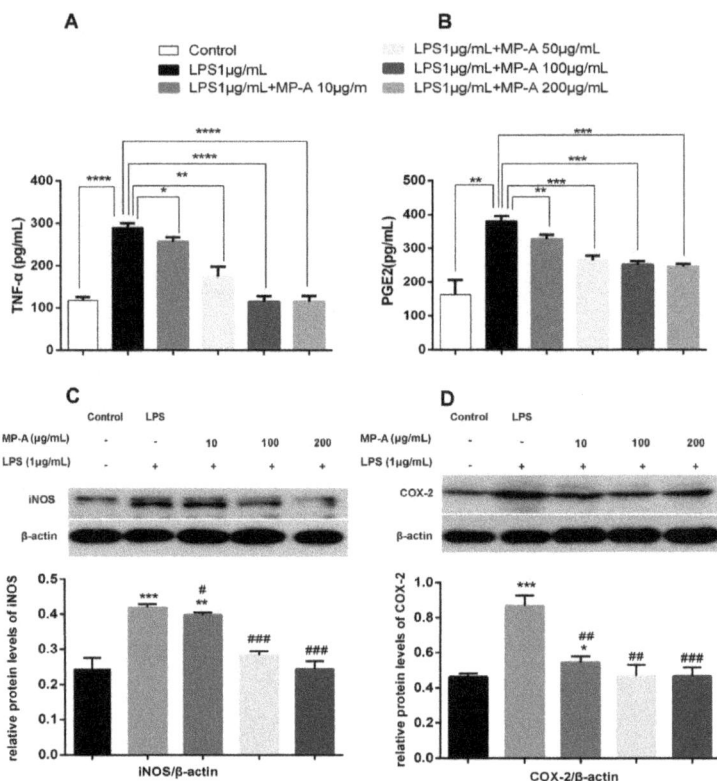

Figure 3. Effect of MP-A on TNF-α and PGE2 production and iNOS and COX-2 protein expression in LPS-stimulated THP-1 cells. (**A,B**) MP-A inhibition of TNF-α and PGE2 production in LPS-stimulated THP-1 cells. TNF-α (6-h stimulation) and PGE2 (24-h stimulation) were measured via an ELISA. The data represent three independent experiments. * $p < 0.05$, ** $p < 0.01$, *** $p < 0.001$, and **** $p < 0.0001$ compared to the LPS group. (**C,D**) MP-A inhibition of iNOS and COX-2 protein expression, as assessed by western blotting analysis in LPS-stimulated THP-1 cells. * $p < 0.05$, ** $p < 0.01$, and *** $p < 0.001$, when compared to controls; # $p < 0.05$, ## $p < 0.05$, and ### $p < 0.001$ compared to the LPS group ($n = 3$).

3.5. MP-A Inhibits iNOS and COX-2 Expression in LPS-Stimulated THP-1 Cells

A western blot analysis was conducted to investigate the effect of MP-A treatment on iNOS and COX-2 expression in LPS-stimulated THP-1 macrophages. As depicted in Figure 3C,D, COX-2 and iNOS protein expression were both dramatically increased by treatment with LPS alone compared to control group, whereas pre-treatment with MP-A decreased protein levels of COX-2 and iNOS in a dose-dependent manner. The reduction of iNOS and COX-2 protein expression was consistent with the above descried observed inhibition of NO and PGE$_2$ (Figures 1C and 3B).

3.6. MP-A Treatment Inhibits LPS-Induced Phosphorylation of MAPKs and NF-κB in THP-1 Cells

LPS from Gram-negative bacteria is known to stimulate inflammatory responses via TLR4-initiation of several distinct signaling pathways, including the MAPK and NF-κB pathways. To determine whether either of these pathways was affected by MP-A treatment, cytoplasmic cell lysates were analyzed by western blotting with specific phosphor-antibodies against P65 (NF-κB), ERK1/2, JNK1/2, and p38 (MAPK). The results of this analysis showed MP-A to dose-dependently inhibit the LPS-induced phosphorylation of P65, ERK1/2, JNK1/2, and p38 in the THP-1 cells (Figure 4).

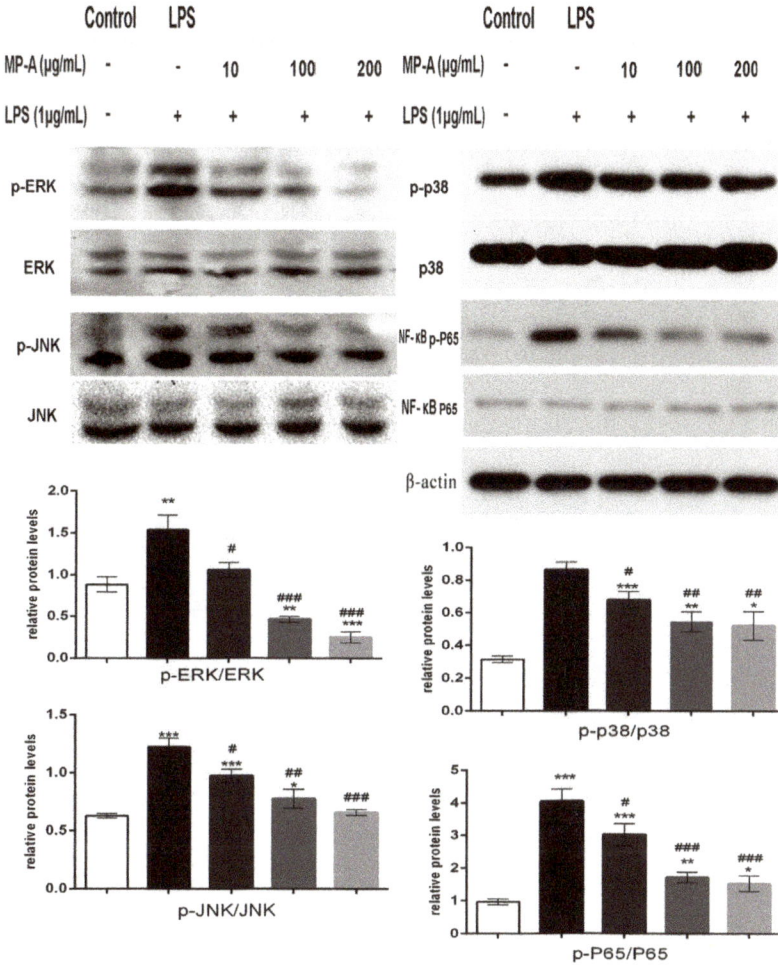

Figure 4. MP-A significantly attenuated LPS-induced activation of the mitogen-activated protein kinases (MAPK) and NF-κB signaling pathways in THP-1 cells. The ratios of p-p38/p38, p-JNK/JNK, p-ERK1/2/ERK1/2, and p-P65 /P65 were analyzed by western blot analysis. * $p < 0.05$, ** $p < 0.01$, *** $p < 0.001$, and **** $p < 0.0001$, when compared to controls; # $p < 0.05$, ## $p < 0.05$, ### $p < 0.001$, and #### $p < 0.0001$ compared to the LPS group ($n = 3$).

3.7. MP-A Prevented LPS-Induced Activation and the Nuclear Translocation of NF-κB in THP-1 Cells

NF-κB regulates many molecules of the various stages of the inflammatory response. In unstimulated control cells, NF-κB retains its original state as an inactive cytoplasmic complex by its inhibitor IκB. Upon LPS stimulation, the phosphorylation and degradation of IκB release NF-κB for nuclear translocation. We studied the NF-κB translocation using a primary antibody against the p65 subunit of NF-κB and the nuclei dye DAPI (Figure 5). When comparing with the control (Figure 5A(a–c)), NF-κB p65 traveled from the cytosol to the nucleus in macrophages by 1 μg/mL LPS treatment (Figure 5B(d–f)), however, 200 µg/mL MP-A obviously prevented LPS-induced activation and the nuclear translocation of p65 (Figure 5C(g–i)).

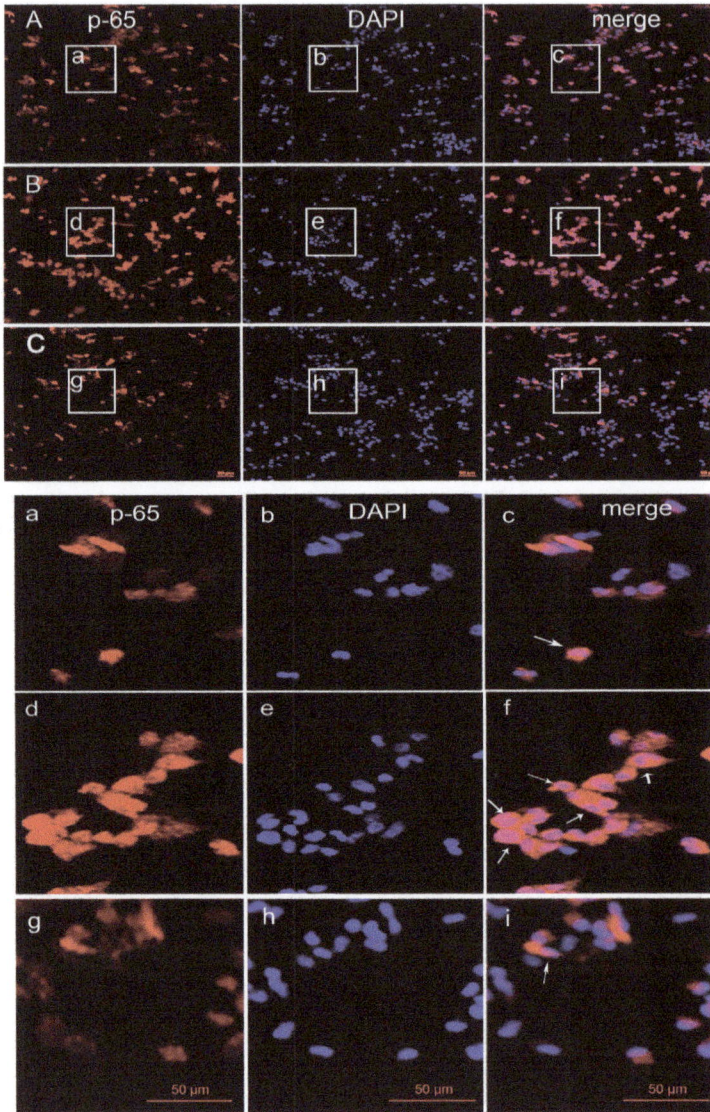

Figure 5. MP-A prevented LPS-induced activation and the nuclear translocation of NF-κB p65. THP-1 cells labeled with NF-κB subunit p65 (red) and DAPI (blue) were imaged simultaneously and merged (pink). (**A**) Control cells were treated with neither MP-A nor LPS solution. (**B**) Cells were treated with 1 µg/mL LPS for 24 h (**C**) Cells were treated with 200 µg/mL MP-A and 1 µg/mL LPS for 2 h. (a–i) Magnification imaging corresponding to the white boxes in Figure 5A–C. The images were obtained by confocal laser microscopy and overlay; the pink fluorescence (as white arrows show above) indicates location of p65 protein in nuclei.

3.8. Affinity of MP-A for Recombinant Human TLR4, TLR2, and Dectin-1

SPR technology (with a BIAcore 3000 biosensor system) was applied to analyze the affinity of MP-A for recombinant human TLR4, TLR2, and Dectin-1 proteins. Each of the proteins was immobilized on a CM5 chip (Figure 6A,C,E). The RU for TLR4, TLR2, and Dectin-1 bound to the CM5 chip surface was, respectively, 5022.4, 8333.8, and 1131.7. The sensorgrams of MP-A for TLR4, TLR2, and Dectin-1 demonstrated that MP-A exhibited a high binding affinity for TLR4 (KD = 5.07×10^{-5} M), but hardly any affinity for TLR2 and Dectin-1 even up to a concentration of 2500 μg/mL (Figure 6B,D,F).

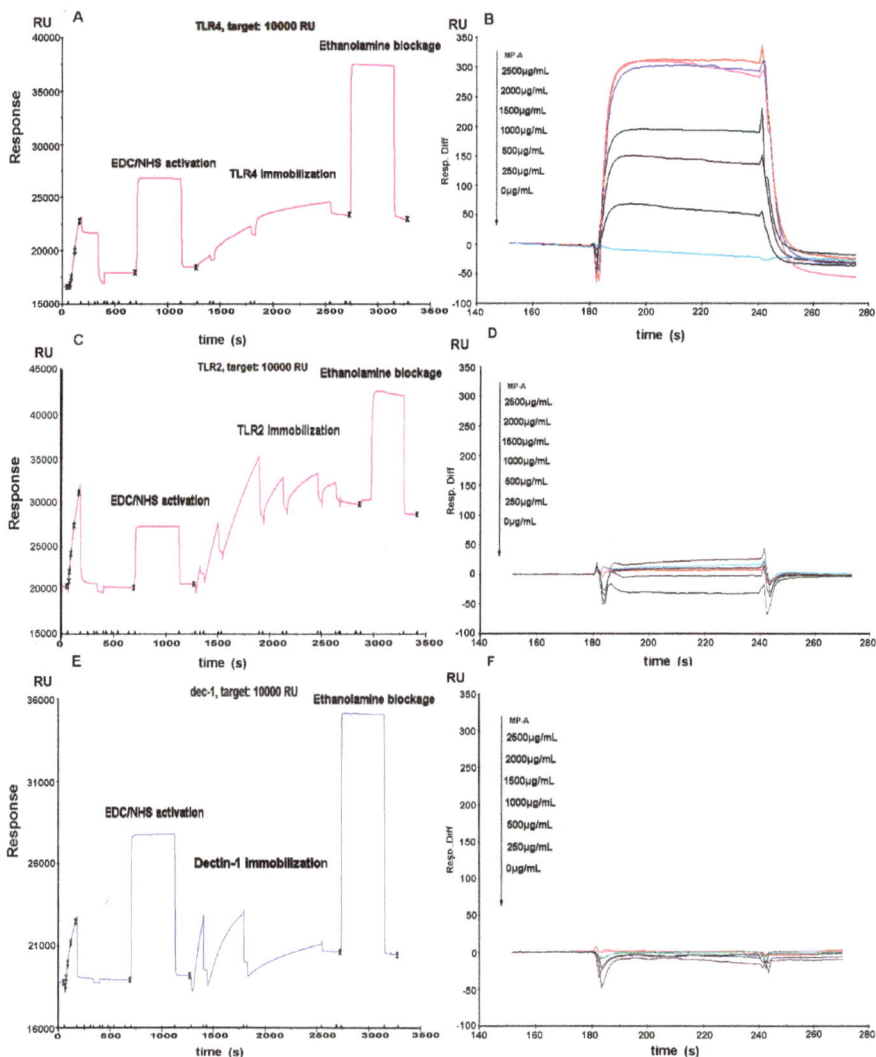

Figure 6. Binding affinity of MP-A for TLR4, TLR2, and Dectin-1, as evaluated by surface plasmon resonance (SPR) analysis. Cumulative MP-A concentrations were injected at 30 μL/min over 60-second association periods, with the concentrations shown next to the arrows. (**A,C,E**) TLR4, TLR2, and Dectin-1 immobilization on CM5 sensor chips, respectively. (**B,D,F**) Kinetic-binding responses of MP-A to TLR4, TLR2, and Dectin-1, respectively.

4. Discussion

The preset study used THP-1 macrophages as an in vitro cell model to investigate the effect of MP-A on immune modulation. Given that LPS has been previously shown to activate multiple signaling pathways in macrophages, and to thereby induce the production of pro-inflammatory mediators and cytokines such as NO, TNF-α, and interleukins, we chose LPS-stimulation as the method for inducing experimental inflammation of the THP-1 cells. The results of the present study demonstrate MP-A to exert an anti-inflammatory effect in LPS-stimulated THP-1 cells, via the inhibition of the TLR4/NFκB and MAPK pathways.

An increase in phagocytic activity is one of the most characteristic features of macrophage activation, and the phagocytosis and subsequent destruction of microorganisms is the most important function of monocytes and macrophages in maintaining the immune response against infection. LPS has been previously reported to suppress the phagocytosis of immunoglobulin G-opsonized sheep red blood cells (SRBCs) by peritoneal macrophages. LPS suppresses phagocytosis of SRBCs by altering the distribution of microfilaments and microtubules, and this suppression is independent of cytokine (IL-1, IL-6, TNF- or IFN α/β) production [27,28]. LPS has been reported to increase obviously the phagocytic activity in RAW264.7 macrophages [29,30]. The data generated in the present study suggest that LPS treatment markedly increased phagocytic activity in THP-1 macrophage cells, and furthermore, these effects were synergistically increased by combined treatment with LPS and MP-A. While the molecular mechanism underlying the increased phagocytosis induced by MP-A is unknown, we hypothesize that it is likely to be independent of cytokine production in a similar manner to LPS, since cytokine production was observed to be reduced by MP-A treatment in LPS-simulated THP-1 cells.

NO is a key molecule in immune function, and has been shown to exert beneficial biological effects in a variety of cell types involved in immunomodulatory, inflammatory, and/or other physiological processes [31,32]. NO is synthesized by a family of enzymes known as NOS, comprising three main isoforms, constitutive NOS (nNOS), endothelial constitutive NOS (eNOS), and inducible NOS (iNOS). Of these, iNOS is the pro-inflammatory enzyme that is most critical for upregulating the levels of NO production in response to pro-inflammatory stimuli. For example, LPS macrophage stimulation induces NO production via iNOS [33,34]. In the present study, MP-A treatment was shown to effectively inhibit NO production in LPS-activated THP-1 macrophages via the inhibition of iNOS protein expression, without affecting cell viability. In contrast, MP-A treatment alone was found to be insufficient to affect NO production.

Cyclooxygenase-1 (COX-1) and Cyclooxygenase-2 (COX-2) can regulate the production of prostaglandins [35]. COX-2 mediates the conversion of arachidonic acid to prostaglandin H2, a precursor of PGE$_2$, in activated macrophages. Overexpression of iNOS and COX-2 has been previously found to lead to the overproduction of NO and PGE$_2$, and this results in the development of inflammatory diseases. The results of the present study suggest that MP-A significantly suppresses COX-2 expression in LPS-stimulated THP-1 macrophages. Since one of the current strategies to mitigate inflammatory disorders is the modulation of iNOS and COX-2 expression, MP-A may be a promising potential therapeutic candidate for controlling inflammatory mediator overproduction.

TNF-α has been reported to trigger the downstream activation of inflammatory gene expression, and to cause rheumatoid arthritis, inflammatory bowel disease, psoriasis, and refractory asthma [36–39]. The present study demonstrated MP-A treatment of THP-1 cells to significantly attenuate TNF-α production in a dose-dependent manner. We previously observed a similar phenomenon to occur while treating RAW264.7 cells with curdlan sulfate (CS3) [29]. In the previous study, treatment with CS3 or curdlan alone was found to stimulate TNF-α production, whereas treatment of LPS-stimulated RAW264.7 cells with CS3 or curdlan instead attenuated TNF-α production to some extent. Another β-Glucan, LNT-S, that was isolated from *Lentinus edodes*, has also been determined to suppress NO and TNF-α production in LPS-stimulated RAW264.7 cells [15]. Interestingly, CS3, curdlan, and LNT-S have a β-glucan structure, while MP-A instead exhibits an α-glucan structure. Nevertheless, the results of the present study indicate that MP-A is similar to those β-glucans, and is a promising potential therapeutic agent for use in controlling diseases associated with pro-inflammatory mediator overproduction. β-glucans such as CS3 and LNT-S have been identified to bind the key macrophage surface receptor, Dectin-1 [15,28,29]. This receptor has been documented to be required for β-glucan recognition, and can collaborate with TLR2 to mediate the biological effects of β-glucans [40,41]. To determine whether MP-A binds to TLR2, TLR4, and/or Dectin-1 receptors, we evaluated potential interactions between MP-A and each of the three receptors using an SPR analysis. The results of this analysis show that MP-A can strongly bind TLR4, but not TLR2 nor Dectin-1, thus, TLR4, but not TLR2 or Dectin-1, can recognize the water-soluble α-glucan, MP-A.

TLR4 alone is not sufficient for LPS signaling, and indeed a secretory protein, MD-2, has also been shown to be an essential to this process [42]. TLR4 recognizes LPS in conjunction with MD-2 and CD14, such that they have been shown to form a physical complex on LPS-responsive cell surfaces [43,44]. We recently demonstrated LPS to exhibit a poor binding affinity for recombinant TLR4 using SPR technology, and provided more evidence for LPS signaling via TLR4 as a receptor is required for an additional molecule [30].

Various inflammatory diseases upregulate pro-inflammatory cytokines (such as TNF-α and IL-1β) and inflammatory mediators (such as NO and PGE$_2$) via the NF-κB and MAPKs signaling pathways in macrophages [45,46]. The present study aimed to elucidate the way in which MP-A interacts in these processes. The results show that MP-A can prevent LPS-induced activation via regulating the phosphorylation of MAP kinase and/or NF-κB p65 signaling pathway components (Figures 4 and 5). Specifically, MP-A inhibited LPS-induced iNOS and COX-2 expression, and subsequent NO and PGE$_2$ production, via the selective suppression of the phosphorylation of ERK1/2, JNK, and p38 in the MAPK signaling pathway, and the nuclear translocation of P65 in the NF-κB signaling pathway. The mechanism by which MP-A exerts this anti-inflammatory activity in LPS-stimulated THP-1 cells is likely due to competitive binding to TLR4 at the cell membrane, leading to the inhibition of the LPS-TLR4 signaling pathway, and thus inhibiting the downstream phosphorylation of MAPK and the nuclear translocation of NF-κB pathway components. Other molecules involved in the inhibition mechanism will be further studied in detail in our future work.

5. Conclusions

In summary, the high-molecular-weight α-D-Glucan MP-A, isolated from the hard-shelled mussel (*Mytilus coruscus*), has been observed to exert an anti-inflammatory effect, and thus represents a promising therapeutic candidate for the control of disease-associated pro-inflammatory mediator overproduction. The current study provides a preliminary pharmacological basis, and underlying molecular mechanism, for the use of MP-A in the control of inflammatory disorders.

Acknowledgments: The authors are grateful to Xiaonan Du and Jiawei Wu at the General Electric Co for the technical assistance with SPR. We also acknowledge funding from the National 863 Program (No. 2014AA093603). All authors have read and approved the final manuscript.

Author Contributions: The author contributions are as follows: Peixue Ling, Fengshan Wang, Xiqiang Zhu and Fuyan Liu conceived and designed the experiments; Fuyan Liu, XiaoFeng Zhang, Yuqiu Li, Qixin Chen, Xinlei Song and Fei Liu performed the experiments; Fuyan Liu, Li Mei and Xia Liu analyzed the data; Jinhua Zhang, Zhigang Song and Wen Zhang contributed reagents/material/analysis tools; Fuyan Liu wrote the paper.

Conflicts of Interest: The authors declare no conflict of interest.

Abbreviations

LPS	lipopolysaccharide
TLR4	Toll-like receptor 4
TLR2	Toll-like receptor 2
TLRs	toll like receptors
TNF-α	tumor necrosis factor α

iNOS	inducible nitric oxide synthase
COX-2	cyclooxygenase-2
PGE$_2$	prostaglandin E2
SPR	surface plasmon resonance
CCK-8	Cell Counting Kit-8
PMA	phorbol-12-myristate-13-acetate
DAPI	2-(4-amidinophenyl)-6-indolecarbamidine dihydrochloride
MAPK	mitogen-activated protein kinase
ERK	extracellular signal regulated kinase
JNK	c-Jun N terminal kinase
NF-κB	nuclear factor-kappa B

References

1. Xu, H.; Guo, T.; Guo, Y.F.; Zhang, J.; Li, Y.; Feng, W.; Jiao, B. Characterization and protection on acute liver injury of a polysaccharide mp-i from *mytilus coruscus*. *Glycobiology* **2008**, *18*, 97–103. [CrossRef] [PubMed]
2. Kim, E.-K.; Oh, H.-J.; Kim, Y.-S.; Hwang, J.-W.; Ahn, C.-B.; Lee, J.S.; Jeon, Y.-J.; Moon, S.-H.; Sung, S.H.; Jeon, B.-T.; et al. Purification of a novel peptide derived from *mytilus coruscus* and in vitro/in vivo evaluation of its bioactive properties. *Fish Shellfish Immunol.* **2013**, *34*, 1078–1084. [CrossRef] [PubMed]
3. Kim, Y.S.; Ahn, C.B.; Je, J.Y. Anti-inflammatory action of high molecular weight mytilus edulis hydrolysates fraction in lps-induced raw264.7 macrophage via nf-kappab and mapk pathways. *Food Chem.* **2016**, *202*, 9–14. [CrossRef] [PubMed]
4. Li, G.; Fu, Y.; Zheng, J.; Li, D. Anti-inflammatory activity and mechanism of a lipid extract from hard-shelled mussel (*mytilus coruscus*) on chronic arthritis in rats. *Mar. Drugs* **2014**, *12*, 568–588. [CrossRef] [PubMed]
5. Tzianabos, A.O. Polysaccharide immunomodulators as therapeutic agents: Structural aspects and biologic function. *Clin. Microbiol. Rev.* **2000**, *13*, 523–533. [CrossRef] [PubMed]
6. Cavaillon, J.M. Cytokines and macrophages. *Biomed. Pharmacother.* **1994**, *48*, 445–453. [CrossRef]
7. Miller, T.E.; Ormrod, D.J.; Geddes, R. Anti-inflammatory activity of glycogen extracted from perna canaliculus (nz green-lipped mussel). *Agents Actions* **1993**, *38*, 139–142. [CrossRef]
8. Cesaretti, M.; Luppi, E.; Maccari, F.; Volpi, N. Isolation and characterization of a heparin with high anticoagulant activity from the clam tapes phylippinarum: Evidence for the presence of a high content of antithrombin iii binding site. *Glycobiology* **2004**, *14*, 1275–1284. [CrossRef] [PubMed]
9. Luan, J.; Xin, T.; Chu, Z.Y.; Wang, J.C.; Zhang, S.; Shen, Y. Immunomodulation of mytihus edulis linnaeus polysaccharides in mice. *Chin. J. Mar. Drugs* **2010**, *29*, 39–41.
10. Mao, J.; Hou, Z.; Chen, D.; Zhang, W. Anti-hyperlipi-demic effects of polysaccharide ma from *mytilus coruscus* on experimental atherosclerosis in rabitts. *J. Pharm. Pract.* **2014**, *32*, 27–30.
11. Czop, J.K. The role of beta-glucan receptors on blood and tissue leukocytes in phagocytosis and metabolic activation. *Pathol. Immunopathol. Res.* **1986**, *5*, 286–296. [CrossRef] [PubMed]
12. Williams, D.L. Overview of (1→3)-β-D-glucan immunobiology. *Mediat. Inflamm.* **1997**, *6*, 247–250. [CrossRef] [PubMed]
13. Ross, G.D.; Vetvicka, V.; Yan, J.; Xia, Y.; Vetvickova, J. Therapeutic intervention with complement and beta-glucan in cancer. *Immunopharmacology* **1999**, *42*, 61–74. [CrossRef]
14. Muller, A.; Rice, P.J.; Ensley, H.E.; Coogan, P.S.; Kalbfleish, J.H.; Kelley, J.L.; Love, E.J.; Portera, C.A.; Ha, T.; Browder, L.W.; et al. Receptor binding and internalization of a water-soluble (1→3)-β-D-glucan biologic response modifier in two monocyte/macrophage cell lines. *J. Immunol.* **1996**, *156*, 3418–3425. [PubMed]
15. Xu, X.; Yasuda, M.; Nakamura-Tsuruta, S.; Mizuno, M.; Ashida, H. Beta-glucan from lentinus edodes inhibits nitric oxide and tumor necrosis factor-alpha production and phosphorylation of mitogen-activated protein kinases in lipopolysaccharide-stimulated murine raw 264.7 macrophages. *J. Biol. Chem.* **2012**, *287*, 871–878. [CrossRef] [PubMed]
16. Yang, X.B.; Gao, X.D.; Han, F.; Xu, B.S.; Song, Y.C.; Tan, R.X. Purification, characterization and enzymatic degradation of ycp, a polysaccharide from marine filamentous fungus phoma herbarum ys4108. *Biochimie* **2005**, *87*, 747–754. [CrossRef] [PubMed]

17. Zhu, R.; Zhang, X.; Liu, W.; Zhou, Y.; Ding, R.; Yao, W.; Gao, X. Preparation and immunomodulating activities of a library of low-molecular-weight alpha-glucans. *Carbohydr. Polym.* **2014**, *111*, 744–752. [CrossRef] [PubMed]

18. Chanput, W.; Mes, J.J.; Wichers, H.J. Thp-1 cell line: An in vitro cell model for immune modulation approach. *Int. Immunopharmacol.* **2014**, *23*, 37–45. [CrossRef] [PubMed]

19. Beutler, B.; Rietschel, E.T. Innate immune sensing and its roots: The story of endotoxin. *Nat. Rev. Immunol.* **2003**, *3*, 169–176. [CrossRef] [PubMed]

20. Lee, S.H.; Soyoola, E.; Chanmugam, P.; Hart, S.; Sun, W.; Zhong, H.; Liou, S.; Simmons, D.; Hwang, D. Selective expression of mitogen-inducible cyclooxygenase in macrophages stimulated with lipopolysaccharide. *J. Biol. Chem.* **1992**, *267*, 25934–25938. [PubMed]

21. Buchanan, M.M.; Hutchinson, M.; Watkins, L.; Yin, H. Toll-like receptor 4 in cns pathologies. *J. Neurochem.* **2010**, *114*, 13–27. [CrossRef] [PubMed]

22. Uto, T.; Fujii, M.; Hou, D.-X. 6-(methylsulfinyl)hexyl isothiocyanate suppresses inducible nitric oxide synthase expression through the inhibition of janus kinase 2-mediated jnk pathway in lipopolysaccharide-activated murine macrophages. *Biochem. Pharmacol.* **2005**, *70*, 1211–1221. [CrossRef] [PubMed]

23. Zar, P.P.K.; Morishita, A.; Hashimoto, F.; Sakao, K.; Fujii, M.; Wada, K.; Hou, D.-X. Anti-inflammatory effects and molecular mechanisms of loquat (eriobotrya japonica) tea. *J. Funct. Foods* **2014**, *6*, 523–533. [CrossRef]

24. Zhou, J.; Zhu, P.; Jiang, J.L.; Zhang, Q.; Wu, Z.B.; Yao, X.Y.; Tang, H.; Lu, N.; Yang, Y.; Chen, Z.N. Involvement of cd147 in overexpression of mmp-2 and mmp-9 and enhancement of invasive potential of pma-differentiated thp-1. *BMC Cell Biol.* **2005**, *6*, 25. [CrossRef] [PubMed]

25. Zhuang, X.; Pang, X.; Zhang, W.; Wu, W.; Zhao, J.; Yang, H.; Qu, W. Effects of zinc and manganese on advanced glycation end products (ages) formation and ages-mediated endothelial cell dysfunction. *Life Sci.* **2012**, *90*, 131–139. [CrossRef] [PubMed]

26. Xu, Z.; Lin, S.; Wu, W.; Tan, H.; Wang, Z.; Cheng, C.; Lu, L.; Zhang, X. Ghrelin prevents doxorubicin-induced cardiotoxicity through tnf-alpha/nf-kappab pathways and mitochondrial protective mechanisms. *Toxicology* **2008**, *247*, 133–138. [CrossRef] [PubMed]

27. Wonderling, R.S.; Ghaffar, A.; Mayer, E.P. Lipopolysaccharide-induced suppression of phagocytosis: Effects on the phagocytic machinery. *Immunopharmacol. Immunotoxicol.* **1996**, *18*, 267–289. [CrossRef] [PubMed]

28. De Lima, T.M.; Sampaio, S.C.; Petroni, R.; Brigatte, P.; Velasco, I.T.; Soriano, F.G. Phagocytic activity of lps tolerant macrophages. *Mol. Immunol.* **2014**, *60*, 8–13. [CrossRef] [PubMed]

29. Li, P.; Zhang, X.; Cheng, Y.; Li, J.; Xiao, Y.; Zhang, Q.; Zong, A.; Zhong, C.; Wang, F. Preparation and in vitro immunomodulatory effect of curdlan sulfate. *Carbohydr. Polym.* **2014**, *102*, 852–861. [CrossRef] [PubMed]

30. Liu, F.; Zhang, X.; Ling, P.; Liao, J.; Zhao, M.; Mei, L.; Shao, H.; Jiang, P.; Song, Z.; Chen, Q.; et al. Immunomodulatory effects of xanthan gum in lps-stimulated raw 264.7 macrophages. *Carbohydr. Polym.* **2017**, *169*, 65–74. [CrossRef] [PubMed]

31. Davis, K.L.; Martin, E.; Turko, I.V.; Murad, F. Novel effects of nitric oxide. *Annu. Rev. Pharmacol. Toxicol.* **2001**, *41*, 203–236. [CrossRef] [PubMed]

32. Nathan, C. Nitric oxide as a secretory product of mammalian cells. *FASEB J.* **1992**, *6*, 3051–3064. [PubMed]

33. Ohno, N.; Hashimoto, T.; Adachi, Y.; Yadomae, T. Corrigendum to: "Conformation dependency of nitric oxide synthesis of murine peritoneal macrophages by β-glucans in vitro" [immunol. Lett. 52 (1996) 1–7]. *Immunol. Lett.* **1996**, *53*, 157–163. [CrossRef]

34. Gupta, S.C.; Sundaram, C.; Reuter, S.; Aggarwal, B.B. Inhibiting nf-kappab activation by small molecules as a therapeutic strategy. *Biochim. Biophys. Acta* **2010**, *1799*, 775–787. [CrossRef] [PubMed]

35. Iezzi, A.; Ferri, C.; Mezzetti, A.; Cipollone, F. Cox-2: Friend or foe? *Curr. Pharm. Des.* **2007**, *13*, 1715–1721. [CrossRef] [PubMed]

36. Han, G.; Wang, G.; Zhu, X.; Shao, H.; Liu, F.; Yang, P.; Ying, Y.; Wang, F.; Ling, P. Preparation of xanthan gum injection and its protective effect on articular cartilage in the development of osteoarthritis. *Carbohydr. Polym.* **2012**, *87*, 1837–1842. [CrossRef]

37. Kim, Y.S.; Ko, H.M.; Kang, N.I.; Song, C.H.; Zhang, X.; Chung, W.C.; Kim, J.H.; Choi, I.H.; Park, Y.M.; Kim, G.Y. Mast cells play a key role in the development of late airway hyperresponsiveness through tnf-α in a murine model of asthma. *Eur. J. Immunol.* **2007**, *37*, 1107–1115. [CrossRef] [PubMed]

38. Roux, C.H.; Brocq, O.; Breuil, V.; Albert, C.; Euller-Ziegler, L. Safety of anti-tnf-alpha therapy in rheumatoid arthritis and spondylarthropathies with concurrent b or c chronic hepatitis. *Rheumatology* **2006**, *45*, 1294–1297. [CrossRef] [PubMed]

39. Stokkers, P.; Camoglio, L.; Van Deventer, S. Tumor necrosis factor (tnf) in inflammatory bowel disease: Gene polymorphisms, animal models, and potential for anti-tnf therapy. *J. Inflamm.* **1994**, *47*, 97–103.

40. Brown, G.D. Dectin-1: A signalling non-tlr pattern-recognition receptor. *Nat. Rev. Immunol.* **2006**, *6*, 33–43. [CrossRef] [PubMed]

41. Gantner, B.N.; Simmons, R.M.; Canavera, S.J.; Akira, S.; Underhill, D.M. Collaborative induction of inflammatory responses by dectin-1 and toll-like receptor 2. *J. Exp. Med.* **2003**, *197*, 1107–1117. [CrossRef] [PubMed]

42. Takeuchi, A.; Kamiryou, Y.; Yamada, H.; Eto, M.; Shibata, K.; Haruna, K.; Naito, S.; Yoshikai, Y. Oral administration of xanthan gum enhances antitumor activity through toll-like receptor 4. *Int. Immunopharmacol.* **2009**, *9*, 1562–1567. [CrossRef] [PubMed]

43. Shimazu, R.; Akashi, S.; Ogata, H.; Nagai, Y.; Fukudome, K.; Miyake, K.; Kimoto, M. Md-2, a molecule that confers lipopolysaccharide responsiveness on toll-like receptor 4. *J. Exp. Med.* **1999**, *189*, 1777–1782. [CrossRef] [PubMed]

44. Fujimoto, T.; Yamazaki, S.; Eto-Kimura, A.; Takeshige, K.; Muta, T. The amino-terminal region of toll-like receptor 4 is essential for binding to md-2 and receptor translocation to the cell surface. *J. Biol. Chem.* **2004**, *279*, 47431–47437. [CrossRef] [PubMed]

45. Moynagh, P.N. The nf-κb pathway. *J. Cell Sci.* **2005**, *118*, 4589–4592. [CrossRef] [PubMed]

46. Tak, P.P.; Firestein, G.S. Nf-κb: A key role in inflammatory diseases. *J. Clin. Investig.* **2001**, *107*, 7–11. [CrossRef] [PubMed]

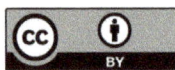

marine drugs

MDPI

Article

Protective Effect of Pyrogallol-Phloroglucinol-6,6-Bieckol from *Ecklonia cava* on Monocyte-Associated Vascular Dysfunction

Seyeon Oh [1,†], Myeongjoo Son [1,2,†], Hye Sun Lee [1,3], Hyun-Soo Kim [4], You-Jin Jeon [4,*] and Kyunghee Byun [1,2,3,*]

[1] Functional Cellular Networks Laboratory, Lee Gil Ya Cancer and Diabetes Institute, Gachon University, Incheon 21999, Korea; seyeon8965@gachon.ac.kr (S.O.); mjson@gachon.ac.kr (M.S.); 201740538@gc.gachon.ac.kr (H.S.L.)
[2] Department of Anatomy & Cell Biology, Graduate School of Medicine, Gachon University, Incheon 21936, Korea
[3] Department of Health Sciences and Technology, GAIHST, Gachon University, Incheon 21999, Korea
[4] Department of Marine Life Science, Jeju National University, Jeju 63243, Korea; gustn783@naver.com
* Correspondence: youjinj@jejunu.ac.kr (Y.-J.J.); khbyun1@gachon.ac.kr (K.B.); Tel.: +82-64-754-3475 (Y.-J.J.); +82-32-899-6511 (K.B.)
† These authors contributed equally to this work.

Received: 23 October 2018; Accepted: 6 November 2018; Published: 9 November 2018

Abstract: *Ecklonia cava* (*E. cava*) can alleviate vascular dysfunction in diseases associated with poor circulation. *E. cava* contains various polyphenols with different functions, but few studies have compared the effects of these polyphenols. Here, we comparatively investigated four major compounds present in an ethanoic extract of *E. cava*. These four major compounds were isolated and their effects were examined on monocyte-associated vascular inflammation and dysfunctions. Pyrogallol-phloroglucinol-6,6-bieckol (PPB) significantly inhibited monocyte migration in vitro by reducing levels of inflammatory macrophage differentiation and of its related molecular factors. In addition, PPB protected against monocyte-associated endothelial cell death by increasing the phosphorylations of PI3K-AKT and AMPK, decreasing caspase levels, and reducing monocyte-associated vascular smooth muscle cell proliferation and migration by decreasing the phosphorylations of ERK and AKT. The results of this study show that four compounds were effective for reduction of monocyte-associated vascular inflammation and dysfunctions, but PPB might be more useful for the treatment of vascular dysfunction in diseases associated with poor circulation.

Keywords: poor blood circulation; *Ecklonia cava*; phlorotannins; pyrogallol-phloroglucinol-6,6-bieckol; functional ingredients; endothelial cell death; vascular smooth muscle cell proliferation and migration; inflammation

1. Introduction

Weight gain has been intimately associated with diseases associated with poor circulation, such as stroke, atherosclerosis and high blood pressure [1,2]. Most obese individuals have elevated blood levels of glucose, low-density lipoprotein (LDL) or free fatty acids (FFA), and these changes can alter blood functions and blood vessel construction.

In blood vessel walls, endothelial cells (ECs) and vascular smooth muscle cells (VSMCs) influence vessel tone. ECs form vessel barriers, regulating blood flow and inflammatory response, whereas VSMCs have proliferative, contractile and biosynthetic roles in vessel walls. Alterations in the differentiated states of these cells play critical roles in the pathogeneses disease associated with poor circulation. Saturated free fatty acids (FFA), elevated glucose or LDL lead to EC and VSMC dysfunction.

Furthermore, these abnormal changes induce bioavailable nitric oxide (NO) deficiency, reduce vascular relaxation, induce the overproductions of growth factors, increase adhesion and inflammatory molecule expressions, induce the generation of reactive oxygen species (ROS) in ECs [3–5], adversely influence glucose metabolism, and promote the abnormal proliferation and migration of VSMCs [6,7].

High glucose, LDL and FFA can also indirectly affect ECs and VSMCs via the inflammation induction of monocytes. Obesity affects the activations of circulating monocytes. In particular, high glucose levels increase monocyte adhesion and trans-endothelial migration by activating the AKT-GSK axis [8], which leads to the inductions of inflammatory factors, such as tumor necrosis factor-alpha (TNF-α), monocyte chemoattractant protein-1 (MCP-1), interleukin-beta (IL-1β) and Toll-like receptors (TLRs) via oxidant stress [9–11].

Edible marine plants have emerged as a potential source of bioactive compounds for the developments of cosmeceutical ingredients [12]. *Ecklonia cava* (*E. cava*) is an edible marine brown alga, and it is one of nature's richest sources of phlorotannins, and phlorotannin derivatives which do not exist in land-originating plants. The phlorotannins are a sub-classification of polyphenolic compounds that are confirmed by dibenzo-1,4-dioxin backbone which is this backbone linkage can make the structure tight and strongly interact with various biological molecules [13,14]. *E. cava* extracts have been shown to suppress the production of inflammatory cytokines and the activation of NF-κB in lipopolysaccharide (LPS) challenged human ECs and to reduce vascular inflammation by preventing oxidation [13,15].

Some studies have shown these compounds have different beneficial effects of various *E. cava* phlorotannins, but the efficacies of these compounds have not been previously compared. In a previous study [16], we successfully isolated four phlorotannins from an ethanoic extract of *E. cava*, that is, dieckol, 2,7-phloroglucinol-6,6-bieckol (PHB), phlorofucofuroeckol-A (PFFA), and pyrogallol-phloroglucinol-6,6-bieckol (PPB), by centrifugal partition chromatography. In the present study, we sought to determine which compound most effectively inhibits monocyte migration and differentiation to inflammatory macrophages and monocyte-associated vascular cell dysfunction in vitro.

2. Results and Discussion

2.1. Structures of the Four Compounds Isolated from E. cava

The four compounds were isolated and purified using centrifugal partition chromatography in one step [16]. The peaks a-d on the high-performance liquid chromatography (HPLC) shown in Figure S1 were assigned to DK, PHB, PFFA and PPB, respectively by mass spectrometry analysis (Figure S2). They show a single peak in the HPLC chromatogram and had a purity of 90% or more. Our previous study shown the 4 compounds identified using ^{1}H NMR and ^{13}C NMR and HPLC–DAD–ESI/MS (negative ion mode) analyses [16] and each chemical structure shown in Figure 1. Previous studies on various biological properties of phlorotannins including anti-oxidant [17], anti-inflammation [18], anti-neurodegeneration [19], anti-cancer [20,21], and anti-cardiovascular diseases [22] of *E. cava* extract have shown. Among numerous properties, anti-oxidant activities of *E. cava* phlorotannins extract on reactive oxygen species (ROS) have shown it exhibits radical scavenging activity against oxidized low-density lipoprotein (ox-LDL), 1,1-diphenyl-2-picrylhydrazyl (DPPH) radicals, and peroxynitrite [14,16,17] and these anti-oxidant activities closely related with other beneficial effects of *E. cava*.

Interestingly, the difference in anti-oxidant effect between various *E. cava* phlorotannins is related to the number of hydroxyl groups present. According to a study by Li and colleagues, dieckol and 6,6'-bieckol (more than 10 OH groups) had higher anti-oxidant efficacy than phloroglucinol and eckol (less than 10 OH groups) [14]. The PPB used in this study is also expected to have anti-inflammatory effects, including monocyte migration and macrophage polarization, because of the presence of 15 OH groups.

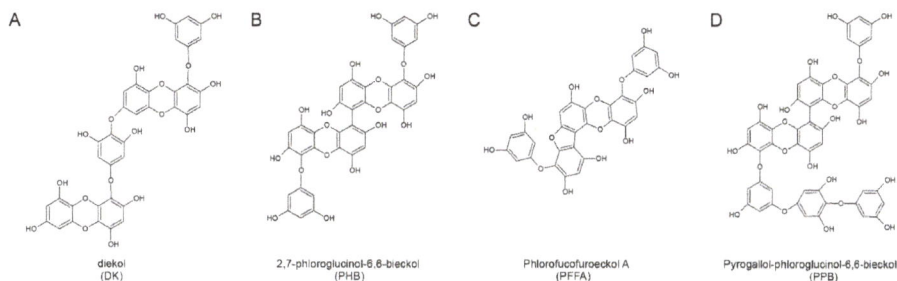

Figure 1. The chemical structures of the four major compounds isolated from *E. cava*. (**A–D**) Chemical structures of dieckol (DK), 2,7-phloroglucinol-6,6-bieckol (PHB), phlorofucofuroeckol-A (PFFA), and pyrogallol-phloroglucinol-6,6-bieckol (PPB).

2.2. Analysis of the Effects of 4 Compounds on Monocyte Migration and Macrophage Polarization

In diseases associated with inadequacy of blood flow in organs [23], monocyte migration is important and closely related to vascular inflammation. Figure 2A provides a schematic of the inhibitory effects of these four compounds on palmitic acid conjugated bovine serum albumin (PA-BSA) induced monocyte trans-migration and macrophage polarization (Figure 2A). Experiments were performed on two monocyte cell lines (P388D1 and Raw 264.7). Numbers of trans-migrating monocytes were greatest for PA-BSA-treated monocytes, and all four compounds significantly reduced numbers of migrating cells (Figure 2B) and the results were similar in Raw 264.7 (Figure S3A). Trans-migrating monocytes differentiated to macrophages of the pro-inflammatory (M1 type macrophages) or anti-inflammatory (M2 type macrophages) types (Figure 2C–F). Furthermore, PA-BSA-treated monocytes contained elevated levels of inflammatory factors, including inducible nitric oxide synthase (iNOS), CD80, TNF-α and interleukin-1β (IL-1β) (Figure 2C,D) and low levels of anti-inflammatory like arginase-1 (Arg-1), CD206, transforming growth factor beta 1 (TGF-β) and interleukin-10 (IL-10) (Figure 2E,F) and the results were similar in Raw 264.7 (Figure S3B–E). Interestingly, when monocytes were treated with four compounds with PA-BSA and these inductions were reduced, PPB had the greatest effect. As well as its anti-oxidant effects, *E. cava* extract has anti-inflammatory effects. For example, an ethanoic extract of *E. cava* was found to contain large amounts of phlorotannins and to inhibit the productions of prostaglandin-E2 (PGE2) and nitric oxide (NO) and suppress cyclooxygenase-2 (COX-2) and iNOS expressions in LPS-stimulated Raw 264.7 cells [24]. In inflammatory lung diseases, *E. cava* extract was found to significantly reduce inflammatory reactions, such as eosinophil migration to lungs, inflammatory cell and cytokine increases, and to reduce airway epithelial hyperplasia, lung fibrosis and smooth muscle cell thickness [14,15,17,25].

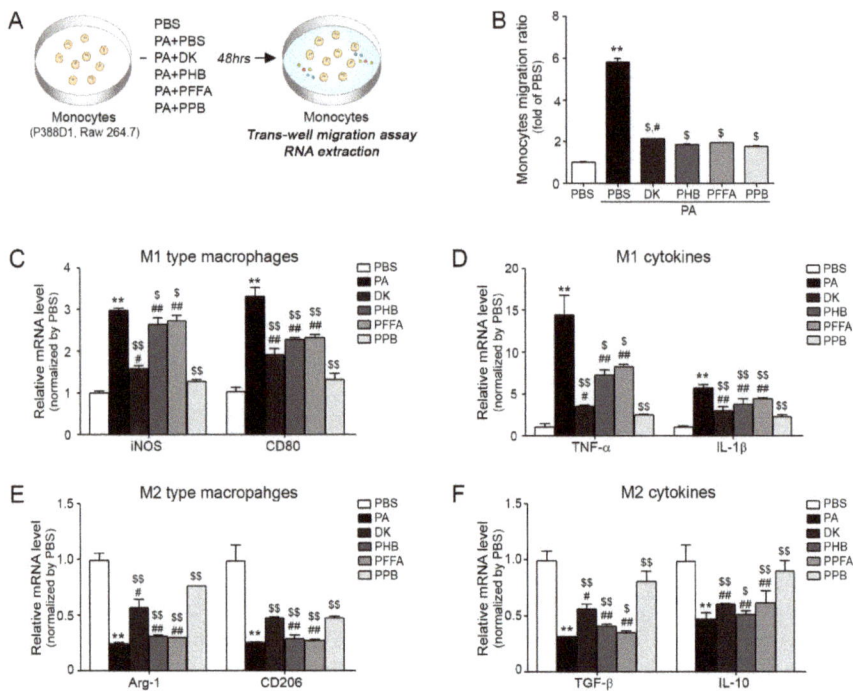

Figure 2. Inhibitory effects of PPB on monocyte polarization and related cytokines and EC dysfunction. (**A**) Illustration showing the palmitic acid conjugated bovine serum albumin (PA-BSA)-treated monocyte trans-migration model. (**B**) Migrating monocytes levels in 4 compounds with PA-BSA as determined by the trans-well migration assay. (**C,D**) mRNA expression levels of M1 type macrophages (inducible nitric oxide synthase (*iNOS*) and *Cd80*) and M2 type macrophages (arginase-1 (*Arg-1*) and *Cd206*) as determined by quantitative real-time polymerase chain reaction (qRT-PCR). (**E,F**) mRNA expression levels of M1 related cytokines (tumor necrosis factor-alpha (*TNF-α*) and interleukin-beta (*IL-1β*)) and M2 related cytokines (transforming growth factor beta 1 (*TGF-β*) and interleukin-10 (*IL-10*)) by qRT-PCR. Kruskal–Wallis tests were used to determine differences between groups and post-hoc comparisons were made with the Mann–Whitney U test **, $p < 0.01$, ***, $p < 0.001$, vs. PBS; $, $p < 0.05$, $$, $p < 0.01$, vs. PA-BSA; #, $p < 0.05$, ##, $p < 0.01$, vs. PA-BSA with PPB, DK; dieckol, PHB; 2,7-phloroglucinol-6,6-bieckol, PFFA; phlorofucofuroeckol-A, PPB; pyrogallol-phloroglucinol-6,6-bieckol.

2.3. Effects of Four Compounds on Monocyte-Induced Endothelial Cell Death

The inhibiting effects of four compounds on PA-BSA treated ECs and VSMCs dysfunctions induced by monocytes are summarized in Figure 3 and Figure 4. Monocytes were treated four compounds with PA-BSA respectively, and then each conditioned medium (CM) from the four compounds treated monocytes was incubated with ECs or VSMCs for 24 h (Figure 3A and Figure 4B). Adhesion molecule expressions (E-selectin, intercellular adhesion molecule 1; ICAM-1, vascular cell adhesion molecule 1; VCAM-1 and von Willebrand factor; vWF) in ECs were significantly higher when they were treated with PA-BSA CM than BSA CM, but the expression was significantly lowest when ECs were treated with PPB CM (Figure 3B). The various adhesion molecules are related to vascular inflammation, and these molecules are regulated by mast cells, macrophages, and neutrophils, which also secrete pro-inflammatory cytokines, such as TNF-α, interferon gamma (IFN-γ), and IL-6. These pro-inflammatory cytokines induce the expressions of adhesion molecules in ECs and recruit leukocytes, which are important components of the pathogenesis of vascular inflammation [26,27].

Adhesion molecules are also related to EC survival [21]. In addition to the abovementioned adhesion molecule changes, all four compounds improved the survival ratios of PA-BSA CM treated ECs, and PPB CM treated cells had the lowest levels of caspases 3 and 8 and it was related with the phosphorylated PI3K-AKT-eNOS and AMPK signaling pathways (Figure 3C,E and Figure S4). In addition, although the AKT inhibitor A6730 was treated, the expression of pAKT was increased in the single compounds treated group (Figure 3D). In ECs, the PI3K-AKT pathway is essential for mediating cell survival, migration, proliferation, and angiogenesis [28,29]. In particular, high glucose-induced EC apoptosis depends on Akt de-phosphorylation and activation of the PI3K/AKT/eNOS signaling pathway protects ECs from apoptosis [30].

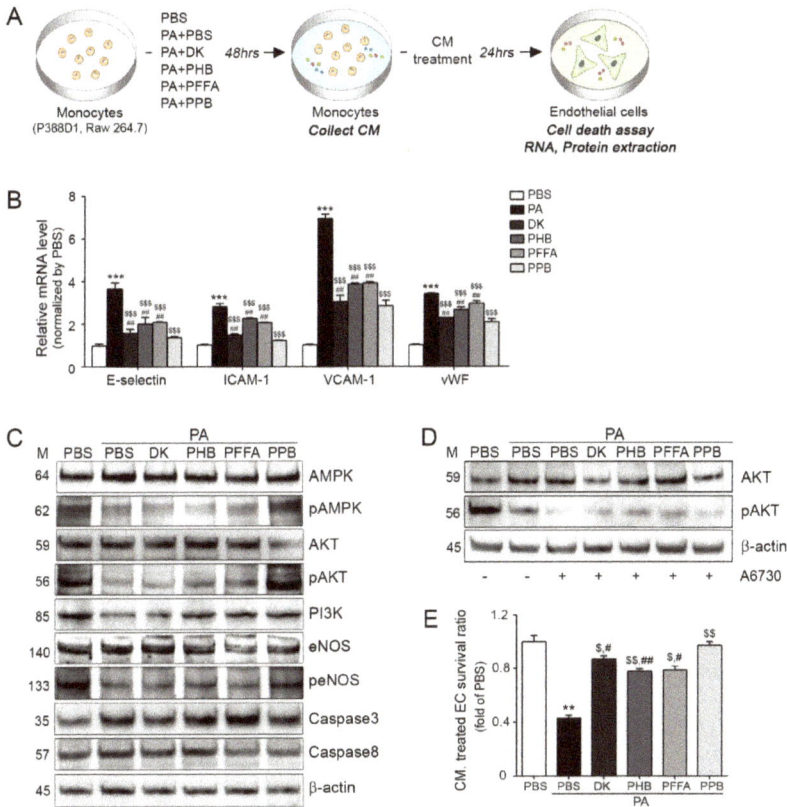

Figure 3. Prevention of monocyte-induced endothelial cell death by DK, PHB, PFFA or PPB. (**A**) Endothelial cells (ECs) were treated with conditioned medium (CM) collected from PA-BSA induced transmigrating monocytes. (**B**) mRNA expression levels of adhesion molecules (*E-selectin*, *ICAM-1*, *VCAM-1* and *vWF*) in CM treated ECs were measured by qRT-PCR. (**C**) Protein levels of cell-death related molecules, that is, AMPK, pAMPK, AKT, pAKT, PI3K eNOS, peNOS, Caspase 3, and Caspase 8 in CM treated endothelial cells were determined by western blotting. (**D**) The AKT inhibitor (A6370) was treated to monocyte and collected CM was treated EC. The ECs determined by western blotting. (**E**) Survival levels of CM treated ECs were measured using a cell survival assay. Kruskal–Wallis tests were used to determine differences between groups and post-hoc comparisons were made with the Mann–Whitney U test. **, $p < 0.01$, ***, $p < 0.001$, vs. PBS; $, $p < 0.05$, $$, $p < 0.01$, $$$, $p < 0.001$, vs. PA-BSA; #, $p < 0.05$, ##, $p < 0.01$ vs. PA-BSA with PPB, DK; dieckol, PHB; 2,7-phloroglucinol-6,6-bieckol, PFFA; phlorofucofuroeckol-A, PPB; pyrogallol-phloroglucinol-6,6-bieckol.

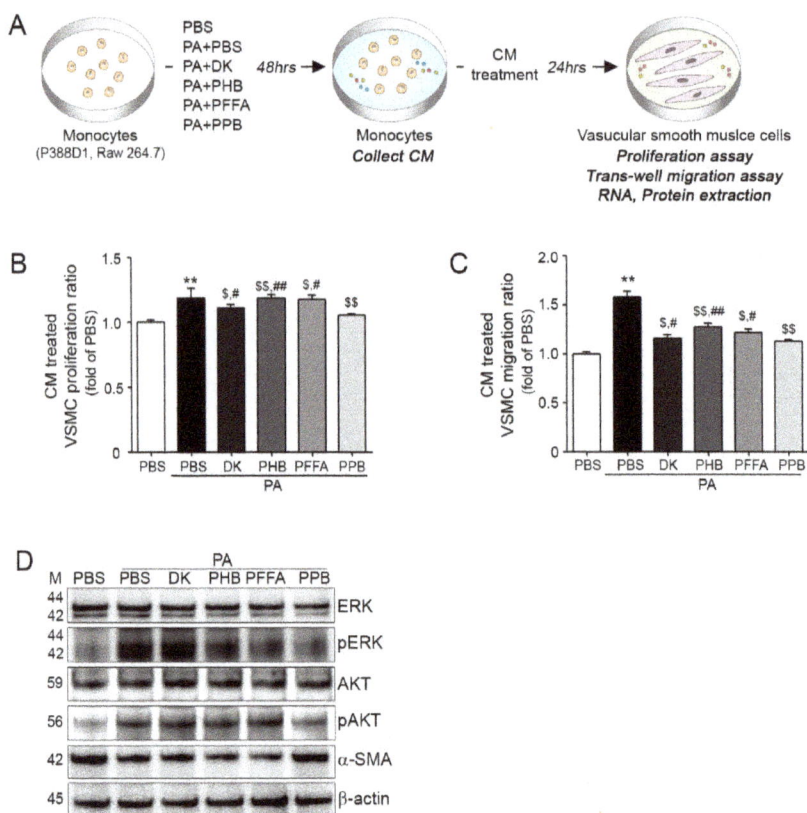

Figure 4. DK, PHB, PFFA or PPB inhibited monocytes migration and prevented monocyte-associated vascular smooth muscle cell proliferation and migration. (**A**) Illustration of the CM-induced vascular smooth muscle cells (VSMCs) proliferation and trans-migration model. (**B**) VSMC proliferation after CM treatments were measured using a proliferation assay. (**C**) Trans-migrating VSMC numbers were measured using a trans-migration assay. (**D**) Protein levels of proliferation and migration related molecules, that is, ERk, pERK, AKT, pAKT, α-SMA in CM treated VSMCs were determined by western blotting. Kruskal–Wallis tests were used to determine differences between groups and post-hoc comparisons were made with the Mann–Whitney U test. **, $p < 0.01$, vs. PBS; $, $p < 0.05$, $$, $p < 0.01$, vs. PA-BSA; #, $p < 0.05$, ##, $p < 0.01$, vs. PA-BSA with PPB, DK; Dieckol, PHB; 2,7-phloroglucinol-6,6-bieckol, PFFA; phlorofucofuroeckol-A, PPB; pyrogallol-phloroglucinol-6,6-bieckol.

2.4. Effects of All Four Compounds on Monocyte-Induced VSMC Proliferation and Migration

DK, PHB, PFFA and PPB CM treated VSMCs proliferated and migrated significantly less than PA-BSA CM treated VSMCs, and PPB CM was related with phosphorylations of the AKT and ERK pathways (Figure 4B–D), and the results were similar in Raw 264.7 (Figure S5). In addition, PA-BSA CM treated VSMCs had the highest α-SMA levels, and PPB CM had greatest effect, suggesting VSMCs would be closer to the contractile phenotype (Figure 4D and Figure S5C). Phenotype switching of VSMCs is important for the maintenance of vascular tone and alpha-smooth muscle actin (α-SMA) promotes the synthetic phenotype. In previous studies, higher expression of α-SMA in PA-BSA than in BSA treated VSMCs was found to reduce the contractile phenotype and increase proliferation and migration rates via the AKT and ERK pathways [31–33]. VSMCs can perform both contractile and synthetic functions, which are associated with the maintenance of vascular tone. The synthetic VSMCs phenotype has characteristics that include increased proliferation and migration rates, extensive ECM degradation/synthesis abilities, and an increased cell size, which is closely related with neo-intima hyperplasia formation [31–34].

3. Materials and Methods

3.1. Materials

3.1.1. *E. cava* Extraction

E. cava powder (2.5 g) was soaked in 50% ethanol (100 mL) and stirred at 130 rpm for 1 h at room temperature. The mixture was then centrifuged at ~3667× *g* for 10 min, and the supernatant was filtered through 3M paper and concentrated under vacuum. The crude extract was stored at −20 °C until required.

3.1.2. Isolation of Compounds from *E. cava* Extract

Compounds were isolated, as previously described [16]. Briefly, centrifugal partition chromatography (CPC) was performed using a two-phase solvent system comprised of n-hexane/ethyl acetate/methanol/water (2:7:3:7, *v/v/v/v*). The CPC column was first filled with the organic stationary phase and the mobile phase was pumped into the column in descending mode at the same flow rate used for separation (2 mL/min).

3.1.3. Experimental Cell Models

To prepare PA-BSA, 2.267 g of fatty acid-free BSA (Sigma-Aldrich; St. Louis, MO, USA) was thawed in pre-warmed 100 mL of 150 mM NaCl. The mixture was stirred at 37 °C (no higher than 40 °C) in a water bath until completely dissolved. The BSA solution was from a filtered new bottle and it was stirred at 37 °C. While the BSA was being stirred in the water bath, 30.6 mg of Sodium palmitate was thawed in 150 mM NaCl 50 mL in a water bath at 70 °C.

The PA-BSA was divided into 5 mL portions and transferred to the BSA solution, stirred at 37 °C for 1 h, and adjusted to a final volume of 100 mL with 150 mM NaCl and pH 7.4 with 1N NaOH. The solution was stored −20 °C until required and thawed in a 37 °C water bath for 10 min prior to use.

3.2. Cell Culture and Treatment

3.2.1. Monocytes

Monocytes (P388D1 cells) were purchased from ATCC (Washington, DC, USA). RPMI 1640 (Gibco; Grand island, NY, USA), 10% fetal bovine serum (FBS), 25 mM hydroxyethyl-piperazineethane-sulfonic acid buffer (HEPES) buffer and 1% penicillin-streptomycin were used as growth medium. To investigate the inhibitory effects of DK, PHB, PFFA and PPB in 0.25 mM PA-BSA treated monocytes, we used the same concentration (2.5 µg/mL) for a treatment time of 48 h. To collect conditioned medium (CM), monocytes were treated with PA-BSA with or without DK, PHB, PFFA or PPB for 48 h.

3.2.2. Vascular Endothelial Cells (ECs)

ECs (SVEC 4–10 cells) were also purchased from ATCC. Dulbecco's Modified Eagle's medium (DMEM; Gibco) and 1% penicillin-streptomycin (Gibco) were used as growth medium.

3.2.3. Vascular Aortic Smooth Muscle Cells (VSMCs)

VSMCs (MOVAS cells) were also obtained from ATCC. DMEM, 10% FBS and antibiotics G-418 were used as growth medium.

3.3. Extraction and Isolation

3.3.1. RNA Extraction and cDNA Synthesis

The cells were homogenized in ice using a disposable pestle in 1 mL of RNisol (TAKARA; Kusatsu, Japan), and homogenates were added to 0.2 mL of chloroform, mixed, and centrifuged at $12,000 \times g$ for 15 min at 4 °C. Aqueous phases were collected, placed in cleaned tubes, mixed with 0.5 mL of isopropanol, and centrifuged using the same conditions. Isolated RNA was then washed with 70% ethanol and dissolved in 50 μL of diethyl pyrocarbonate (DEPC) treated water. To perform quantitative real-time polymerase chain reaction (qRT-PCR), cDNA was synthesized from 1 μg of total RNA using a Prime Script 1st strand cDNA Synthesis Kit (TAKARA, Japan).

3.3.2. Protein Isolation

Cell proteins were extracted using the EzRIPA lysis kit (ATTO; Tokyo, Japan). Initially, tissues were homogenized with lysis buffer containing proteinase and phosphatase inhibitors and briefly sonicated for 10 s in a cold bath sonicator. After centrifuging at $14,000 \times g$ for 20 min at 4 °C, supernatants were collected and protein concentrations were determined using a Bicinchoninic acid assay kit (BCA kit; Thermo Fisher Scientific, Inc.; Waltham, MA, USA).

3.4. Monocyte Trans-Well Migration Assay

Monocytes were seeded at a density of 10^6 per well onto 8-μm Transwell inserts (Thermo Fisher Scientific). The lower chamber was filled with 500 μL low serum medium containing DK, PHB, PFFA or PPB and 0.25 mM PA-BSA and incubated for 48 h at 5% CO_2 incubator. Migration activities were evaluated using water-soluble tetrazolium salts (WST; Daeil Lab Service Co.; Seoul, Korea) and optical densities were measured.

3.5. Monocyte-Associated EC Viability Assay

To analyze monocyte-associated EC viability, 5000 ECs were seeded in the wells of a 96-well culture plate (Thermo Fisher Scientific) and incubated for 24 h in a 5% CO_2 humidified incubator at 37 °C. The WST was mixed with serum free DMEM (1:9, v/v, 200 μL/well) and the mixture was incubated for 4 h in ECs. Optical densities were measured using a plate reader at 450 nm (Spectra max plus, Molecular devices).

3.6. Monocyte-Associated VSMC Proliferation Assay

To analyze monocyte-associated VSMC proliferation, VSMCs were seeded in a 96-well culture plate (Thermo Fisher Scientific Inc.; Waltham, MA, USA) at 5000 per well and incubated for 24 h in 5% CO_2 humidified incubator at 37 °C. VSMC proliferations were determined using the WST assay as described above.

3.7. Monocyte-Associated VSMC Trans-Well Migration Assay

VSMCs were seeded at 5×10^4 per well onto 8-μm Transwell inserts (Corning Inc.; Corning, NY, USA). Lower chambers were filled with 500 μL of containing each CM and incubated for 48 h in a 5% CO_2 atmosphere. Migration activities were evaluated using the WST assay as described above.

3.8. Western Blotting

Inhibitory effects of DK, PHB, PFFA and PPB on monocyte-associated EC survival and VSMC proliferation and migration were investigated by western blotting. Cell lysates were prepared as described above. Equal amounts of proteins were separated by 8–12% sodium dodecyl sulfate polyacrylamide gel electrophoresis (SDS-PAGE) and then transferred to polyvinylidene fluoride (PVDF) membranes, which were incubated with appropriate diluted primary antibodies at 4 °C overnight.

Membranes were then washed with tris buffered saline containing 1% Tween 20 (TTBS) three times and incubated with secondary antibodies for 1 h at room temperature. Primary and secondary antibodies are listed in Table S1. Membranes were developed by enhanced chemiluminescence (ECL) on LAS-4000s (GE Healthcare; Chicago, IL, USA).

AKT Inhibition Study

EC were seeded at a density of 10^5 per well in 100 mm culture dish (SPL Life Science; Pocheon, Korea) and incubated for 24 h in 5% CO_2 humidified incubator at 37 °C. Then ECs were treated with A6730 (Sigma) 40 μM for 1 h. 1 h later, the supernatant of monocyte was treated for 48 h. Then EC were isolated EzRIPA lysis kit (ATTO).

3.9. Quantitative Real Time Polymerase Chain Reaction (qRT-PCR)

qRT-PCR was performed using the CFX384 TouchTM Real-Time PCR detection system and reaction efficiencies and threshold cycle numbers were determined using CFX ManagerTM Software. Primers are detailed in Table S2.

3.10. Statistical Analysis

Non-parametric analysis was used given the small samples available. Comparisons were made using the Mann-Whitney U test. Significant differences are indicated as follows; by an asterisk (*) versus PBS, $ versus PA-BSA, and # versus PA-BSA with PPB. Results are presented as means $\pm$ SDs and experiments were performed in triplicate. The analysis was conducted using SPSS version 22 (IBM Co.; Armonk, NY, USA).

4. Conclusions

Four major phlorotannins, that is, DK, PHB, PFFA and PPB, were isolated for the ethanoic extraction of *E. cava*. Monocyte trans-migration and inflammatory macrophage differentiation by monocytes were effectively reduced by PPB, which also modulated vascular tone by protecting monocyte-associated EC death, by increasing phosphorylations of PI3K-AKT and AMPK and reducing monocyte-induced VSMC proliferation and migration via the phosphorylations of ERK and AKT in PPB treated the cells. The study suggests PPB be considered as a component in healthy functional foods to ameliorate vascular dysfunction in diseases associated with poor circulation.

Supplementary Materials: The following are available online at http://www.mdpi.com/1660-3397/16/11/441/s1, Materials and methods: High-performance liquid chromatography (HPLC) chromatogram, Raw 264.7 cell cultivation and quantification of Western blotting; Figure S1: HPLC chromatograms and purity of four compounds from *E. cava* extract; Figure S2: Mass spectrometry analysis of four compounds from *E. cava* extract; Figure S3: Inhibitory effects of PPB in monocyte polarization and related cytokines; Figure S4: Inhibitory effects of PPB in Raw 264.7 cell-associated endothelial cell death; Figure S5: Inhibitory effects of PPB in Raw 264.7-associated VSMC proliferation and migration. Table S1: List of antibodies for western blotting; Table S2: List of primer for qRT-PCR.

Author Contributions: K.B. and Y.-J.J. were responsible for study conceptualization and methodology. Formal analysis and data collection were implemented by S.O. and M.S.; Data analysis and interpretation by H.S.L.; Draft preparation by S.O. and M.S.; and supervision and provision of funding acquisition K.B. and Y.-J.J.

Funding: This research was a part of a project entitled 'Development of functional food products with natural materials derived from marine resources' (no. 20170285), funded by the Ministry of Oceans and Fisheries, Korea.

Acknowledgments: The author would like to thank the Aqua green technology Co. Ltd. for assistance in collecting samples.

Conflicts of Interest: The authors have no conflict of interest to declare.

References

1. Haslam, D. Obesity: A medical history. *Obes. Rev.* **2007**, *8*, 31–36. [CrossRef] [PubMed]
2. Lavie, C.J.; Milani, R.V.; Ventura, H.O. Obesity and cardiovascular disease: Risk factor, paradox, and impact of weight loss. *J. Am. Coll. Carrdiol.* **2009**, *53*, 1925–1932. [CrossRef] [PubMed]
3. Hempel, A.; Maasch, C.; Heintze, U.; Lindschau, C.; Dietz, R.; Luft, F.C.; Haller, H. High glucose concentrations increase endothelial cell permeability via activation of protein kinase C alpha. *Circ. Res.* **1997**, *81*, 363–371. [CrossRef] [PubMed]
4. Laughlin, M.H.; Newcomer, S.C.; Bender, S.B. Importance of hemodynamic forces as signals for exercise-induced changes in endothelial cell phenotype. *J. Appl. Physiol.* **2008**, *104*, 588–600. [CrossRef] [PubMed]
5. Popov, D. Endothelial cell dysfunction in hyperglycemia: Phenotypic change, intracellular signaling modification, ultrastructural alteration, and potential clinical outcomes. *Int. J. Diabetes Mellit.* **2010**, *2*, 189–195. [CrossRef]
6. Chiong, M.; Morales, P.; Torres, G.; Gutierrez, T.; Garcia, L.; Ibacache, M.; Michea, L. Influence of glucose metabolism on vascular smooth muscle cell proliferation. *Vasa* **2013**, *42*, 8–16. [CrossRef] [PubMed]
7. Wang, K.; Deng, X.; Shen, Z.; Jia, Y.; Ding, R.; Li, R.; Liao, X.; Wang, S.; Ha, Y.; Kong, Y.; et al. High glucose promotes vascular smooth muscle cell proliferation by upregulating proto-oncogene serine/threonine-protein kinase Pim-1 expression. *Oncotarget* **2017**, *8*, 88320–88331. [CrossRef] [PubMed]
8. Nandy, D.; Janardhanan, R.; Mukhopadhyay, D.; Basu, A. Effect of Hyperglycemia on Human Monocyte Activation. *J. Investig. Med.* **2011**, *59*, 661–667. [CrossRef] [PubMed]
9. Dasu, M.R.; Devaraj, S.; Jialal, I. High glucose induces IL-1β expression in human monocytes: Mechanistic insights. *Am. J. Physiol. Endocrinol. Metab.* **2007**, *293*, E337–E346. [CrossRef] [PubMed]
10. Dasu, M.R.; Devaraj, S.; Zhao, L.; Hwang, D.H.; Jialal, I. High Glucose Induces Toll-Like Receptor Expression in Human Monocytes: Mechanism of Activation. *Diabetes* **2008**, *57*, 3090–3098. [CrossRef] [PubMed]
11. Shanmugam, N.; Reddy, M.A.; Guha, M.; Natarajan, R. High glucose-induced expression of proinflammatory cytokine and chemokine genes in monocytic cells. *Diabetes* **2003**, *52*, 1256–1264. [CrossRef] [PubMed]
12. Kiuru, P.; D'Auria, M.V.; Muller, C.D.; Tammela, P.; Vuorela, H.; Yli-Kauhaluoma, J. Exploring marine resources for bioactive compounds. *Planta Med.* **2014**, *80*, 1234–1246. [CrossRef] [PubMed]
13. Shin, H.C.; Kim, S.H.; Park, Y.; Lee, B.H.; Hwang, H.J. Effects of 12-week oral supplementation of *Ecklonia cava* polyphenols on anthropometric and blood lipid parameters in overweight Korean individuals: A double-blind randomized clinical trial. *Phytother. Res.* **2012**, *26*, 363–368. [CrossRef] [PubMed]
14. Li, Y.; Qian, Z.J.; Ryu, B.; Lee, S.H.; Kim, M.M.; Kim, S.K. Chemical components and its antioxidant properties in vitro: An edible marine brown alga, *Ecklonia cava*. *Bioorg. Med. Chem.* **2009**, *17*, 1963–1973. [CrossRef] [PubMed]
15. Kim, T.H.; Bae, J.S. *Ecklonia cava* extracts inhibit lipopolysaccharide induced inflammatory responses in human endothelial cells. *Food Chem. Toxicol.* **2010**, *48*, 1682–1687. [CrossRef] [PubMed]
16. Lee, J.H.; Ko, J.Y.; Oh, J.Y.; Kim, C.Y.; Lee, H.J.; Kim, J.; Jeon, Y.J. Preparative isolation and purification of phlorotannins from *Ecklonia cava* using centrifugal partition chromatography by one-step. *Food Chem.* **2014**, *158*, 433–437. [CrossRef] [PubMed]
17. Athukorala, Y.; Kim, K.N.; Jeon, Y.J. Antiproliferative and antioxidant properties of an enzymatic hydrolysate from brown alga, *Ecklonia cava*. *Food Chem. Toxicol.* **2006**, *44*, 1065–1074. [CrossRef] [PubMed]
18. Yang, Y.I.; Shin, H.C.; Kim, S.H.; Park, W.Y.; Lee, K.T.; Choi, J.H. 6,6'-Bieckol, isolated from marine alga *Ecklonia cava*, suppressed LPS-induced nitric oxide and PGE$_2$ production and inflammatory cytokine expression in macrophages: The inhibition of NFκB. *Int. Immunopharmacol.* **2012**, *12*, 510–517. [CrossRef] [PubMed]
19. Kang, I.J.; Jang, B.G.; In, S.; Choi, B.; Kim, M.; Kim, M.J. Phlorotannin-rich *Ecklonia cava* reduces the production of beta-amyloid by modulating alpha- and gamma-secretase expression and activity. *Neurotoxicology* **2013**, *34*, 16–24. [CrossRef] [PubMed]
20. Park, S.J.; Kim, Y.T.; Jeon, Y.J. Antioxidant dieckol downregulates the Rac1/ROS signaling pathway and inhibits Wiskott-Aldrich syndrome protein (WASP)-family verprolin-homologous protein 2 (WAVE2)-mediated invasive migration of B16 mouse melanoma cells. *Mol. Cells* **2012**, *33*, 363–369. [CrossRef] [PubMed]

21. Kong, C.S.; Kim, J.A.; Yoon, N.Y.; Kim, S.K. Induction of apoptosis by phloroglucinol derivative from *Ecklonia cava* in MCF-7 human breast cancer cells. *Food Chem. Toxicol.* **2009**, *47*, 1653–1658. [CrossRef] [PubMed]

22. Wijesinghe, W.A.; Ko, S.C.; Jeon, Y.J. Effect of phlorotannins isolated from *Ecklonia cava* on angiotensin I-converting enzyme (ACE) inhibitory activity. *Nutr. Res. Pract.* **2011**, *5*, 93–100. [CrossRef] [PubMed]

23. Norgre, L.; Hiatt, W.R.; Dormandy, J.A.; Nehler, M.R.; Harris, K.A.; F.G.R. Fowkes on behalf of the TASC II Working Group. Inter-Society Consensus for the Management of Peripheral Arterial Disease (TASC II). *J. Vasc. Surg.* **2007**, *45*, S5–S67. [CrossRef] [PubMed]

24. Wijesinghe, W.; Ahn, G.; Lee, W.W.; Kang, M.C.; Kim, E.A.; Jeon, Y.J. Anti-inflammatory activity of phlorotannin-rich fermented *Ecklonia cava* processing by-product extract in lipopolysaccharide-stimulated RAW 264.7 macrophages. *J. Appl. Phycol.* **2013**, *25*, 1207–1213. [CrossRef]

25. Kim, S.K.; Lee, D.Y.; Jung, W.K.; Kim, J.H.; Choi, I.; Park, S.G.; Seo, S.K.; Lee, S.W.; Lee, C.M.; Yea, S.S. Effects of *Ecklonia cava* ethanolic extracts on airway hyperresponsiveness and inflammation in a murine asthma model: Role of suppressor of cytokine signaling. *Biomed. Pharmacother.* **2008**, *62*, 289–296. [CrossRef] [PubMed]

26. Zhang, J.; Alcaide, P.; Liu, L.; Sun, J.; He, A.; Luscinskas, F.W.; Shi, G.P. Regulation of endothelial cell adhesion molecule expression by mast cells, macrophages, and neutrophils. *PLoS ONE* **2011**, *6*, e14525. [CrossRef] [PubMed]

27. Smith, C.W. Endothelial adhesion molecules and their role in inflammation. *Can. J. Physiol. Pharmacol.* **1993**, *71*, 76–87. [CrossRef] [PubMed]

28. Chavakis, E.; Dimmeler, S. Regulation of endothelial cell survival and apoptosis during angiogenesis. *Arterioscler. Thromb. Vasc. Biol.* **2002**, *22*, 887–893. [CrossRef] [PubMed]

29. Abid, M.R.; Guo, S.; Minami, T.; Spokes, K.C.; Ueki, K.; Skurk, C.; Walsh, K.; Aird, W.C. Vascular endothelial growth factor activates PI3K/Akt/forkhead signaling in endothelial cells. *Arterioscler. Thromb. Vasc. Biol.* **2004**, *24*, 294–300. [CrossRef] [PubMed]

30. Ho, F.M.; Lin, W.W.; Chen, B.C.; Chao, C.M.; Yang, C.R.; Lin, L.Y.; Lai, C.C.; Liu, S.H.; Liau, C.S. High glucose-induced apoptosis in human vascular endothelial cells is mediated through NF-κB and c-Jun NH2-terminal kinase pathway and prevented by PI3K/Akt/eNOS pathway. *Cell Signal.* **2006**, *18*, 391–399. [CrossRef] [PubMed]

31. Allard, D.; Figg, N.; Bennett, M.R.; Littlewood, T.D. Akt Regulates the Survival of Vascular Smooth Muscle Cells via Inhibition of FoxO3a and GSK3. *J. Biol. Chem.* **2008**, *283*, 19739–19747. [CrossRef] [PubMed]

32. Nelson, P.R.; Yamamura, S.; Mureebe, L.; Itoh, H.; Kent, K.C. Smooth muscle cell migration and proliferation are mediated by distinct phases of activation of the intracellular messenger mitogen-activated protein kinase. *J. Vasc. Surg.* **1998**, *27*, 117–125. [CrossRef]

33. Hayashi, K.I.; Takahashi, M.; Kimura, K.; Nishida, W.; Saga, H.; Sobue, K. Changes in the balance of phosphoinositide 3-kinase/protein kinase B (Akt) and the mitogen-activated protein kinases (ERK/p38MAPK) determine a phenotype of visceral and vascular smooth muscle cells. *J. Cell Biol.* **1999**, *145*, 727–740. [CrossRef] [PubMed]

34. Bhattacharyya, A.; Lin, S.; Sandig, M.; Mequanint, K. Regulation of Vascular Smooth Muscle Cell Phenotype in Three-Dimensional Coculture System by Jagged1-Selective Notch3 Signaling. *Tissue Eng. Part A* **2014**, *20*, 1175–1187. [CrossRef] [PubMed]

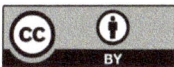

marine drugs

MDPI

Article

6-Bromoindole Derivatives from the Icelandic Marine Sponge *Geodia barretti*: Isolation and Anti-Inflammatory Activity

Xiaxia Di [1,2], **Caroline Rouger** [3,†], **Ingibjorg Hardardottir** [2,4], **Jona Freysdottir** [2,4], **Tadeusz F. Molinski** [5], **Deniz Tasdemir** [3,6] and **Sesselja Omarsdottir** [1,*]

[1] Faculty of Pharmaceutical Sciences, University of Iceland, Hagi, Hofsvallagata 53, IS-107 Reykjavik, Iceland; xid1@hi.is

[2] Department of Immunology and Centre for Rheumatology Research Landspitali-The National University Hospital of Iceland, Hringbraut, IS-101 Reykjavik, Iceland; ih@hi.is (I.H.); jonaf@landspitali.is (J.F.)

[3] GEOMAR Centre for Marine Biotechnology (GEOMAR-Biotech), Marine Natural Products Chemistry Research Unit, GEOMAR Helmholtz Centre for Ocean Research Kiel, Am Kiel-Kanal 44, 24106 Kiel, Germany; caroline.rouger@u-bordeaux.fr (C.R.); dtasdemir@geomar.de (D.T.)

[4] Faculty of Medicine, Biomedical Center, University of Iceland, Vatnsmyrarvegur 16, IS-101 Reykjavik, Iceland

[5] Department of Chemistry and Biochemistry and Skaggs School of Pharmacy and Pharmaceutical Sciences, University of California, San Diego, La Jolla, CA 92093, USA; tmolinski@ucsd.edu

[6] Faculty of Mathematics and Natural Sciences, Kiel University, Christian-Albrechts-Platz 4, 24118 Kiel, Germany

[*] Correspondence: sesselo@hi.is; Tel.: +354-8424514

[†] Current address: Univ. de Bordeaux, UFR des Sciences Pharmaceutiques, Unité de recherche Œnologie EA 4577, USC 1366 INRA, ISVV, 210 Chemin de Leysotte, CS 50008, 33882 Villenave d'Ornon, France.

Received: 18 October 2018; Accepted: 6 November 2018; Published: 8 November 2018

Abstract: An UPLC-qTOF-MS-based dereplication study led to the targeted isolation of seven bromoindole alkaloids from the sub-Arctic sponge *Geodia barretti*. This includes three new metabolites, namely geobarrettin A–C (**1–3**) and four known compounds, barettin (**4**), 8,9-dihydrobarettin (**5**), 6-bromoconicamin (**6**), and L-6-bromohypaphorine (**7**). The chemical structures of compounds **1–7** were elucidated by extensive analysis of the NMR and HRESIMS data. The absolute stereochemistry of geobarrettin A (**1**) was assigned by ECD analysis and Marfey's method employing the new reagent L-N^α-(1-fluoro-2,4-dinitrophenyl)tryptophanamide (L-FDTA). The isolated compounds were screened for anti-inflammatory activity using human dendritic cells (DCs). Both **2** and **3** reduced DC secretion of IL-12p40, but **3** concomitantly increased IL-10 production. Maturing DCs treated with **2** or **3** before co-culturing with allogeneic CD4$^+$ T cells decreased T cell secretion of IFN-γ, indicating a reduction in Th1 differentiation. Although barettin (**4**) reduced DC secretion of IL-12p40 and IL-10 (IC$_{50}$ values 11.8 and 21.0 µM for IL-10 and IL-12p40, respectively), maturing DCs in the presence of **4** did not affect the ability of T cells to secrete IFN-γ or IL-17, but reduced their secretion of IL-10. These results indicate that **2** and **3** may be useful for the treatment of inflammation, mainly of the Th1 type.

Keywords: 6-bromoindole; *Geodia barretti*; anti-inflammatory activity; dendritic cells; T cell differentiation

1. Introduction

Many chronic illnesses, including cancer, neurological diseases, diabetes, and autoimmune diseases, exhibit dysregulation of pathways that have been linked to inflammation [1,2]. A vast number of unique marine natural products possessing in vitro and in vivo anti-inflammatory activity have been isolated [3,4], however, no marine-derived anti-inflammatory agent is currently on the market. Therefore, the search and development of new natural products to treat chronic inflammatory diseases is of great importance [5,6]. Marine sponges, due to their phenomenal biological and chemical diversity, are considered as a notable source of natural products with potential anti-inflammatory activity [5,7,8].

Geodia barretti Bowerbank (family Geodiidae, class Demospongiae, order Astrophorida) is an abundant cold-water sponge with a wide geographic distribution, including the Icelandic waters. *G. barretti* has been reported to contain 6-bromoindole alkaloids [9–13], including barettin (**4**) [10], 8,9-dihydrobarettin (**5**) [11], bromobenzisoxazolone barettin [12], 6-bromoconicamin (**6**) [14], and 2-(6-bromo-1*H*-indol-3-yl)-2-hydroxy-*N*,*N*,*N*-trimethylethanaminium [13], as well as nucleosides [15], peptides [16], sterols and fatty acids [17].

The chemical structure of barettins isolated from *G. barretti* feature a diketopiperazine (DKP)-type cyclic dipeptide, a condensation product of arginine (Arg) and 6-bromo-8-en-tryptophan residues in a "head-to-tail" fashion [11,18]. The DKP core, present in many bioactive compounds, is a relevant scaffold for drug discovery and development [19]. Barettins display interesting biological activities, such as anti-inflammatory, antioxidant, antifouling, acetylcholinesterase (AChE) inhibitory, and selective serotonin (5-HT) receptor ligand effects [11–13,20,21]. In particular, barettin (**4**), the major compound in *G. barretti* has shown potent antifouling, antioxidant, and anti-inflammatory activities [11,12,20], making it a potential lead compound in prevention of chronic inflammatory diseases. Therefore, the search for new barettins is of great interest for investigation of their anti-inflammatory effects and structure–activity relationships.

The present study was undertaken to isolate 6-bromoindole derivatives from the Icelandic sponge *G. barretti* and to evaluate their anti-inflammatory activity on human monocyte-derived dendritic cells (DCs) and their ability to activate T cell responses. DCs play an important role in initiation of adaptive immune responses by activating naïve T cells and inducing their differentiation by cytokine secretion [22]. The naïve CD4$^+$ T cells differentiate into different T helper (Th) effector cells, such as Th1, Th2, Th9, or Th17 phenotypes, which participate in various inflammatory diseases [23–25] or, if the DCs secrete anti-inflammatory cytokines, such as IL-10, into T regulatory cells (Tregs) [26]. In this study, we describe (i) the isolation and structure elucidation of three new 6-bromoindole derivatives, geobarrettin A–C (**1–3**) and four known 6-bromoindole alkaloids (**4–7**), (ii) the absolute stereoassignment of geobarrettin A (**1**) using the Marfey's method employing the new reagent L-*N*$^\alpha$-(1-fluoro-2,4-dinitrophenyl)tryptophanamide (L-FDTA) followed by HPLC comparison with standards, and (iii) the re-evaluation of the stereochemical configuration of barettin (**4**).

2. Results

The sponge *G. barretti* was collected at the west of Iceland (−388 m) and kept frozen until work-up. The CH$_2$Cl$_2$:CH$_3$OH (*v/v*, 1:1) soluble extract of the sponge was partitioned into five subextracts (hexane, chloroform, dichloromethane, *n*-butanol, and water) using a modified Kupchan solvent partitioning method [27,28]. The crude extracts and subextracts were chemically profiled by UPLC-qTOF-MS for selective and sensitive detection of bromoindoles and other trace components [29,30]. The bromoindole containing chloroform and dichloromethane subextracts were combined and purified by a combination of RP-VLC and HPLC to afford three new 6-bromoindole derivatives geobarrettin A–C (**1–3**) and four known alkaloids **4–7** (Figure 1).

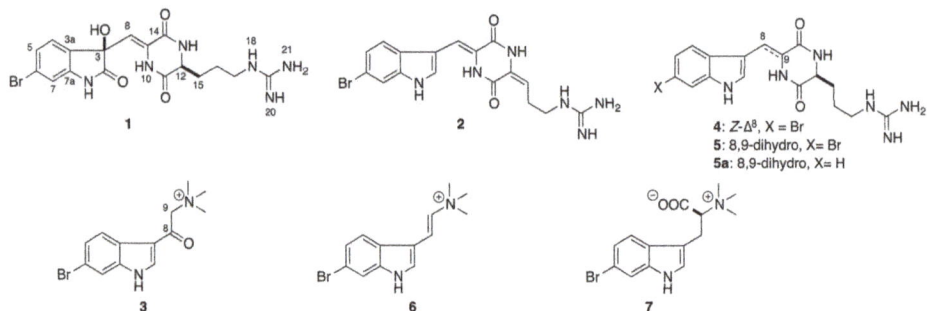

Figure 1. Chemical structures of compounds 1–7 and 5a.

2.1. Structural Elucidation

Compound **1** was obtained as a yellow solid. Its UV spectrum was characteristic for an oxindole skeleton with absorption λ_{max} at 217 and 263 nm [31,32], while the IR spectrum showed the presence of OH (ν_{max} 3352 cm^{-1}), NH$_2$ (ν_{max} 3285, 3214, and 1614 cm^{-1}), and lactam (ν_{max} 1679 cm^{-1}) functionalities. The characteristic isotope pseudo-molecular ion peaks at m/z 451.0728:453.0732 ([M + H]$^+$) in a 1:1 ratio in the HRESIMS spectrum of **1** suggested the presence of a bromine atom in the molecule. The HRESIMS data indicated the molecular formula of C$_{17}$H$_{20}$^{79}BrN$_6$O$_4$, corresponding to eleven degrees of unsaturation. This formula was supported by the ^{1}H, ^{13}C NMR, and HSQC data, indicating the presence of three methylenes (δ_C 42.0, 32.6 and 24.8), three aromatic methines (δ_C 127.1, 126.9 and 115.0), one aliphatic methine (δ_C 56.0), an isolated olefinic methine (δ_C 112.8), four quaternary aromatic carbons (δ_C 143.9, 132.4, 132.2, and 124.7), one tertiary alcohol (δ_C 78.3), and four quaternary heteroatom-bounded sp^2 carbons (δ_C 179.3, 167.2, 160.5 and 158.7). The ^{1}H NMR spectrum in CD$_3$OD contained three aromatic resonances, including a broad singlet at δ_H 7.11 (1H) and an overlapped 2H broad singlet at δ_H 7.25 (Table 1). When acquired in DMSO-d_6, these aromatic signals were resolved into a well-separated ABX system at δ_H 7.26 (1H, d, J = 7.9 Hz, H-4), 7.23 (1H, dd, J = 7.9, 1.5 Hz, H-5), and 7.03 (1H, d, J = 1.5 Hz, H-7), suggesting the presence of a trisubstituted benzene ring. The chemical shift of the quaternary aromatic carbon C-7a (δ_C 143.9) indicated that C-7a was substituted by an NH group. The characteristic resonances of the amide carbonyl C-2 at δ_C 179.3 and the oxygenated carbon (C-3, δ_C 78.3), as well as the HMBC correlations observed from H-4 to C-3, C-6, and C-7a, and from H-7 to C-3a, assisted the construction of a 3-hydroxy-2-oxindole skeleton. The chemical shifts for carbon atoms were in good agreement with those of previously published 3-hydroxy-2-oxindole scaffolds [33,34]. The position of the bromine atom at C-6 was determined based on the HMBC correlations H-4/C-3, H-4/C-6, and H-4/C-7a; H-5/C-3a and H-5/C-7; as well as H-7/C-3a, H-7/C-5, and H-7/C-6. This was supported by the NOE correlations between H-4/H-8 observed in spectrum run in CD$_3$OD and a weak cross peak between H-7/NH-1 in spectrum run in DMSO-d_6, in combination with characteristic coupling constant values, namely $J_{4,5}$ (7.9 Hz) and $J_{5,7}$ (1.5 Hz). A similar weak cross peak between H-7/NH-1 has previously been observed for 6-bromoindole cyclic guanidine alkaloids [35]. The presence of two amide carbonyl signals C-11 (δ_C 167.2) and C-14 (δ_C 160.5) suggested the presence of a DKP moiety attached to the oxindole skeleton and the chemical shift of C-14 indicated that this carbon was conjugated to a double bond (Δ^8). Cross correlations observed in the HMBC spectrum between H-12/C-11, H-12/C-14, H-8/C-14, H-8/C-3, and H-8/C-9 supported this assumption. ^{1}H-^{1}H COSY spectrum indicated the presence of an additional linear spin system starting from H-12 (δ_H 4.28, 1H, t, J = 6.0 Hz) and including three aliphatic methylene signals H$_2$-15 (δ_H 1.89, 1H, m; δ_H 2.01, 1H, m), H$_2$-16 (δ_H 1.67, 1H, m; 1.74, 1H, m), and H$_2$-17 (δ_H 3.24, 2H, t, J = 6.0 Hz). The molecular fragments described above account for all atoms except three nitrogen atoms and one quaternary carbon atom (δ_C 158.7, C-19) and for 10 of 11 degrees of unsaturation. The position of the remaining three nitrogen atoms and the carbon atom was assigned to a guanidine group connected to the linear spin system at C-17 based on the HMBC correlation between H_2-17/C-19 (Figure 2). This suggested that the aliphatic side chain linked to the DKP moiety was an Arg residue. Further examination of the NMR data revealed that spectroscopic data of compound **1** were very similar to those of compound **4** [10], with the main differences being the upfield shift of the H-7 resonance (δ_H 7.03 (1H d, *J* = 1.5 Hz) in compound **1**; δ_H 7.67 (1H d, *J* = 1.6 Hz) in compound **4**) and the replacement of the indole Δ^2 double bond by a hydroxyl group at C-3 and a carbonyl group at C-2. The latter was confirmed by the HMBC correlation observed between H-8 and C-2 (Figure 2). The structure proposed for compound **1** is consistent with its molecular formula (*m/z* 451.0728 [M + H]$^+$, $C_{17}H_{20}{}^{79}BrN_6O_4$) in comparison to that of compound **4** (*m/z* 419.0830 [M + H]$^+$, $C_{17}H_{20}{}^{79}BrN_6O_2$). The geometry of the exocyclic double bond Δ^8 was defined as Z based on NOESY correlations observed in H-8/H-4 and NH-10/NH-1.

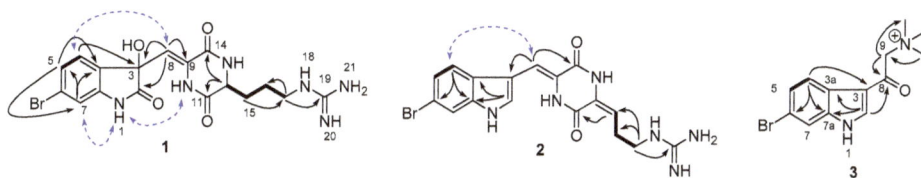

Figure 2. Key HMBC (H→C), ^{1}H-^{1}H COSY (−) and NOESY (H↔H, in dashed blue) correlations of compounds **1**–**3**.

Table 1. NMR spectroscopic data for compounds 1–3 (δ in ppm, 600 MHz for ^1H NMR and 150 MHz for ^{13}C NMR).

No.	1 — δ_H, Mult. (*J* in Hz) [a]	1 — δ_H, Mult. (*J* in Hz) [b,c]	1 — δ_C, Type [a]	2 — δ_H, Mult. (*J* in Hz) [a]	2 — δ_C, Type [a]	3 — δ_H, Mult. (*J* in Hz) [a]	3 — δ_C, Type [a]
1		10.76, br s	179.3, C	7.83, s	127.6, CH	8.27, s	135.9, CH
2			78.3, C		110.0, C		116.1, C
3			132.4, C		127.5, C		125.7, C
3a							
4	7.25, br s	7.26, d (7.9)	126.9, CH	7.61, d (8.5)	120.9, CH	8.16, d (8.5)	124.1, CH
5	7.25, br s	7.23, dd (7.9, 1.5)	127.1, CH	7.27, dd (8.5, 2.0)	124.7, CH	7.39, dd (8.5, 2.0)	127.1, CH
6			124.7, C		117.2, C		118.3, C
7	7.11, br s	7.03, d (1.5)	115.0, CH	7.62, d (2.0)	115.7, CH	7.68, d (2.0)	116.3, CH
7a			143.9, C		138.5, C		139.2, C
8	5.61, s	5.37, s	112.8, CH	7.22, s	111.0, CH		186.0, C
9		9.88, s	132.2, C		123.5, C	4.92, s	67.8, CH$_2$
10							
11			167.2, C		159.3, C		
12	4.28, t (6.0)	4.19, td (5.4, 1.9)	56.0, CH		130.5, C		
13		8.58, d (1.9)					
14			160.5, C		160.3, C		
15	1.89, m; 2.01, m	1.76, m	32.6, CH$_2$	5.98, t (7.8)	114.9, CH	3.42, s	54.9, CH$_3$
16	1.67, m; 1.74, m	1.49, m; 1.55, m	24.8, CH$_2$	2.57, q (7.8)	26.2, CH$_2$	3.42, s	54.9, CH$_3$
17	3.24, t (6.0)	3.12, m	42.0, CH$_2$	3.37, t (7.2)	41.4, CH$_2$	3.42, s	54.9, CH$_3$
18		7.49, br t (5.5)					
19			158.7, C		158.8, C		
20,21	6.60–7.65, br						
3-OH	7.28, br s						

[a] Recorded in CD$_3$OD. [b] Recorded in DMSO-*d$_6$*. [c] The complete assignment of proton chemical shifts was in accordance with the literature for similar DKP-indole alkaloids [10,36].

The configurations of two chiral centers at C-3 and C-12 in compound **1** were determined using a combination of techniques. The absolute configuration of C-3 was determined by comparison of the ECD spectra (Figure 3) of the hydrogenolysis product of compound **1** with the compound (*R*)-3-propyldioxindole (**8**), which share the dioxindole core structure. (*R*)-**8** was obtained by hydrogenolysis of *R*-dioxindole (**8a**, a gift from Dr. Annaliese K. Franz (University of California, Davis)) (Scheme 1) [37]. The CD spectra of (*R*)-**8** (EtOH, 23 °C) revealed Cotton effects (λ 208 nm (Δε +13.1), 232 (−10.7), 259 (+3.5)) similar to dioxindoles recently investigated [38]. Hydrogenolysis of geobarretin A (**1**) (Scheme 1) gave debromodihydrogeobarrettin A (**1a**) with a CD spectrum identical to that of (*R*)-**8** (Figure 3). Given the identical CD spectra of **1a** and (*R*)-**8**, whose absolute configuration was established by X-ray crystallography, and the similarity of their Cotton effects with those of (*R*)-5-methyldioxindole [39] and the natural product (+)-trikentramide I [38], the C-3 configuration of compound **1** was assigned as *R*, unambiguously.

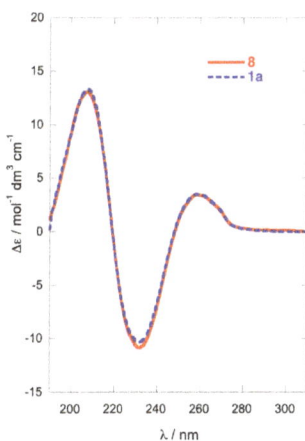

Figure 3. Comparison of CD of model compound (*R*)-3-propyldioxindole (**8**) and debromodihydrogeobarrettin A (**1a**). Red line: (*R*)-**8**; Blue line: **1a**.

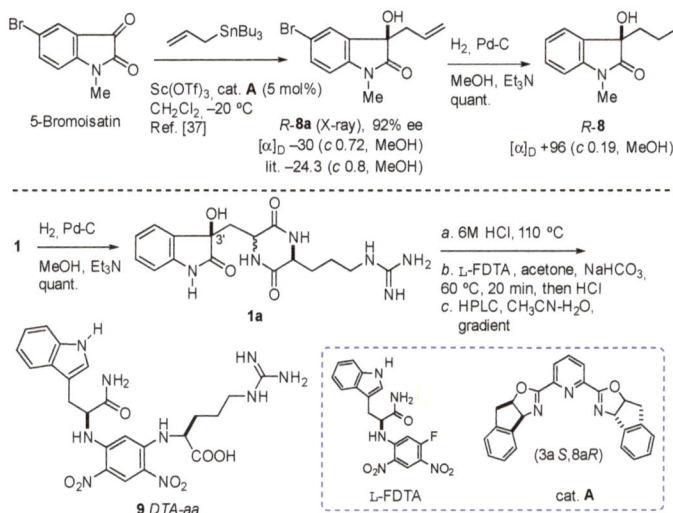

Scheme 1. Hydrogenolysis of (*R*)-(**8a**) to (*R*)-(**8**) and hydrogenation, hydrolysis, and L-FDTA-derivatization of geobarrettin A (**1**) to **9**.

Determination of amino acid configuration using Marfey's method and chiral derivatizing agents (CDAs) such as L-fluoro-2-4-dinitrophenyl-5-L-alanine amide (FDAA, Marfey's reagent) or the homolog, L-fluoro-2,4-dinitrophenyl-5-L-leucineamide (FDLA), are popular and effective [40]. Compound **1a** was hydrolyzed (6 M HCl, 110 °C) and the product was derivatized with the new CDA, L-FDTA [41], to produce **9**. Comparison with standards D- and L-Arg-DTA derivatives was then achieved using HPLC (Figure S32) and UPLC-MS analyses. D- and L-Arg-DTA derivatives were observed with integral values of 19:81 suggesting either natural **1** is partially racemic at C-12, or that Arg underwent partial racemization under the conditions of hydrolysis. The latter possibility is ruled out by precedence; Arg essentially is stable to the conditions of hydrolysis. In a careful systematic study Kaiser and Benner (2005) demonstrated that the amount of D-Arg produced during acid hydrolysis of L-Arg (110 °C, 6 M HCl, 20 h) is not more than $1.0 \pm 0\%$ of the total for free amino acid, or $2.8 \pm 0.4\%$ when bonded in lysozyme [42]. We conclude that compound **1** is a cryptic mixture of diastereomers with stereofidelity at C-3, but partial epimerization at C-12. Therefore, the configuration of geobarrettin A (**1**) is 3R, 8Z, 12S.

Geobarrettin B (**2**) was isolated as a yellow solid. The UV spectrum showed the characteristic indole chromophore with absorptions at λ_{max} 230, 270, and 289 nm [43]. Its molecular formula $C_{17}H_{18}{}^{79}BrN_6O_2$ was deduced by HRESIMS (m/z 417.0675/419.0685 1:1, [M + H]$^+$), indicating the presence of a bromine atom and 12 degrees of unsaturation. Detailed analysis of the ^{1}H, ^{13}C NMR (Table 1) and HSQC data suggested the planar structure of compound **2** to be very similar to that of the known compound barettin (**4**). Comparison of the 1D NMR spectra of compounds **2** and **4** suggested that the only difference was the presence of a double bond in the Arg side chain of **2**, namely between C-12 (δ_C 130.5) and C-15 (δ_C 114.9). The HMBC correlations from H-15 (δ_H 5.98, t, J = 7.8 Hz) to C-11 and C-17, and from H-16 (δ_H 2.57, q, J = 7.8 Hz) to C-12, as well as COSY correlations between H-15/H$_2$-16 and H$_2$-16/H$_2$-17 supported the position of the unsaturation at Δ^{12}. Finally the two mass units difference between the molecular formulae of **2** and **4**, as determined by HRESIMS data, clearly supported **2** being the Δ^{12} unsaturated analog of **4**. The geometry of Δ^{12} in α,β-dehydroamino-acids was determined by analyzing the reported trends in chemical shift differences of vinyl protons in E- and Z-isomers. Comparison of the chemical shift of H-15 (δ_H 5.98) in compound **2** with that of alkylidene-2,5-piperazinedione derivatives reported in the literature [44,45] therefore supports an E-Δ^{12} configuration. Hence compound **2** is the Δ^{12} dehydro-derivative of barettin (**4**), which we named as geobarrettin B.

Geobarrettin C (**3**) was obtained as a yellow oil. The molecular formula $C_{13}H_{16}BrN_2O^+$ was assigned to compound **3** by its HRESIMS data. Analysis of the ^{1}H and ^{13}C NMR spectra pointed out the presence of a substituted 6-bromoindole scaffold. The substituent was identified as *N,N,N*-trimethyl-2-oxoethanaminium salt, based on the 1D NMR spectra that possessed resonances of a methylene group at δ_C 67.8 and δ_H 4.92 (2H, s, H-9), a conjugated keto group at δ_C 186.0 (C-8), and three methyl signals at δ_C 54.9; δ_H 3.42 (9H, s, -N(CH$_3$)$_3$). The HMBC correlations observed between CH$_3$-N/C-9, H$_2$-9/C-8, and H-2/C-8 indicated the *N,N,N*-trimethyl-2-oxoethanaminium moiety to be attached to 6-bromoindole at C-3 position (δ_C 116.1). A literature search showed that **3** is an oxidation product of a previously isolated secondary alcohol 2-(6-bromo-1*H*-indol-3-yl)-2-hydroxy-*N,N,N*-trimethylethanaminium ($C_{13}H_{18}BrN_2O^+$) [13]. Thus, compound **3** was identified as the quaternary ammonium salt 2-(6-bromo-1*H*-indol-3-yl)-*N,N,N*-trimethyl-2-oxoethanaminium and named as geobarrettin C (**3**).

The gross structures of the remaining known compounds, barettin (**4**) [10], 8,9-dihydrobarettin (**5**) [11], 6-bromoconicamin (**6**) [14], and L-6-bromohypaphorine (**7**) [46] were identified by comparison of their NMR, HRMS, and specific rotation data with those reported in the literature.

The sole chiral amino acid residue in barettin (**4**), first reported in 1986 from a deep-water specimen of *G. barretti* collected in Sweden, presumably from Koster fjord [12], was assigned as Pro, but the configuration was not determined at that time. A second report of **4** in 2004 from a Norwegian deep-water sample of *G. barretti* [11] corrected the structure to an Arg-containing DKP, but also omitted the specific rotation. Finally, the configuration of **4** was established as L-Arg by comparison of optical rotations of natural and synthetic **4** [42]. Although they had similar signs, the specific rotations of synthetic and natural **4** were different ($[\alpha]_D^{26}$ −32.5 (*c* 2, MeOH) [18]; natural **4** $[\alpha]_D$ −25 (*c* 3, MeOH)) [9]. In the present study, the rotation of **4** was found to be even higher ($[\alpha]_D^{25}$ −84 (*c* 0.5, MeOH)). In order to resolve this paradox, the L-FDTA method was applied to the hydrolysate as described above for **1**. HPLC analysis detected the presence of D-Arg-DTA and L-Arg-DTA in a ratio of 19:81 suggesting L-Arg was predominant, but—as with **3**—our sample of **4** was also partially racemic. Assuming no racemization occurred during the synthesis of **4** [42], our finding would be consistent with partially racemic natural **4** in the Swedish sample. The hydrolysis was repeated on debromo-8,9-dihydrobarettin (**5a**) (Figure 1), obtained by hydrogenolysis of **4**, and the product was again converted to L-DTA derivatives and analyzed by HPLC as before to give D-Arg-DTA and L-Arg-DTA (19:81).

The structure of compound **7** was assigned as 6-bromohypaphorine by comparing the recorded and published NMR data [46]. The sign of optical rotation of compound **7** ($[\alpha]_D^{23}$ +36, *c* 0.2, EtOH) was similar to that of L-6-bromohypaphorine ($[\alpha]_D$ +58, *c* 0.25, EtOH) [46] and opposite to that of the D-6-bromohypaphorine ($[\alpha]_D^{17}$ −27, *c* 0.80, MeOH-CF$_3$COOH, 8:1) [47]. Hence, compound **7** was assigned as L-6-bromohypaphorine.

2.2. Anti-Inflammatory Activity

To evaluate the potential anti-inflammatory activity of compounds **1**–**7**, their effects on DC secretion of the pro-inflammatory cytokine IL-12p40 and the anti-inflammatory cytokine IL-10 was determined. The tested compounds did not show cytotoxic effects on the DCs, with the cell viability being more than 90% in the presence of the compounds at 10 μg/mL (data not shown). Compound **4** inhibited by more than 50% secretion of both IL-12p40 and IL-10. Compounds **2** and **6** decreased DC secretion of IL-12p40 by 29 and 32%, respectively, without affecting secretion of IL-10, which suggests an overall anti-inflammatory activity of these compounds. Compound **3** slightly decreased DC secretion of IL-12p40 (13%) but increased secretion of the anti-inflammatory cytokine IL-10 by 40%, which also suggests an anti-inflammatory activity. Compounds **1**, **5**, and **7** did not affect DC secretion of IL-12p40 or IL-10 (Figure 4).

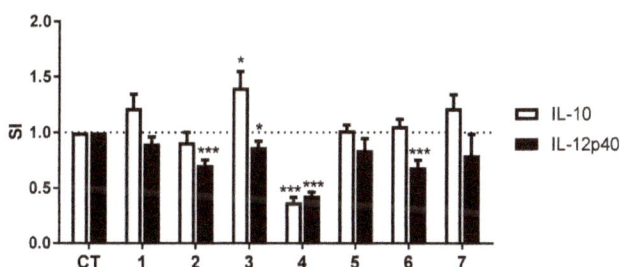

Figure 4. The effects of compounds **1**–**7** on dendritic cell (DC) secretion of IL-12p40 and IL-10. DCs were matured and activated by TNF-α, IL-1β and LPS in the absence (solvent control (CT)) or presence of compounds **1**–**7** at 10 μg/mL for 24 h. The supernatants were collected and the concentrations of IL-12p40 and IL-10 were determined by ELISA. The data are presented as SI, i.e., the concentration of each cytokine in the supernatant of cells matured and activated in the presence of compounds divided by the concentration of the cytokine in the supernatant of cells matured and activated in the presence of solvent control. The results are shown as mean + standard error of the mean (SEM), *n* = 7–11, except for compound **7**, *n* = 3. Different from CT: * *p* < 0.05, *** *p* < 0.001.

We next examined whether compounds **2**, **3**, and **4** affected cytokine secretion by the DCs in a dose-dependent manner. The effects of compounds **2** and **3** on IL-12p40 and IL-10 secretion by DCs were not dose-dependent although for compound **2** there was a tendency towards an increasing effect on IL-12p40 secretion at higher concentrations. Compound **4** inhibited secretion of IL-12p40 and IL-10 in a dose-dependent manner with IC_{50} being 21.04 µM for IL-12p40 and 11.80 µM for IL-10 (Figure 5), with IL-12p40 and IL-10 secretion decreasing at the lowest concentrations tested, i.e., 5.96 µM (2.5 µg/mL) and 11.93 µM (5 µg/mL), respectively.

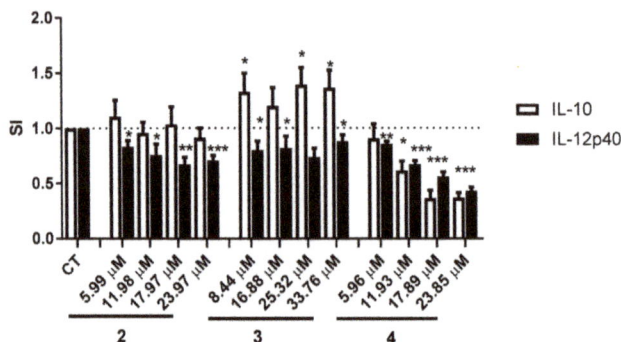

Figure 5. Dose-dependent inhibition of cytokines IL-12p40 and IL-10 by compounds **2–4**. DCs were matured and activated by TNF-α, IL-1β, and LPS in the absence (solvent control (CT)) or presence of indicated concentration of compound **2** (5.99, 11.98, 17.97, and 23.97 µM), compound **3** (8.44, 16.88, 25.32, and 33.76 µM), and compound **4** (5.96, 11.93, 17.89, and 23.85 µM). The levels of IL-12p40 and IL-10 in the supernatants were determined by ELISA. The data are presented as SI. The results are shown as mean + SEM, $n = 5$–11. Different from CT: * $p < 0.05$, ** $p < 0.01$, *** $p < 0.001$.

To further elucidate the anti-inflammatory activity of compounds **2–4**, DCs matured in their presence were co-cultured with allogeneic CD4$^+$ T cells and the differentiation of the T cells investigated by determining secretion of the cytokines IL-10, IL-17, and IFN-γ. T cells co-cultured with DCs matured in the presence of compounds **2** or **3** secreted less IL-10 and IFN-γ than T cells co-cultured with DCs matured in the absence of the compounds, but maturing DCs in the presence of compounds **2** or **3** did not affect T cell secretion of IL-17 (Figure 6). Co-culturing T cells with DCs matured in the presence of compound **4** resulted in a substantial decrease in secretion of IL-10 with no effect on secretion of either IL-17 or IFN-γ.

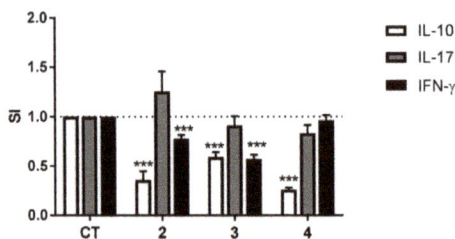

Figure 6. The effects of compounds **2–4** on the ability of DCs to induce cytokine secretion by allogeneic CD4$^+$ T cells. DCs matured and activated in the absence (solvent control (CT)) or presence of compounds **2–4** at a concentration of 10 µg/mL for 24 h were co-cultured with isolated allogeneic CD4$^+$ T cells for six days and the concentrations of IFN-γ, IL-17, and IL-10 in the supernatants were determined by ELISA. The data are presented as SI, i.e., the concentration of each cytokine in the supernatant of co-cultures containing DCs treated with compounds divided by the concentration of each cytokine in the supernatant of co-cultures containing DCs treated with solvent control. The results are shown as mean + SEM, $n = 9$–12. Different from CT: *** $p < 0.001$.

3. Discussion

Three new 6-bromoindole derivatives were isolated from *G. barretti*, including a dioxindole featuring a DKP-type cyclic dipeptide, geobarrettin A (**1**); a 6-bromoindole possessing DKP system, geobarrettin B (**2**); and a new 6-bromoindole alkaloid, geobarrettin C (**3**).

Compounds **2** and **3** inhibited IL-12p40 production by DCs and DCs treated with compounds **2** and **3** reduced IFN-γ secretion by co-cultured T cells, hence reduced Th1 responses, which are linked to inflammatory disorders and many chronic inflammatory diseases [48,49]. As IL-12 is the main inducer of Th1 polarization of T cells with subsequent IFN-γ secretion [50], the down-regulation of IFN-γ observed in the co-culture of T cells with DCs is most likely resulting from a reduced ability of the DCs matured in the presence of compounds **2** and **3** to secrete IL-12p40 (one of the two chains that form the IL-12 molecule). Compound **2** did not affect IL-10 secretion by DCs but compound **3** increased IL-10 secretion by DCs. Therefore, the decreased concentration of IL-10 in co-cultures of T cells and DCs matured in the presence of compounds **2** and **3** was unexpected. The reduced IL-10 levels observed in the co-cultures were most likely the result of reduced secretion by the T cells but not the DCs, but whether it is so needs to be confirmed, e.g., by intracellular staining for IL-10 on T cells and DCs in the co-culture experiments. Although the decreased secretion of IL-10 in the co-cultures may hamper the anti-inflammatory effect of compounds **2** and **3**, the downregulation of IFN-γ secretion is strongly suggestive of inhibition of inflammatory Th1 response and subsequently that compounds **2** and **3** may have the potential of being a starting point for development of new anti-inflammatory drugs.

The anti-inflammatory effect of compound **4**, shown previously in a monocytic cell line [6], was confirmed in the present study as it downregulated secretion of IL-12p40 by the DCs. However, compound **4** also downregulated IL-10 production, which could interfere with the anti-inflammatory effect observed by reduced IL-12p40 secretion. This seemed to be the case as, when DCs treated with compound **4** were co-cultured with T cells, the effect of compound **4** was not anti-inflammatory as neither Th1 nor Th17 cytokines were affected. These results were unexpected and suggest that the effect of compound **4** to decrease IL-10 secretion by the DCs seems to be the determining factor, overriding the effect of downregulation of IL-12p40 and subsequently leading to a reduction in IL-10 in the co-culture of the two cell types.

Despite structural similarities of compounds **1**, **2**, **4**, and **5**, which all possess the structure of a DKP-type cyclic dipeptide, there were remarkable differences in their anti-inflammatory effects. Oxidation of the indole ring in compound **1** as compared with compound **4** caused the disappearance of the anti-inflammatory activity, indicating that the indole skeleton is important in inhibition of cytokine secretion by the DCs. Both the number and the position of double bonds on the DKP-type cyclic dipeptide may affect the anti-inflammatory activity (**2** vs. **4** vs. **5**). The disappearance of the double bond at C-8 could decrease the anti-inflammatory activity, as compound **5** did not affect cytokine secretion by the DCs whilst compounds **4** and **2** did, suggesting that the double bond at C-8 is required for the activity. However, the double bond at C-12 may be responsible for the reduction of anti-inflammatory activity when comparing compound **2** with compound **4**. Considering these observations, the bromotryptophan containing the double bond at C-8 may be important for the activity. The double bond at the *N,N,N*-trimethylethanaminium group increased the suppression of IL-12p40 production and increased the IL-10 secretion (**6** vs. **7**). Collectively, 6-bromoindole derivatives may have anti-inflammatory activity that depends on the bromotryptophan nucleus (**1**, **2**, **4**, and **5**) or the side chain at C-3 position of the 6-bromoindole (**3**, **6**, and **7**), suggesting that there may be more than one potential target site or mode of action.

The observations described above indicate that *G. barretti* is a prolific source of 6-bromoindoles with potential anti-inflammatory activities, which may be a starting point for the development of new drug s with a potential for being used in the treatment of inflammatory diseases in the future.

4. Materials and Methods

4.1. General Produres

Optical rotations were measured on a P-2000 polarimeter (Jasco, OK, USA) equipped with a 10 mm pathlength cell. UV spectra were recorded on a NanoVue™ spectrophotometer (GE Healthcare Life Science, Little Chalfont, UK). ECD spectra were measured on a JASCO J-810 spectropolarimeter in quartz cells (1 or 5 mm pathlength) at 23 °C. IR spectra were measured on a Spectrum Two™ FTIR spectrometer (Perkin Elmer, Waltham, MA, USA). NMR spectra were recorded on a Bruker AM-400 spectrometer (proton frequency 400.13 MHz and carbon frequency 100.62 MHz, respectively) for compounds **4–7** (in CD_3OD and/or DMSO-d_6) using TMS as an internal standard or a Bruker Avance 600 spectrometer (proton frequency 600.13 MHz and carbon frequency 150.76 MHz, respectively) for compounds **1** (in CD_3OD and DMSO-d_6), **2–3** (in CD_3OD), and **7** (in DMSO-d_6). The ^{1}H NMR spectrum of compound **8** (in $CDCl_3$) was recorded on a Varian Mercury 400 spectrometer and the ^{13}C NMR spectrum was measured on a Varian Xsens 500 spectrometer equipped with a $^{13}C\{^1H\}$ cryoprobe at 125 MHz. High-resolution mass spectra were obtained on a Waters G1 Synapt qTOF mass spectrometer. An UHPLC system (ACQUITY UPLC Waters) was coupled in line with a qTOF mass spectrometer (Synapt G1, Waters) operating in the positive mode. HPLC was performed on a Dionex 3000 HPLC system equipped with a G1310A isopump, a G1322A degasser, a G1314A VWD detector (210 nm), a 250 × 21.2 mm Phenomenex Luna C18(2) column (5 μm), and a 250 × 4.6 mm Phenomenex Gemini-NX C18 column (5 μm). Alkaloids were detected by TLC on Merck silica gel F254 plates by immersing the plates in Dragendorff's reagent. VLC chromatography was performed on C_{18} adsorbent (LiChroprep RP-18, 40–63 μm, Merck Inc., Darmstadt, Germany). All organic solvents were purchased from Sigma-Aldrich and were HPLC grade or the highest degree of purity.

4.2. Animal Materials

The sponge material *Geodia barretti* was collected in the west of Iceland (65°27.6′ N–30°46.6′ W) at 388 m depth in September 2010. The sponge was identified by Dr. Hans Tore Rapp, University of Bergen (Norway). A voucher specimen was deposited at the Department of Natural Products Chemistry, Faculty of Pharmaceutical Sciences, University of Iceland. The collected specimens (six in total) (wet weight, 1.8 kg) were immediately frozen and stored at −20 °C.

4.3. Extraction and Isolation

The frozen sponge material was cut into small pieces and lyophilized prior to extraction with CH_2Cl_2:CH_3OH (*v*/*v*, 1:1) mixture (3 × 20 L, each for 24 h) at room temperature. The combined extracts were concentrated under *vacuum* to yield a dark gum and stored at −20 °C. The crude extract (1.8 g) was submitted to a modified Kupchan partition to yield five subextracts, namely hexane (fraction A), chloroform (fraction B), dichloromethane (fraction C), *n*-butanol (fraction D), and water (fraction E). Each fraction was analyzed by UPLC-qTOF-MS before preparative-scale isolation work commenced and the data were processed and analyzed by MassLynx programme and compared to available references in ChemSpider database [51] and SciFinder Scholar (Chemical Abstracts Service, Columbus, OH, USA). The fractions B and C showed similar patterns on TLC and the analysis of qTOF-MS data revealed similar chemical compositions. Thus, they were combined and fractionated by VLC on a C18 reversed-phase column using gradient elution of MeOH-H_2O (10:90→ 100:0) mixtures to obtain nine fractions (F2.1−F2.9). F2.2 (750 mg) was purified by preparative HPLC (28:72:0.1 CH_3CN-H_2O-TFA, 8.0 mL/min) to afford compounds **3** (3.5 mg), **4** (7.3 mg), and **6** (1.5 mg) and two impure fractions (F2.2.1 and F2.2.2). F2.2.1 (78.9 mg) was purified by semi-preparative HPLC using CH_3CN-H_2O-TFA (27:73:0.1) to yield compounds **1** (1.8 mg) and **5** (1.2 mg). F2.2.2 (10.1 mg) was also re-chromatographed by semi-preparative HPLC (ACN-H_2O-TFA, 31:69:1) to give compound **7** (5.3 mg). F2.4 (12.1 mg) was purified by semi-preparative HPLC (30:70:0.1 MeOH-H_2O-TFA, 2.2 mL/min) to yield compound **2** (3.0 mg).

Geobarrettin A (**1**): yellow solid (1.8 mg); $[\alpha]_D^{27}$ +7 (*c* 0.2, MeOH); UV (MeOH) λ_{max} (log ε) nm: 217 (3.17), 263 (2.64); IR ν_{max} cm^{-1}: 3352, 3214, 1679, 1441, 1205, 1138, 1057, 841, 802, 724; ^{1}H and ^{13}C NMR data, see Table 1; HRESIMS *m/z* 451.0728 [M + H]$^+$ (calcd for $C_{17}H_{20}{}^{79}BrN_6O_4$, 451.0729).

Geobarrettin B (**2**): yellow solid (3.0 mg); UV (MeOH) λ_{max} (log ε) nm: 231 (3.62), 270 (3.39), 289 (3.41), 372 (3.51); IR ν_{max} cm^{-1}: 3297, 1677, 1438, 1206, 1139, 843, 803, 725; ^{1}H and ^{13}C NMR data, see Table 1; HRESIMS *m/z* 417.0675 [M + H]$^+$ (calcd for $C_{17}H_{18}{}^{79}BrN_6O_2$, 417.0675).

Geobarrettin C (**3**): yellow solid (3.5 mg); UV (MeOH) λ_{max} (log ε) nm: 211 (3.42), 247 (3.17), 269 (3.12), 283 (2.95); IR ν_{max} cm^{-1}: 3207, 1676, 1523, 1445, 1203, 1134, 892, 802, 722; ^{1}H and ^{13}C NMR data, see Table 1; HRESIMS *m/z* 295.0440 [M]$^+$ (calcd for $C_{13}H_{16}{}^{79}BrN_2O^+$, 295.0446).

Barettin (**4**): dark yellow solid (7.3 mg); $[\alpha]_D^{25}$ −84 (*c* 0.5, MeOH), lit. $[\alpha]_D^{26}$ −32.5 (*c* 2, MeOH) [18], lit. $[\alpha]$ −25 (*c* 3, MeOH); HRESIMS *m/z* 419.0830 [M + H]$^+$ (calcd for $C_{17}H_{20}{}^{79}BrN_6O_2$, 419.0831); all remaining spectroscopic data are in good agreement with those previously published [9].

8,9-Dihydrobarettin (**5**): yellowish solid (1.2 mg); $[\alpha]_D^{25}$ −12.5 (*c* 0.096, MeOH), lit. $[\alpha]_D^{21}$ −24 (*c* 0.096, MeOH); HRESIMS *m/z* 421.0987 [M + H]$^+$ (calcd for $C_{17}H_{22}{}^{79}BrN_6O_2$, 421.0988); all remaining spectroscopic data are in good agreement with those previously published [11].

6-Bromoconicamin (**6**): colorless amorphous solid (1.5 mg); HRESIMS *m/z* 279.0495 [M]$^+$ ($C_{13}H_{16}{}^{79}BrN_2^+$, 279.0497); all remaining spectroscopic data are in good agreement with those previously published [14].

L-6-Bromohypaphorine (**7**): yellow solid (5.3 mg); $[[\alpha]_D^{23}$ +36 (*c* 0.2, EtOH); HRESIMS *m/z* 325.0550 [M + H]$^+$ (calcd for $C_{14}H_{18}{}^{79}BrN_2O_2$, 325.0546); all remaining spectroscopic data are in good agreement with those previously published [46].

4.4. Hydrogenolysis of R-Dioxindole (**8a**) to (R)-3-Propyldioxindole (**8**)

To a solution of (*R*)-dioxindole (**8a**) (16.7 mg, 59 μmol) (92% ee, $[\alpha]_D$ −30 (*c* 0.72, MeOH); lit. (88% ee) −24.3 (*c* 0.8, MeOH) [37]) in MeOH (5.0 mL) containing Et$_3$N (3 drops) was added 10% Pd-C (10 mg). The mixture was evacuated-purged with H$_2$ and allowed to hydrogenate (1 atm, H$_2$) for 7 h. Filtration of the mixture (Celite), followed by concentration of the eluate and passage through a short plug of silica (1:1 EtOAc-hexanes) to remove Et$_3$N•HBr gave (*R*)-3-propyldioxindole (**8**) as a colorless solid. UV (CF$_3$CH$_2$OH) λ_{max} (log ε) nm: 208 (3.10), 257 (3.32), 268 (sh), 286 (2.74). CD (CF$_3$CH$_2$OH) λ_{max} ($\Delta\varepsilon$) nm: 208 (+13.1), 219 (0), 232 (−10.7), 249 (0), 259 (+3.5). $[\alpha]_D$ + 96 (*c* 0.19, MeOH); + 50 (*c* 0.21, CF$_3$CH$_2$OH). IR (ZnSe) ν_{max} 3404, 2962, 1703, 1609, 1495, 1470, 1377, 1119, 1082, 754 cm^{-1}; ^{1}H NMR (CDCl$_3$, 400 MHz) δ 7.37 (1H, d, *J* = 7.2 Hz, H-4), 7.33 (1H, t, *J* = 7.6 Hz, H-6), 7.10 (1H, t, *J* = 7.6 Hz, H-5), 6.83 (1H, d, *J* = 7.6 Hz, H-7), 3.19 (3H, s, *N*-Me), 1.93 (2H, m, CH$_2$-1′), 1.12 (2H, m, CH$_2$-2′); 0.84 (3H, t, *J* = 7.2 Hz, C-*CH$_3$*-3′); ^{13}C NMR (CDCl$_3$, 125 MHz) δ 178.4 (C, C-2), 143.6 (C, C-7a), 130.1 (C, C-3a), 129.7 (CH, C-6), 124.0 (CH, C-5), 123.2 (CH, C-4), 108.5 (CH, C-7), 76.8 (C, C-3), 40.9 (CH$_2$, C-1′), 26.3 (CH$_3$, *N*-Me), 16.8 (CH$_2$, C-2′), 14.2 (CH$_3$, C-3′); HRESIMS *m/z* 228.0992 [M + Na]$^+$ (calcd for $C_{12}H_{15}NO_2Na^+$, 228.0995) (Figures S26–S30).

4.5. Hydrogenolysis of Geobarrettin A (**1**) to Debromodihydrogeobarrettin A (**1a**)

A sample of compound **1** was hydrogenated (1 atm H$_2$, MeOH, 20 equiv. Et$_3$N) for 15 h. The mixture was filtered and concentrated to give a colorless solid (~0.4 mg) consisting of an equimolar mixture of debromodihydrogeobarrettin A (**1a**) and Et$_3$N•HBr that was used, directly, for CD measurements and subsequent hydrolysis-DTA derivatization. UV-vis (CF$_3$CH$_2$OH) λ_{max} (log ε) nm: 207 (4.15), 269 (3.65), 281 (sh) (Figure S31); CD (CF$_3$CH$_2$OH) λ_{max} ($\Delta\varepsilon$) nm: 208 (+13.1), 232 (−10.7), 259 (+3.5). Identical with that of (*R*)-(**8**) (Figure 3).

4.6. Acid Hydrolysis of Debromodihydrogeobarrettin B (1a)

Approximately 0.31 mg of compound **1a** was separately hydrolyzed with 6 M HCl (0.8 mL) for 15 h at 110 °C, dried under a stream of N_2 followed by high vacuum to remove volatiles, and the resulting material subjected to further derivatization (see below).

4.7. Absolute Configuration of the Amino Acid of Geobarrettin A (1)

The determination of absolute configuration of the amino acids was performed as previously described [41]. After hydrolysis of **1a**, the residue was dissolved in acetone (50 µL) and treated with L-FDTA (25 mM in acetone, 50 µL) and 1 M NaHCO$_3$ (50 µL) and heated to 80 °C for 20 min. After cooling to 23 °C, the sample was quenched with 1 M HCl (50 µL), centrifuged, and the supernatant analyzed by RP HPLC (10 µL injection, Phenomenex Luna C18, 4.6 × 250 mm, gradient elution profile (15/85–65/35 CH$_3$CN-H$_2$O-0.1 M NH$_4$OAc-0.1% TFA, over 40 min, 0.7 mL/min). The L-FDTA derivatives were detected by UV-vis (λ_{max} 335 nm). Two peaks were eluted with retention times (ratio 19:81), coinciding with authentic L-DTA derivatives of D-Arg (25.33 min), L-Arg (26.78 min), respectively.

4.8. Absolute Configuration of the Amino Acid of Barettin (4)

A sample of barettin (**4**, 1.7 mg) was hydrogenated (1 atm H$_2$, 10% Pd-C, MeOH) for 19 h. The mixture was filtered and concentrated to give debromo-8,9-dihydrobarettin (**5a**) as a colorless solid (1.4 mg) consisting of an equimolar mixture of C-3 epimers. HRESIMS m/z 343.1874 [M + H]$^+$ (calcd for C$_{17}$H$_{23}$N$_6$O$_2$, 343.1877). The residue was hydrolyzed under standard conditions (6 M HCl, 15 h, see above) and the hydrolysate converted to the L-DTA derivatives and analyzed by RP HPLC as before. Two peaks, A and B, were eluted with retention times of t_R = 25.33 and 26.78 min (ratio A:B = 19:81), respectively, coinciding with authentic L-DTA derivatives of D- and L-Arg (25.33 and 26.78 min, respectively). When the same procedures were conducted on **4** without prior hydrogenation, D- and L-Arg-L-DTA derivatives were obtained in a ratio of 19:81 indicating partially racemic **4** (62% ee).

4.9. Maturation and Activation of DCs

DCs were developed and matured from human monocytes as previously described [52,53]. CD14$^+$ monocytes were isolated from peripheral blood mononuclear cells obtained from healthy human donors using CD14 Microbeads (Miltenyi Biotech, Bergisch Gladbach, Germany). Immature DCs were obtained by culturing CD14$^+$ monocytes at 5 × 10^5 cells/mL for 7 days in the presence of IL-4 at 12.5 ng/mL and GM-CSF at 25 ng/mL (both from R&D Systems, Abingdon, England), with fresh medium and cytokines added at day 3. The immature DCs were matured and activated by culturing them at 2.5 × 10^5 cells/mL for 24 h with IL-1β at 10 ng/mL, TNF-α at 50 ng/mL (both from R&D Systems), and lipopolysaccharide (LPS) at 500 ng/mL (Sigma-Aldrich, Munich, Germany). Pure compounds were dissolved in DMSO at the concentration of 10 µg/mL and added to the DCs at the same time as the cytokines and LPS. The final concentration of DMSO in the medium of DCs cultured with the pure compounds was 0.002% and the same concentration of DMSO was used as solvent control. In order to determine whether the effects of compounds **2–4** were dose-dependent, the concentrations of 2.5, 5, 7.5, 10 µg/mL were used. After 24 h the mature and activated DCs were harvested and the effects of the pure compounds on DC maturation and activation determined by measuring cytokine concentration in the culture medium by ELISA. Cell viability was determined by counting cells following staining with trypan blue and calculating the percentage of live cells.

4.10. Co-Culture of DCs and Allogeneic CD4$^+$ T Cells

DCs matured in the presence/absence of a pure compound at 10 µg/mL or solvent control only were co-cultured with allogeneic CD4$^+$ T cells at DC:T cell ratio of 1:10 (2 × 10^5 DCs/mL: 2 × 10^6 T cells/mL) for 6 days. CD4$^+$ T cells were obtained from PBMCs using CD4 Microbeads

Mar. Drugs **2018**, *16*, 437

(Miltenyi Biotec). The effects of the pure compounds on the ability of the DCs to differentiate the CD4⁺ T cells were determined by measuring cytokine concentrations in the co-culture supernatants by ELISA.

4.11. Determination of Cytokine Concentration by ELISA

The concentrations of IL-12p40 and IL-10 in culture supernatants from DCs and of IFN-γ, IL-17 and IL-10 in supernatants from co-cultures of DCs and allogeneic CD4⁺ T cells were measured by sandwich ELISA using DuoSets from R&D Systems according to the manufacturer's protocol. The results were expressed as secretion index (SI), which was calculated by dividing the cytokine concentration in supernatants from DCs cultured with pure compound or co-cultures of these DCs with allogeneic CD4⁺ T cells by the cytokine concentration in supernatants of DCs cultured with solvent only or co-cultures of these DCs with allogeneic CD4⁺ T cells.

4.12. Statistical Analysis

Data are presented as the mean values $\pm$ standard error of the mean (SEM). As the data were not normally distributed, Mann-Whitney U test or Kruskal Wallis one-way ANOVA with Tukey's post-hoc test were used to determine statistical differences between treatments (SigmaStat 3.1, Systat Software, San Jose, CA, USA) and $p < 0.05$ was considered as statistically significant.

5. Conclusions

In conclusion, three new 6-bromoindole derivatives, geobarrettin A–C (**1**–**3**), and four known ones (**4**–**7**) were obtained from the marine sponge *G. barretti* collected from west of Iceland. Compounds **2**, **3** and **4** showed anti-inflammatory properties by inhibiting DC secretion of IL-12p40 with varying effects on IL-10, and the anti-inflammatory effect of compounds **2** and **3** was confirmed by inhibition of IFN-γ secretion in co-cultures of T cells and DCs matured in the presence of the compounds. It is increasingly being recognized that low-grade, subclinical inflammation is a significant pathogenic factor in many chronic diseases that have not, until now, been considered inflammatory in nature. Importantly, this includes most diseases that today are the main cause of morbidity and mortality in Western countries, such as atherosclerotic diseases, cancers, chronic pain disorders, and Alzheimer's disease [54]. Therefore, the discovery of the two new 6-bromoindole derivatives with anti-inflammatory effects is important as they could be used in the development of treatments for diseases with inflammatory components.

Supplementary Materials: The following are available online at http://www.mdpi.com/1660-3397/16/11/437/s1, The 1D and 2D NMR, HRESIMS, and IR spectra of the new compounds **1**–**3**. The 1D NMR, UV, IR and HRESIMS spectra of **8**. The UV spectrum and HPLC chromatogram of L-DPT derivative of the hydrolysate **1a**.

Author Contributions: Methodology and formal analysis, X.D., C.R., I.H., J.F., T.F.M., D.T., and S.O.; Writing—original draft preparation, X.D.; Writing—review and editing, C.R., I.H., J.F., T.F.M., D.T., and S.O.; Supervision, I.H., J.F., D.T., and S.O.; Funding Acquisition, I.H., J.F., and S.O.

Funding: This research was funded by University of Iceland Research Fund (Doctoral Grant and Project Grant), AVS R&D Fund of Ministry of Fisheries and Agriculture in Iceland, the Landspitali University Hospital Research Fund, and the Memory Fund of Helga Jonsdottir and Sigurlidi Kristjansson. Funding from the National Institutes of Health (to T.F.M, R21 AT009783-01) is acknowledged.

Acknowledgments: The authors would like to thank Hans Tore Rapp at the University of Bergen for the identification of animal material, Nathalie Kringlstein for technical assistance, Annaliese Franz at University of California, Davis, for the generous gift of **8a**, Sigridur Jonsdottir at University of Iceland for running NMR spectra on a Bruker AM-400 spectrometer, Finnur Freyr Eiriksson and Margret Thorsteinsdottir for running UPLC-qTOF-MS and Kare Telnes for giving the permission to use the sponge picture in the Graphical abstract.

Conflicts of Interest: The authors declare no conflict of interest. The funders had no role in the design of the study; in the collection, analyses, or interpretation of data; in the writing of the manuscript, or in the decision to publish the results.

References

1. Dubois, R.N. The Jeremiah Metzger Lecture: Inflammation, immune modulators, and chronic disease. *Trans. Am. Clin. Climatol. Assoc.* **2015**, *126*, 230–236. [PubMed]
2. Chen, L.; Deng, H.; Cui, H.; Fang, J.; Zuo, Z.; Deng, J.; Li, Y.; Wang, X.; Zhao, L. Inflammatory responses and inflammation-associated diseases in organs. *Oncotarget* **2018**, *9*, 7204–7218. [CrossRef] [PubMed]
3. Mayer, A.M.S.; Rodriguez, A.D.; Taglialatela-Scafati, O.; Fusetani, N. Marine pharmacology in 2012–2013: Marine compounds with antibacterial, antidiabetic, antifungal, anti-inflammatory, antiprotozoal, antituberculosis, and antiviral activities; Affecting the immune and nervous systems, and other miscellaneous mechanisms of action. *Mar. Drugs* **2017**, *15*, 273. [CrossRef]
4. Malve, H. Exploring the ocean for new drug developments: Marine pharmacology. *J. Pharm. Bioallied. Sci.* **2016**, *8*, 83–91. [CrossRef] [PubMed]
5. Senthilkumar, K.; Kim, S.K. Marine invertebrate natural products for anti-inflammatory and chronic diseases. *Evid. Based Complement. Alternat. Med.* **2013**, *2013*, 572859. [CrossRef] [PubMed]
6. Yuan, G.; Wahlqvist, M.L.; He, G.; Yang, M.; Li, D. Natural products and anti-inflammatory activity. *Asia Pac. J. Clin. Nutr.* **2006**, *15*, 143–152. [PubMed]
7. Gonzalez, Y.; Torres-Mendoza, D.; Jones, G.E.; Fernandez, P.L. Marine diterpenoids as potential anti-inflammatory agents. *Mediat. Inflamm.* **2015**, *2015*, 263543. [CrossRef] [PubMed]
8. Keyzers, R.A.; Davies-Coleman, M.T. Anti-inflammatory metabolites from marine sponges. *Chem. Soc. Rev.* **2005**, *34*, 355–365. [CrossRef] [PubMed]
9. Lidgren, G.; Bohlin, L. Studies of Swedish marine organisms. 7. A novel biologically-active indole alkaloid from the sponge *Geodia baretti*. *Tetrahedron Lett.* **1986**, *27*, 3283–3284. [CrossRef]
10. Solter, S.; Dieckmann, R.; Blumenberg, M.; Francke, W. Barettin, revisited? *Tetrahedron Lett.* **2002**, *43*, 3385–3386. [CrossRef]
11. Sjogren, M.; Goransson, U.; Johnson, A.L.; Dahlstrom, M.; Andersson, R.; Bergman, J.; Jonsson, P.R.; Bohlin, L. Antifouling activity of brominated cyclopeptides from the marine sponge *Geodia barretti*. *J. Nat. Prod.* **2004**, *67*, 368–372. [CrossRef] [PubMed]
12. Hedner, E.; Sjogren, M.; Hodzic, S.; Andersson, R.; Goransson, U.; Jonsson, P.R.; Bohlin, L. Antifouling activity of a dibrominated cyclopeptide from the marine sponge *Geodia barretti*. *J. Nat. Prod.* **2008**, *71*, 330–333. [CrossRef] [PubMed]
13. Olsen, E.K.; Hansen, E.; Moodie, W.; Isaksson, J.; Sepcic, K.; Cergolj, M.; Svenson, J.; Andersen, J.H. Marine AChE inhibitors isolated from *Geodia barretti*: Natural compounds and their synthetic analogs. *Org. Biomol. Chem.* **2016**, *14*, 1629–1640. [CrossRef] [PubMed]
14. Takahashi, Y.; Tanaka, N.; Kubota, T.; Ishiyama, H.; Shibazaki, A.; Gonoi, T.; Fromont, J.; Kobayashi, J. Heteroaromatic alkaloids, nakijinamines, from a sponge *Suberites* sp. *Tetrahedron* **2012**, *68*, 8545–8550. [CrossRef]
15. Lidgren, G.; Bohlin, L.; Christophersen, C. Studies of Swedish marine organisms .10. Biologically-active compounds from the marine sponge *Geodia barretti*. *J. Nat. Prod.* **1988**, *51*, 1277–1280. [CrossRef]
16. Carstens, B.B.; Rosengren, K.J.; Gunasekera, S.; Schempp, S.; Bohlin, L.; Dahlstrom, M.; Clark, R.J.; Goransson, U. Goransson, U. Isolation, characterization, and synthesis of the barrettides: Disulfide-containing peptides from the marine sponge *Geodia barretti*. *J. Nat. Prod.* **2015**, *78*, 1886–1893. [CrossRef] [PubMed]
17. Hougaard, L.; Christophersen, C.; Nielsen, P.H.; Klitgaard, A.; Tendal, O. The chemical-composition of species of *Geodia*, *Isops* and *Stryphnus* (Choristida, Demospongia, Porifera)–a comparative-study with some taxonomical implications. *Biochem. Syst. Ecol.* **1991**, *19*, 223–235. [CrossRef]
18. Johnson, A.L.; Bergman, J.; Sjogren, M.; Bohlin, L. Synthesis of barettin. *Tetrahedron* **2004**, *60*, 961–965. [CrossRef]
19. Borthwick, A.D. 2,5-Diketopiperazines: Synthesis, reactions, medicinal chemistry, and bioactive natural products. *Chem. Rev.* **2012**, *112*, 3641–3716. [CrossRef] [PubMed]
20. Lind, K.F.; Hansen, E.; Osterud, B.; Eilertsen, K.E.; Bayer, A.; Engqvist, M.; Leszczak, K.; Jorgensen, T.O.; Andersen, J.H. Antioxidant and anti-inflammatory activities of barettin. *Mar. Drugs* **2013**, *11*, 2655–2666. [CrossRef] [PubMed]

21. Hedner, E.; Sjogren, M.; Frandberg, P.A.; Johansson, T.; Goransson, U.; Dahlstrom, M.; Jonsson, P.; Nyberg, F.; Bohlin, L. Brominated cyclodipeptides from the marine sponge *Geodia barretti* as selective 5-HT ligands. *J. Nat. Prod.* **2006**, *69*, 1421–1424. [CrossRef] [PubMed]

22. Pooley, J.L.; Heath, W.R.; Shortman, K. Cutting edge: Intravenous soluble antigen is presented to CD4 T cells by CD8- dendritic cells, but cross-presented to CD8 T cells by CD8+ dendritic cells. *J. Immunol.* **2001**, *166*, 5327–5330. [CrossRef] [PubMed]

23. Manetti, R.; Gerosa, F.; Giudizi, M.G.; Biagiotti, R.; Parronchi, P.; Piccinni, M.P.; Sampognaro, S.; Maggi, E.; Romagnani, S.; Trinchieri, G.; et al. Interleukin 12 induces stable priming for interferon gamma (IFN-gamma) production during differentiation of human T helper (Th) cells and transient IFN-gamma production in established Th2 cell clones. *J. Exp. Med.* **1994**, *179*, 1273–1283. [CrossRef] [PubMed]

24. Iyer, S.S.; Cheng, G. Role of interleukin 10 transcriptional regulation in inflammation and autoimmune disease. *Crit. Rev. Immunol.* **2012**, *32*, 23–63. [CrossRef] [PubMed]

25. Schmitt, N.; Ueno, H. Regulation of human helper T cell subset differentiation by cytokines. *Curr. Opin. Immunol.* **2015**, *34*, 130–136. [CrossRef] [PubMed]

26. Workman, C.J.; Szymczak-Workman, A.L.; Collison, L.W.; Pillai, M.R.; Vignali, D.A. The development and function of regulatory T cells. *Cell Mol. Life Sci.* **2009**, *66*, 2603–2622. [CrossRef] [PubMed]

27. Kupchan, S.M.; Tsou, G.; Sigel, C.W. Datiscacin, a novel cytotoxic cucurbitacin 20-acetate from *Datisca glomerata*. *J. Org. Chem.* **1973**, *38*, 1420–1421. [CrossRef] [PubMed]

28. Vanwagenen, B.C.; Larsen, R.; Cardellina, J.H.; Randazzo, D.; Lidert, Z.C.; Swithenbank, C. Ulosantoin, a potent insecticide from the sponge *Ulosa ruetzleri*. *J. Org. Chem.* **1993**, *58*, 335–337. [CrossRef]

29. Jiang, Y.; Liu, F.J.; Wang, Y.M.; Li, H.J. Dereplication-guided isolation of novel hepatoprotective triterpenoid saponins from *Celosiae semen* by high-performance liquid chromatography coupled with electrospray ionization tandem quadrupole-time-of-flight mass spectrometry. *J. Pharm. Biomed. Anal.* **2017**, *132*, 148–155. [CrossRef] [PubMed]

30. Wang, W.G.; Li, A.; Yan, B.C.; Niu, S.B.; Tang, J.W.; Li, X.N.; Du, X.; Challis, G.L.; Che, Y.; Sun, H.D.; et al. LC-MS-guided isolation of penicilfuranone A: A new antifibrotic furancarboxylic acid from the plant endophytic fungus *Penicillium* sp. sh18. *J. Nat. Prod.* **2016**, *79*, 149–155. [CrossRef] [PubMed]

31. Zhang, Z.; Di, Y.T.; Wang, Y.H.; Zhang, Z.; Mu, S.Z.; Fang, X.; Zhang, Y.; Tan, C.J.; Zhang, Q.; Yan, X.H.; et al. Gelegamines A-E: Five new oxindole alkaloids from *Gelsemium elegans*. *Tetrahedron* **2009**, *65*, 4551–4556. [CrossRef]

32. Kamano, Y.; Zhang, H.P.; Ichihara, Y.; Kizu, H.; Komiyama, K.; Pettit, G.R. Convolutamydine A, a novel bioactive hydroxyoxindole alkaloid from marine bryozoan *Amathia Convoluta*. *Tetrahedron Lett.* **1995**, *36*, 2783–2784. [CrossRef]

33. Wu, H.; Xue, F.; Xiao, X.; Qin, Y. Total synthesis of (+)-perophoramidine and determination of the absolute configuration. *J. Am. Chem. Soc.* **2010**, *132*, 14052–14054. [CrossRef] [PubMed]

34. Ghosh, D.; Saravanan, S.; Gupta, N.; Abdi, S.H.R.; Khan, N.U.; Kureshy, R.I.; Bajaj, H.C. Phosphotungstic acid as an efficient catalyst for allylation of isatins and *N*-tert-butyloxycarbonylamido sulfones under solvent-free conditions. *Asian J. Org. Chem.* **2014**, *3*, 1173–1181. [CrossRef]

35. Wei, X.; Henriksen, N.M.; Skalicky, J.J.; Harper, M.K.; Cheatham, T.E., 3rd; Ireland, C.M.; Van Wagoner, R.M. Araiosamines A-D: Tris-bromoindole cyclic guanidine alkaloids from the marine sponge Clathria (Thalysias) araiosa. *J. Org. Chem.* **2011**, *76*, 5515–5523. [CrossRef] [PubMed]

36. Tang, Y.Q.; Sattler, I.; Thiericke, R.; Grabley, S.; Feng, X.Z. Maremycins C and D, new diketopiperazines, and maremycins E and F, novel polycyclic spiro-indole metabolites isolated from *Streptomyces* sp. *Eur. J. Org. Chem.* **2001**, 261–267. [CrossRef]

37. Hanhan, N.V.; Sahin, A.H.; Chang, T.W.; Fettinger, J.C.; Franz, A.K. Catalytic asymmetric synthesis of substituted 3-hydroxy-2-oxindoles. *Angew. Chem. Int. Ed. Engl.* **2010**, *49*, 744–747. [CrossRef] [PubMed]

38. Salib, M.N.; Molinski, T.F. Six trikentrin-like cyclopentanoindoles from *trikentrion flabelliforme*. Absolute structural assignment by NMR and ECD. *J. Org. Chem.* **2018**, *83*, 1278–1286. [CrossRef] [PubMed]

39. Sonderegger, O.J.; Burgi, T.; Limbach, L.K.; Baiker, A. Enantio selective reduction of isatin derivatives over cinchonidine modified Pt/alumina. *J. Mol. Catal. A Chem.* **2004**, *217*, 93–101. [CrossRef]

40. Phyo, Y.Z.; Ribeiro, J.; Fernandes, C.; Kijjoa, A.; Pinto, M.M.M. Marine natural peptides: Determination of absolute configuration using liquid chromatography methods and evaluation of bioactivities. *Molecules* **2018**, *23*, 306. [CrossRef] [PubMed]

41. Salib, M.N.; Molinski, T.F. Cyclic hexapeptide dimers, antatollamides A and B, from the ascidian *Didemnum molle*. A tryptophan-derived auxiliary for L- and D-amino acid assignments. *J. Org. Chem.* **2017**, *82*, 10181–10187. [CrossRef] [PubMed]

42. Kaiser, K.; Benner, R. Hydrolysis-induced racemization of amino acids. *Limnol. Oceanogr.-Meth.* **2005**, *3*, 318–325. [CrossRef]

43. Albinsson, B.; Norden, B. Excited-state properties of the indole chromophore: Electronic-transition moment directions from linear dichroism measurements: Effect of methyl and methoxy substituents. *J. Phys. Chem.* **1992**, *96*, 6204–6212. [CrossRef]

44. Shin, C.G.; Hayakawa, M.; Mikami, K.; Yoshimura, J. Syntheses and configurational assignments of albonoursin and its three geometric isomers. *Tetrahedron Lett.* **1977**, *18*, 863–866. [CrossRef]

45. Shin, C.; Hayakawa, M.; Suzuki, T.; Ohtsuka, A.; Yoshimura, J. α,β-Unsaturated carboxylic-acid derivatives. 13. Synthesis andconfiguration of alkyl 2-acylamino-2-alkenoates and their cyclized 2,5-piperazinedione derivatives. *Bull. Chem. Soc. Jpn.* **1978**, *51*, 550–554. [CrossRef]

46. Kasheverov, I.E.; Shelukhina, I.V.; Kudryavtsev, D.S.; Makarieva, T.N.; Spirova, E.N.; Guzii, A.G.; Stonik, V.A.; Tsetlin, V.I. 6-Bromohypaphorine from marine nudibranch mollusk *Hermissenda crassicornis* is an agonist of human α7 nicotinic acetylcholine receptor. *Mar. Drugs* **2015**, *13*, 1255–1266. [CrossRef] [PubMed]

47. Kondo, K.; Nishi, J.; Ishibashi, M.; Kobayashi, J. Two new tryptophan-derived alkaloids from the Okinawan marine sponge *Aplysina* sp. *J. Nat. Prod.* **1994**, *57*, 1008–1011. [CrossRef] [PubMed]

48. Corthay, A. How do regulatory T cells work? *Scand. J. Immunol.* **2009**, *70*, 326–336. [CrossRef] [PubMed]

49. Romagnani, S. Th1 and Th2 in human diseases. *Clin. Immunol. Immunopathol.* **1996**, *80*, 225–235. [CrossRef] [PubMed]

50. Gee, K.; Guzzo, C.; Che Mat, N.F.; Ma, W.; Kumar, A. The IL-12 family of cytokines in infection, inflammation and autoimmune disorders. *Inflamm. Allergy Drug Targets* **2009**, *8*, 40–52. [CrossRef] [PubMed]

51. Pence, H.E.; Williams, A. ChemSpider: An online chemical information resource. *J. Chem. Educ.* **2010**, *87*, 1123–1124. [CrossRef]

52. Freysdottir, J.; Sigurpalsson, M.B.; Omarsdottir, S.; Olafsdottir, E.S.; Vikingsson, A.; Hardardottir, I. Ethanol extract from birch bark (*Betula pubescens*) suppresses human dendritic cell mediated Th1 responses and directs it towards a Th17 regulatory response in vitro. *Immunol. Lett.* **2011**, *136*, 90–96. [CrossRef] [PubMed]

53. Di, X.; Oskarsson, J.T.; Omarsdottir, S.; Freysdottir, J.; Hardardottir, I. Lipophilic fractions from the marine sponge *Halichondria sitiens* decrease secretion of pro-inflammatory cytokines by dendritic cells and decrease their ability to induce a Th1 type response by allogeneic CD4+ T cells. *Pharm. Biol.* **2017**, *55*, 2116–2122. [CrossRef] [PubMed]

54. Iso, H.; Cui, R.; Date, C.; Kikuchi, S.; Tamakoshi, A.; Group, J.S. C-reactive protein levels and risk of mortality from cardiovascular disease in Japanese: The JACC Study. *Atherosclerosis* **2009**, *207*, 291–297. [CrossRef] [PubMed]

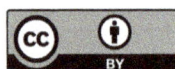

marine drugs

MDPI

Review

Prostaglandins in Marine Organisms: A Review

Federica Di Costanzo, Valeria Di Dato *, Adrianna Ianora and Giovanna Romano

Marine Biotechnology Department, Stazione Zoologica Anton Dohrn Napoli, Villa Comunale, 80121 Napoli, Italy
* Correspondence: valeria.didato@szn.it; Tel.: +39-081-5833-430

Received: 17 June 2019; Accepted: 19 July 2019; Published: 23 July 2019

Abstract: Prostaglandins (PGs) are lipid mediators belonging to the eicosanoid family. PGs were first discovered in mammals where they are key players in a great variety of physiological and pathological processes, for instance muscle and blood vessel tone regulation, inflammation, signaling, hemostasis, reproduction, and sleep-wake regulation. These molecules have successively been discovered in lower organisms, including marine invertebrates in which they play similar roles to those in mammals, being involved in the control of oogenesis and spermatogenesis, ion transport, and defense. Prostaglandins have also been found in some marine macroalgae of the genera *Gracilaria* and *Laminaria* and very recently the PGs pathway has been identified for the first time in some species of marine microalgae. In this review we report on the occurrence of prostaglandins in the marine environment and discuss the anti-inflammatory role of these molecules.

Keywords: prostaglandins; clavulones; punaglandins; thromboxane; inflammation; marine vertebrates; marine invertebrates; diatoms; macroalgae

1. Introduction

Marine organisms have a great potential to produce a vast variety of bioactive molecules with high antibiotic, anti-proliferative, and anti-inflammatory activity [1]. The biodiversity hosted by the oceans is greater than in terrestrial environments [2] but nonetheless, marine bioresources are still underexplored, and many species await to be discovered.

The high probability to find new interesting bioactive molecules from marine organisms has fostered the effort of the scientific community to adopt new technologies and approaches to increase the success of biodiscovery from marine resources, with a main focus on products with antibiotic, antitumor and anti-inflammatory activities. Of particular interest is the search for new anti-inflammatory compounds since inflammation processes are often related to the onset of chronic pathologies and tumors.

Indeed, inflammation processes represent a fundamental way to restore the original equilibrium of a cell or tissue whose physiology has been impaired by damaging stimuli [3]. At the same time, if inflammation is not blocked it can stimulate a cascade of events that eventually lead to serious diseases such as cancer and autoimmune disorders [4]. The inflammation-resolution process can have different features depending on the type of tissue and injurious stimulus [5], therefore, specific types of pro-resolution stimuli or drugs may be necessary [6]. Both the onset and the resolution of the inflammation are active processes that involve a complex interplay of different molecules [7] like chemokines, cell adhesion molecules, proteolytic enzymes, eicosanoids [8], reactive oxygen species (ROS), and reactive nitrogen species (RNS) [9,10]. Among these, eicosanoids deriving from oxidation of polyunsaturated fatty acids (PUFA) through cyclooxygenase (COX) and lipoxygenase (LOX) pathways play a pivotal role both in the onset and in the resolution of inflammation [9]. The main products of COX enzymes are prostaglandins (PGs), fatty acid derivatives with a molecular structure based on 20 carbon atoms that share a prostanoic acid skeleton.

Prostaglandin E$_2$ was the first PGs to be identified in the early 1930s in human seminal plasma by Von Euler [11] and, independently, by Goldblatt [12] although the chemical structures were determined only 30 years later by Bergström, Samuelsson, and co-workers [13].

PGs are very well studied and described in mammals where they are active in a great variety of physiological and pathological processes such as smooth muscle and vaso-tone regulation, signaling, hemostasis sleep-wake regulation, reproduction, and especially inflammation. In these organisms, they are synthetized and released in response to external stimuli [14] and rapidly inactivated by metabolizing enzymes after they have accomplished their function [15].

PGs represent very important and interesting lipid mediators in all vertebrates and in both terrestrial and marine invertebrates [16,17]. Plants utilize chemically related molecules (jasmonic acid) that have a defensive role, similarly to PGs [16,18,19]. Nevertheless, in some plant species like onions and poplar, a few PGs have also been identified [20].

In the marine environment, prostaglandins have been reported both in vertebrates such as carps, sheatfish and leopard sharks, and invertebrates such as sea squirts, mussels, scallops, crawfish, blue crabs, and sea-anemones and in some macroalgae as the red alga *Gracilaria asiatica* C. F. Zhang & B. M. Xia, 1985 and the brown alga *Laminaria digitata* (Hudson) J. V. Lamouroux, 1813.

The earliest report about the presence of prostaglandins in marine invertebrates was by Weinheimer and Spraggins (1969) that discovered 15-epi-prostaglandin A$_2$ and its acetate methyl ester in the gorgonian-type coral *Plexaura homomalla* Esper, 1794 [21]. The discovery of high PGs levels in gorgonians contributed to the rapid growth of the study and application of PGs in the pharmaceutical and biomedical sector [22].

Very recently, Di Dato et al. (2017) described the presence of all the three series of PGs molecules also in diatoms, an ecologically successful group of marine microalgae [23].

In this review, we present a short background on prostaglandin structure and function and give an updated overview of the presence of PGs in marine organisms, discussing the anti-inflammatory role of PGs from the marine environment.

2. Structure, Biosynthesis, and Activity of Prostaglandins in Mammals

Prostaglandins consist of a cyclopentanone nucleus with two side chains. Primary prostaglandins, which include prostaglandin D$_2$ (PGD$_2$), prostaglandin E$_2$ (PGE$_2$), prostaglandin F$_{2\alpha}$ (PGF$_{2\alpha}$), and prostaglandin I$_2$ (PGI$_2$), contain a 15-hydroxyl group with a 13,14-trans double bond (Figure 1).

Currently, three classes of prostaglandins are categorized, based on the number of double bonds present within the molecule and on the fatty acid precursor. Prostaglandins belonging to the series 1 have one double bond and derive from 8,11,14-eicosatrienoic acid (di-homolinolenic acid, ETrA), those of the series 2 have two double bonds and derive from 5,8,11,14-eicosatetraenoic acid (arachidonic acid, ARA), and those of the series 3 have three double bonds and derive from 5,8,11,14,17-eicosapentaenoic acid (EPA).

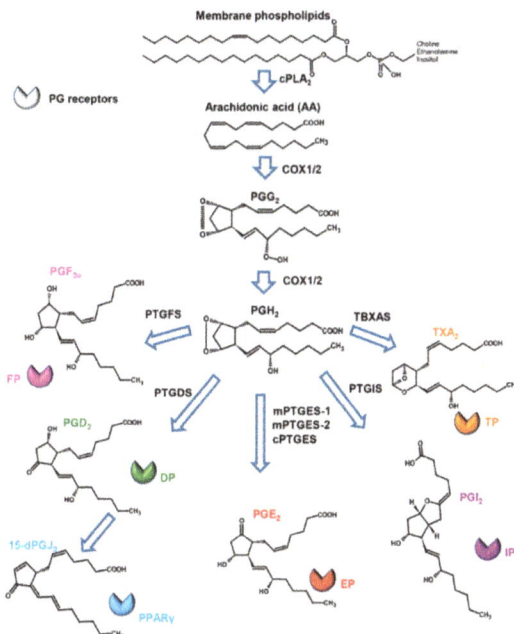

Figure 1. Prostaglandin biosynthetic pathway. Enzymes involved in the pathway are reported next to the arrows. For the abbreviation, refer to the text. Modified from [24].

Their nomenclature comprises 10 specific molecular groups, identified by the letters A through J, that differ by variation in the functional groups attached to positions 9 and 11 of the cyclopentane ring. For PGF, the additional subscript "α" or "β" denotes the spatial configuration of the carbon 9 hydroxyl group. For additional details on the nomenclature of prostaglandins see Lands, 1979 [25].

PGs action is mediated by the interaction with specific receptors present on the plasma membrane. These are transmembrane G-protein coupled receptors (GPCR), named as prostaglandin EP receptor (EP), prostaglandin $F_{2\alpha}$ receptor (FP), prostaglandin DP receptor (DP), and prostacyclin I_2 receptor (IP) receptors, that are highly selective for PGE_2 $PGF_{2\alpha}$, PGD_2, and PGI_2, respectively [26]. The EP family comprises four isoforms (EP_{1-4}) that play a relevant role in inflammation processes [27]. The downstream signaling of this receptor family is responsible for the pleiotropic ability of PGE_2 to activate different processes, including cell proliferation, apoptosis, angiogenesis, inflammation, and immune surveillance in different cell types [24].

Most prostaglandins display a marked structure-activity specificity mainly determined by substitutions in the cyclopentanone ring and the degree of unsaturation of the side chains. They exert their function once secreted into the extracellular medium, where they are rapidly metabolized by 15-hydroxyprostaglandin dehydrogenase (15-OH-PGDH). This enzyme selectively oxidizes the hydroxyl group at carbon 15 into a 15-keto derivative [28] accompanied by a substantial loss of biological activity.

Prostaglandins derive from the sequential actions of highly specific enzymes (Figure 1). Their synthesis is initiated by phospholipases A_2 (PLA_2), a family of enzymes that hydrolyze membrane phospholipids at the sn-2 position, liberating free fatty acid precursors, mainly ARA [15]. These enzymes represent a key step in the PG biosynthetic pathway, being regulated by Ca^{2+} binding and phosphorylation by mitogen-activated protein kinase (MAPK) in response to different stimuli. Membrane-released ARA is then rapidly converted through the cyclization and inclusion of molecular oxygen in the precursor by the action of cyclooxygenase (COXs) enzymes into the unstable metabolite

PGG$_2$, which is subsequently reduced to PGH$_2$ by the same enzyme [14]. Cyclooxygenases exist in a substrate-limiting environment; thus, liberation of fatty acids from esterified stores results in the prompt formation of the products. There are two major COX isoforms; COX-1 is constitutively active and present in most cells in the body; expression of the COX-2 isoform is inducible in many tissues by pro-inflammatory and mitogenic stimuli, such as cytokines [29]. The specific transformation of the first product PGH$_2$ to other PGs and thromboxanes (TXs) by downstream enzymes is complexly orchestrated and is cell specific, since each cell tends to form mainly one of these compounds as the major product. For example, in brain and mast cells, PGH$_2$ is converted to PGD$_2$, whereas it is converted in PGF$_{2\alpha}$ in the uterus; from the same precursor, vascular endothelial cells produce PGI$_2$ (prostacyclin) and platelets release thromboxane A$_2$ (TXA$_2$).

The conversion to PGE$_2$, the most widespread PG, is due to PGE synthase-1, also present in different isoforms in mammals: microsomal PGE synthase-1 (mPTGES-1), mPTGES-2, and cytosolic PGE synthase (cPTGES), the latter of particular interest since frequently associated to the tumorigenic activity of PGE$_2$ [30].

Prostaglandin E$_2$ synthesis is a key event for the development of the three principal signs of inflammation: swelling, redness, pain and fever. Moreover, PGE$_2$ also contributes to the amplification of the inflammatory response by enhancing and prolonging signals produced by pro-inflammatory agents, such as interleukin 1α bradykinin, histamine, neurokinins, and complement [31,32]. These signals, in turn, can increase COX-2 expression thus further increasing PGE$_2$ synthesis. This PG, however, can have a double, inverse role, being also able to act as an immunosuppressant, repressing the differentiation of T helper 1 cells and limiting cytokine release and further prostaglandin synthesis by activating a negative feedback on mPGES-1 (Figure 2a).

PGD$_2$-synthesizing enzymes exist as two distinct genes coding for hematopoietic- and lipocalin-type PGD synthases (H-PTGDS and L-PTGDS, respectively). H-PTGDS is generally localized in the cytosol of immune and inflammatory cells, whereas L-PTGDS has a tissue-based expression [33]. The activity of PGD$_2$ has been mainly associated with inflammatory conditions, being involved in immunologically relevant functions. Its action seems to be mediated by the non-enzymatic production of the PGJ$_2$ family, which occurs through a spontaneous dehydration in aqueous solutions. One of the most studied PGJ$_2$ metabolites, 15-deoxy-Δ12-PGJ$_2$ (15dPGJ$_2$), showed anti-inflammatory properties based on interaction with the intracellular targets Nuclear Factor kappa-light-chain-enhancer of activated B cells (NF-κB), Activator Protein 1 (AP-1), and Peroxisome Proliferator-Activated Receptor gamma (PPAR-γ) [31]. 15dPGJ$_2$ also induces the reduction of neutrophil migration and inhibits the release of Interleukin 6 (IL-6), Interleukin 1β (IL-1β), Interleukin 12 (IL-12), and Tumor Necrosis Factor-α (TNF-α) from macrophages (Figure 2b).

PGD$_2$ can be further metabolized to PGF$_{2\alpha}$, although the latter can also be synthesized from PGH$_2$ via PGF synthase. PGF$_{2\alpha}$ acts via FP receptors, resulting in the elevation of intracellular free calcium concentrations that regulates numerous important physiological functions related to reproduction linking multiple molecular mechanisms that are fine-tuned coordinated events in mammalian physiology [34] (Figure 2c). The emerging role of PGF$_{2\alpha}$ in acute and chronic inflammation has opened new opportunities for the design of novel anti-inflammatory drugs.

A non-enzymatic dehydration reaction is also responsible for the formation of the PGA series from the corresponding PGE. The PG series A and J contain an α,β-unsaturated carbonyl group within the cyclopentenone ring, which seem to contribute to the anti-inflammatory activity of these PGs [35].

The enzyme prostaglandin I synthase (PGIS), a member of the cytochrome P450 superfamily, specifically converts PGH$_2$ to PGI$_2$ [33]. This PG has anti-mitogenic activity and inhibits DNA synthesis through specific IP receptors. It mediates pro-inflammatory stimuli in non-allergic acute inflammation, while acting as an anti-inflammatory mediator in Th2-mediated allergic inflammatory responses. Soon after having exerted its action, PGI$_2$ is rapidly converted by non-enzymatic processes to the inactive product 6-keto-PGF$_{1\alpha}$ (Figure 2d).

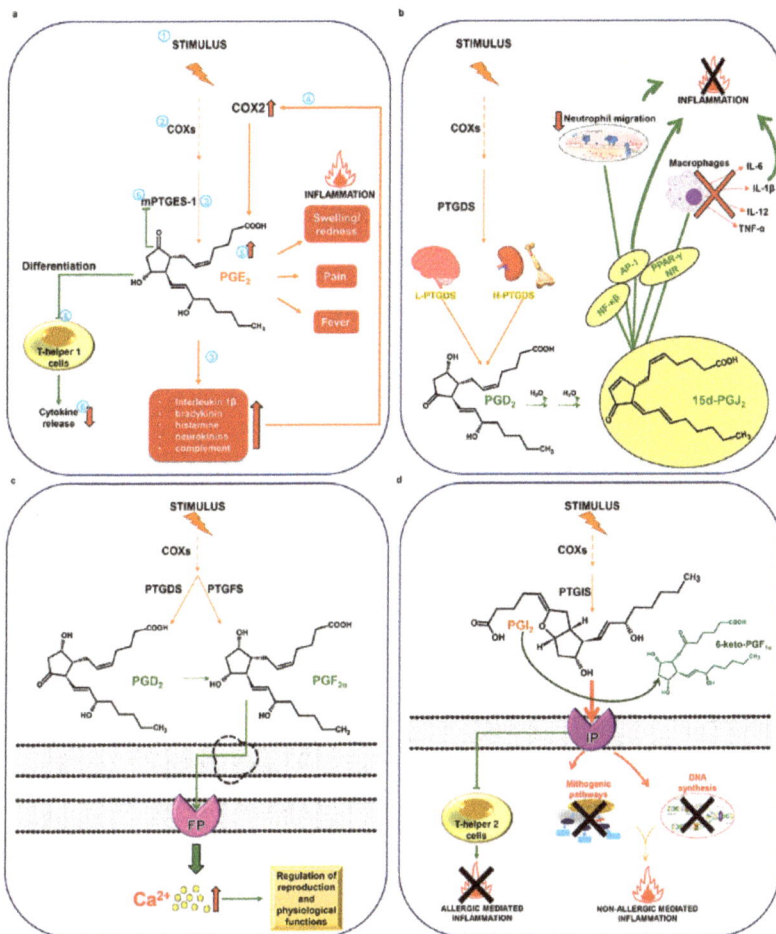

Figure 2. Prostaglandins and inflammation. (**a**) Prostaglandin E_2 (PGE$_2$) stimulation of inflammatory response. Numbers indicate the sequence of events from PGE$_2$ synthesis to stimulation of inflammation trough positive feedback on cyclooxygenase (COX)-2 and negative feedback on microsomal PGE synthase-1 (mPTGES-1); (**b**) The anti-inflammatory role of prostaglandin J$_2$ (PGJ$_2$); (**c**) prostaglandin $F_{2\alpha}$ (PGF$_{2\alpha}$) signaling; (**d**) prostaglandin I$_2$ (PGI$_2$) signaling. For details, refer to the text.

3. Prostaglandins and Derivative Molecules in Marine Organisms

Similar to terrestrial vertebrates, in marine vertebrates prostaglandins are involved in reproduction, osmoregulation, regulation of oxygenation, and cardiovascular system [36]. Marine invertebrates, including sponges, corals, and molluscs, also contain a wide range of prostaglandins, many of which are of the conventional type (PGA$_2$, PGE$_2$, PGD$_2$, PGF$_{2\alpha}$), with similar functions as in mammals (reproduction, ion transport) and are also probably used as defense compounds [17]. Interestingly, in some invertebrates, PGs are able to perform different actions based on the tissue or compartment localization [37].

Complex marine photosynthesizing organisms, like some genera in the brown, green, and red algal groups (respectively, *Laminaria*, *Euglena*, and *Gracilaria* species) express the cyclooxygenase gene synthesizing PGE$_2$, PGF$_{2\alpha}$, and other PGs whose functions are not yet known, but seem to be associated to a defensive role [17].

3.1. Corals

Among marine invertebrates, corals represent a very interesting group producing specific PGs that are not present in mammals. The Caribbean gorgonian *Plexaura homomalla* was indeed the species in which PGs were firstly identified in a marine organism, representing also a major source of these compounds in nature [38] (Figure 3a).

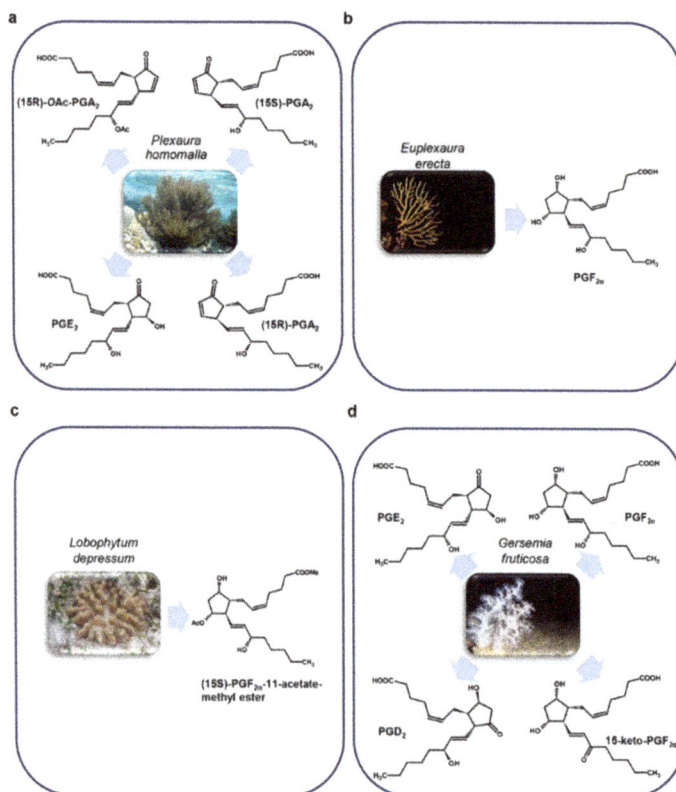

Figure 3. Corals prostaglandins. (**a**) Plexaura homomalla; (**b**) Euplexaura erecta; (**c**) Lobophytum depressum; (**d**) Gersemia fruticosa.

Weinheimer A. and Spraggins R. were the first to perform PGs extraction in *P. homomalla*, identifying in its dry cortex 15-epi-PGA$_2$ and its methyl ester acetate (respectively 0.2% and 1.3%) [15] in an R-configuration on their C-15 asymmetric center, a configuration not present in mammals. In addition to (15R)-epi-PGA$_2$, also (15R)-PGE$_2$, its methyl ester and a complex mixture of other prostaglandins were subsequently found by Light R. and Samuelsson B. [39]. However, these molecules were found also in S configurations [40] and the occurrence of one of the two seems to be related to the geographical distribution of *P. homomalla* [38].

The high PGs concentration in these invertebrates stimulated the attempt to use them as precursors for the chemical synthesis of the biologically active prostaglandins A$_2$, E$_2$, and F$_{2\alpha}$, since their chemical synthesis in large-scale for medical and pharmaceutical purposes was complicated by the necessity of 16 different chemical reactions [41].

The observation that *P. homomalla* present in coral reefs is not commonly eaten by fishes, led Gerhart [42] to hypothesize that the high amount of PGs they contain could be used as chemical defense against potential predators, since it is known that in mammals they can cause vomiting and nausea when administered orally. Indeed, oral doses of both (15R)-PGA$_2$ and (15S)-PGA$_2$ caused vomiting in a test with fishes, while the PGA$_2$ present in the surrounding water did not cause any effect [42]. However, the hypothesized defensive role seems not to be realistic since PGA$_2$ is stored in coral tissues only as acetoxy methyl esters, whose conversion to (15R)-PGA$_2$ (the compound tested by Gerhart) needs about 24 hours [40]. Moreover, while (15R)-PGA$_2$ inhibits fishes from feeding, the acetoxy methyl ester form, orally delivered, does not show any repellent effect. For this reason, as the process of production of the active (15R)-PGA$_2$ seems too slow to provide the coral with an effective defense mechanism, the function of these molecules in corals is still an open question.

The R-prostaglandins extracted from *P. homomalla* collected on the Island of San Andreas, in the Caribbean Ocean, were also tested in vivo on mouse ear edema induced by 12-O-tetradecanoylphorbol-13-acetate (TPA) and in vitro, in anti-inflammatory screenings as leucocyte degranulation, myeloperoxidase (MPO), and elastase enzymatic activity inhibition. The results showed that (15R)-PGE$_2$ and, to a lesser extent, (15R)-O-AcPGA$_2$ had an anti-inflammatory activity in vivo and in vitro (Table 1). In particular, in the leucocyte degranulation assay, (15R)-PGE$_2$ greatly inhibited the release of both MPO and elastase, while the other prostaglandins tested were moderately active in the inhibition of elastase release but not of MPO [43].

Table 1. List of the tested effects of marine prostaglandins, and their derivatives, on mammalian cells.

Prostaglandin	Producer Organism	Activity	Target Cells	Reference
(15R)-PGE$_2$ (15R)-O-AcPGA$_2$	*Plexaura homomalla*	Anti-inflammatory	Leucocyte/TPA-induced mouse-ear edema	Reina et al., 2013 [43]
Clavulones I-III	*Clavularia viridis*	Anti-inflammatory	fertilized chicken eggs	Kikuchi et al., 1983 [44]
Clavulones I-III	*Clavularia viridis*	Anti-cancer	HL-60	Honda et al., 1985 [45]; Huang et al., 2005 [46]
Clavulone II	*Clavularia viridis*	Anti-viral	VSV infected L929	Bader et al., 1991 [47]
Chlorovulone I	*Clavularia viridis*	Anti-proliferative and cytotoxic	HL-60	Iguchi et al., 1985 [48]
PGs Epoxy-prostanoid	*Clavularia viridis*	Anti-proliferative	HL-60	Iguchi et al., 1987 [49]
Bromovulone I and Iodovulone I	*Clavularia viridis*	Anti-proliferative and cytotoxic	HL-60	Iguchi et al., 1986 [50]
Bromovulone III	*Clavularia viridis*	Cytotoxic	PC-3/HT-29	Shen et al., 2004 [51]
Chlorovulones II and III	*Clavularia viridis*	Cytotoxic	PC-3/HT-29	Shen et al., 2004 [51]
Claviridenone F	*Clavularia viridis*	Cytotoxic	A549/HT-29/P-388	Duh et al., 2002 [52]
Claviridenone G	*Clavularia viridis*	Cytotoxic	A549	Duh et al., 2002 [52]
Clavirins I-II	*Clavularia viridis*	Growth-inhibition	HeLa S3	Iwashima et al., 1999 [53]
Clavubicyclone	*Clavularia viridis*	Growth-inhibition	MCF-7/OVCAR-3	Iwashima et al., 2002 [54]
Punaglandins I–IV	*Telesto riisei*	Cytotoxic	L1210	Baker et al., 1985 [55]

Euplexaura erecta Kükenthal, 1908 [56] (Figure 3b), *Lobophytum depressum* Tixier-Durivault, 1966 [57] (Figure 3c), and *Gersemia fruticosa* Sars, 1860 [58] (Figure 3d) also produce PGs. Interestingly, PGF$_{2\alpha}$ and its derivatives were principally found in these species: PGF$_{2\alpha}$ in *E. erecta* [56]; (15S)-PGF$_{2\alpha}$-11-acetate methyl ester, its 18-acetoxy derivative compound and their corresponding free carboxylic acids in *L. depressum* [57]; PGF$_{2\alpha}$ and 15-keto-PGF$_{2\alpha}$ together with PGD$_2$, PGE$_2$ in *G. fruticosa* [58].

In addition to the identification of PGs molecules in corals, also the enzyme responsible for their synthesis, the cyclooxygenase, was isolated and characterized for the first time from *P. homomalla* and *G. fruticosa* [59].

3.2. Other Marine Invertebrates

One of the first studies on marine invertebrates, excluding corals, was a comparative analysis done by Christ E. and Van Dorp D., on representative species in the Mollusca (*Mytilus*), Crustacea (*Homarus*), and Cnidaria (*Cyanea*) phyla versus terrestrial animals [60]. The authors were able to find PGs, particularly $PGF_{1\alpha}$ but only at very low levels. In some cases, the arachidonic acid precursor was also not detectable making it difficult to assert the existence of PGs and their functional role [60]. These results were confirmed in extended studies including more species in the Chordata, Mollusca, Cnidaria, and Crustacea phyla [16,61,62].

With the improvement of instrument sensitivity, it was possible, more than 10 years later, to conduct functional studies on PGs in molluscs (Figure 4a) and crustaceans (Figure 4b).

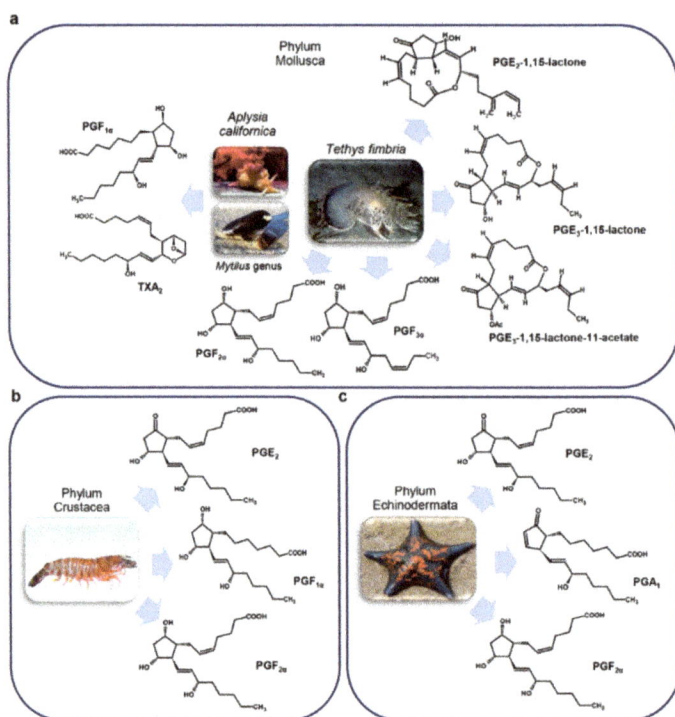

Figure 4. Marine invertebrate prostaglandins. (**a**) Molluscs; (**b**) Crustaceans; (**c**) Echinoderms. Except for *Tethys fimbria* and *Aplysia californica*, pictures show organisms that are only representatives of each phylum. For details, refer to the text.

Results obtained highlighted different roles for PGs in marine invertebrates, like reproduction, regulation of ion flux, and thermoregulation and fever, mediated respectively by $PGF_{2\alpha}$, PGE_2, and PGE_1 (Table 2) [63].

Table 2. Update of prostaglandins and its derivatives, and functional roles in marine organisms.

Compound	Producer Organism	Biological Activities	Reference
PGF2α	*Marsupenaeus japonicus*	Ovarian maturation	Tahara et al., 2004 [64]
	Thunnus thynnus	Contraction of smooth muscles during ejaculation and metabolism of testis	Nomura et al., 1973 [65]
PGE1	Marine Invertebrates	Thermoregulation and fever	Stanley-Samuelson, 1987 [63]
	Laminaria digitata	Protection against stress conditions induced by copper excess	Ritter et al., 2008 [19]
	Salmo sp.	Contraction of smooth muscles during ejaculation and metabolism of testis	Chirst and Van Dorp, 1972 [60]
PGE2	*Marsupenaeus japonicus*	Ovarian maturation	Tahara et al., 2004 [64]
	Paralichthys olivaceus and *Thunnus thynnus*	Contraction of smooth muscles during ejaculation and metabolism of testis	Nomura et al., 1973 [65]
	Gracialaria vermiculophylla	Wounding-activated chemical defense molecules	Nylund et al., 2011 [66]
	Laminaria digitata	Protection against stress conditions induced by copper excess	Ritter et al., 2008 [19]
PGF2α- and PGF3α-1,15-lactones fatty acid esters (PLFE)	*Tethys fimbria*	Reproduction and multiple roles depending on body localization	Cimino et al., 1991 [67]; Di Marzo et al., 1991 [37]
PGF1α	*Oncorhynchus keta*	Contraction of smooth muscles during ejaculation and metabolism of testis	Nomura et al., 1973 [65]
15-keto-PGE2	*Gracialaria vermiculophylla*	Wounding-activated chemical defense molecules	Nylund et al., 2011 [66]
	Laminaria digitata	Protection against stress conditions induced by copper excess	Ritter et al., 2008 [19]
PGE2-1,15-lactone	*Tethys fimbria*	Reproduction and multiple roles depending on body localization	Cimino et al., 1991 [67]; Di Marzo et al., 1991 [37]
PGE3-1,15-lactone-11-acetate	*Tethys fimbria*	Reproduction and multiple roles depending on body localization	Cimino et al., 1991 [67]; Di Marzo et al., 1991 [37]
PGE3-1,15-lactone	*Tethys fimbria*	Reproduction and multiple roles depending on body localization	Cimino et al., 1991 [67]; Di Marzo et al., 1991 [37]
PGD1	*Laminaria digitata*	Protection against stress conditions induced by copper excess	Ritter et al., 2008 [19]
PGA2	*Gracialaria vermiculophylla*	Wounding-activated chemical defense molecules	Nylund et al., 2011 [66]
	Laminaria digitata	Protection against copper stress and trigger of oxidative responses	Zambounis et al., 2012 [68]
PGB2	*Laminaria digitata*	Protection against stress conditions induced by copper excess	Ritter et al., 2008 [19]
PGJ2	*Laminaria digitata*	Protection against stress conditions induced by copper excess	Ritter et al., 2008 [19]
Clavulones	*Clavularia viridis*	Suggested to be hypothetical repellents against other marine organisms	Honda et al., 1985 [45]
iTXB2	*Dayatis sabina*	Blood clotting	Cabrera et al., 2003 [69]
TXB2	*Oncorhynchus mykiss*	Vasodilator agent	Thomson et al., 1998 [70]

In the mollusc *Modiolus demissus* Dillwyn, 1817 the uptake and binding of prostaglandins by gills was investigated, considering that bivalves can both synthetize and accumulate PGs from the surrounding medium [71]. The study revealed the presence of tissue specific, time and pH dependent, PGs binding sites with higher affinity to PGA_2 with respect to PGE_2 or $PGF_{2\alpha}$ [71].

Moreover, three prostaglandin-lactones (PGE_2-1,15-lactone, PGE_3-1,15-lactone, and PGE_3-1,15 -lactone-11-acetate) of the E and F series were identified in the mantle and body, respectively, of the nudibranch mollusc *Tethys fimbria* Linnaeus, 1767 (Figure 4a). High quantities of a complex mixture of $PGF_{2\alpha}$ and $PGF_{3\alpha}$ 1,15-lactones fatty acid esters (PLFE) were found in its eggs, particularly in mature ovotestis but not in immature ones suggesting a role for PLFE in mollusc reproduction [67]. Altogether, these results led to hypothesize a multiple biological role of prostaglandin-lactones, precursors of PGEs, as defense allormones, and involved in the control of smooth muscle contraction, and egg production and fertilization, depending on their body localization (Table 2) [37].

Crustaceans (Figure 4b) also use PGs for physiological functions. Indeed, PGE_2 and $PGF_{2\alpha}$ were identified in the ovary of the prawn *Marsupenaeus japonicus* Spence Bate, 1888 where they participate in ovarian maturation (Table 2) [64] whereas in the crab *Carcinus maenas* Linnaeus, 1758 they are produced in blood cells following a stimulus induced with a calcium ionophore, in the presence of exogenous fatty acids (FA) [72].

Echinoderms (Figure 4c) also represent a source of PGs. Among all the echinoderms analyzed, the starfish *Patinia pectinifera* Muller and Troschel, 1842 had the highest amount of prostaglandins [73]. PGE_2 and $PGF_{2\alpha}$ have been identified from the sea cucumber *Stichopus japonicus* Selenka, 1867 using TLC [73]. A study conducted with PGs-3H evidenced that the sea urchin *Arbacia punctulata* Lamarck, 1816 could accumulate PGs from the surrounding water into its gut or stomach [74], and to accumulate PGA_1 both in fertilized and unfertilized eggs, with fertilized eggs accumulating more PGs than unfertilized eggs [74].

Strongylocentrotus nudus A. Agassiz, 1864 and *S. intermedius* A. Agassiz, 1864 were also reported to have a PGs-like activity in their inner organs [74].

3.3. Marine Vertebrates

As already mentioned, in fish PGs are involved in several processes, such as ovulation, spawning, osmoregulation, regulation of branchial ion fluxes and of the cardiovascular system [36]. Christ and Van Dorp in their comparative studies on PGs considered not only invertebrates, but also fish [60]. They identified moderate yields of PGE_1 in freshwater fish and lower yields in homogenates of gills of *Salmo* sp. [60]. Successively, PGE_2 was identified for the first time in the testis of the flounder *Paralichthys olivaceus* Temminck & Schlegel, 1846, $PGF_{1\alpha}$ in the semen of the salmon *Oncorhynchus keta* Walbaum, 1792 and PGE_2 and $PGF_{2\alpha}$ in the testis of the tuna *Thunnus thynnus* Linnaeus, 1758 [65] (Figure 5a).

In order to explain the reason why prostaglandins are present in these marine animals, although they are oviparous, it was suggested that the identified prostaglandins might be used for the contraction of smooth muscle during ejaculation and for the metabolism of testis in lower animals as in mammals (Table 2) [65]. After this study, PGE_2 was isolated and subsequently identified in the gastrointestinal tract and in the skin of the shark *Triakis scyllia* Müller & Henle, 1839 [16,75] (Figure 5b).

In the brook trout *Salvelinus fontinalis* PGE_2 and $PGF_{2\alpha}$ (Figure 5a) are synthetized in the follicle wall of mature oocytes, but the highest quantity of prostaglandins was found in the extra-follicular tissue [76]. PGE_2 was also found in the skin of *Pleuronectes platessa* Linnaeus, 1758 (Figure 5a) in response to the fungal extract of *Epydermophyton floccosum* (Harz) Langeron & Miloch, 1930 known be an inducer of erythema [77].

Leucocytes of the dogfish *Scyliorhinus canicula* Linnaeus, 1758 secerned high levels of PGE_2, PGD_2 and $PGF_{2\alpha}$ (Figure 5b) when exposed to the Ca^{2+} ionophore A23187 [78]. PGE_2 and $PGF_{2\alpha}$ were found in the red blood cells of the toadfish *Opsanus tau* Linnaeus, 1766 [79] (Figure 5a).

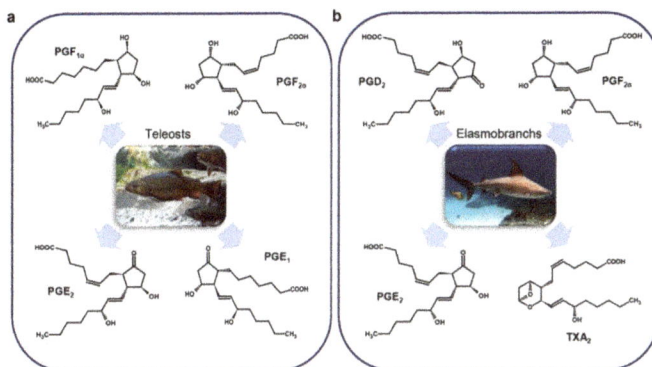

Figure 5. Marine vertebrate prostaglandins. (**a**) Teleosts (Salmo sp., Paralichthys olivaceus, Oncorhynchus keta, Thunnus thynnus, Salvelinus fontinalis, Pleuronectes platessa, Opsanus tau); (**b**) Elasmobranchs (Triakis scyllia, Scyliorhinus canicula). Pictures show organisms that are only representatives of each class. For details, refer to the text.

3.4. Macroalgae

3.4.1. Red Macroalgae

Marine red algae are rich in C20 polyunsaturated fatty acids that, in animals, are precursors of prostaglandins, thromboxane, and other eicosanoids. Although the presence of the prostaglandin-endoperoxide pathway has been demonstrated in non-mammal marine vertebrates and invertebrates, for a long time less was known about these enzymes in non-animal organisms. The first report about the presence of prostaglandins in macroalgae (Figure 6) described the identification of PGE_2 and $PGF_{2\alpha}$ in *Gracilaria lichenoides* Greville, 1830 [80].

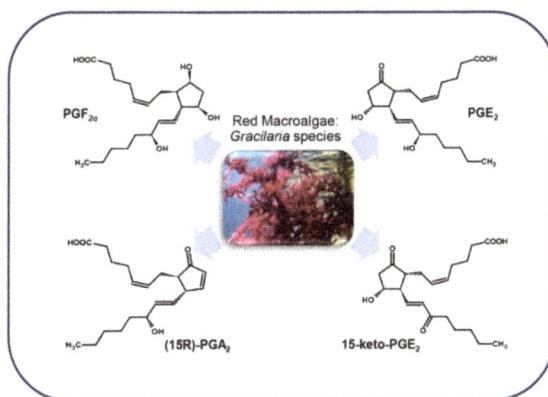

Figure 6. Red algae prostaglandins. The picture shows an organism representative of the genus. For details, refer to the text.

The genus *Gracilaria*, that comprises algae used in the food and cosmetic industry, is very rich in ARA, varying from 45.9% and 62.0% of the total FA depending on the season. Among these, *G. vermiculophylla* (Ohmi) Papenfuss, 1967 is one of the algae with the highest content of ARA [81]. This, with other *Gracilaria* species such as *G. asiatica* and *G. chorda* Holmes, 1896, seem to be responsible for a gastrointestinal disorder known as "onogori" poisoning in Japan when it is eaten raw [18]. The possible reason for this poisoning seems to be the fact that the COX contained in raw seaweeds use the highly unsaturated fatty acids to produce great amounts of PGE$_2$ in the stomach of victims in a short lapse of time [81]. *G. vermiculophylla* is a source of different types of prostaglandins besides PGE$_2$, such as PGA$_2$, PGF$_2$, 15-keto-derivatives of prostaglandins, as well as other eicosanoids [82], whereas the congeneric species *G. asiatica* produces only 15-keto-PGE$_2$ [83]. *G. vermiculophylla* use PGA$_2$, PGE$_2$, 15-keto-PGE$_2$ and other eicosanoids as wounding-activated chemical defense molecules (Table 2) [66], and recently a COX gene producing PGF$_{2\alpha}$ was cloned from this alga and heterologously expressed [84].

Other evidence of prostaglandins as defense molecules in red algae is the fact that gametophytes of the alga *Chondrus crispus* Stackhouse, 1797, when challenged with pathogens, metabolize C20 and C18 PUFAs not only into the corresponding hydroperoxides and derivatives, but also into molecules with mass fragmentation patterns very similar to prostaglandin B$_1$ and B$_2$ [85]. Furthermore, when the crude extract of this alga was treated with 50–100 µM methyl jasmonate for 6 h, PGA$_2$ and 15-keto-PGE$_2$ were identified [86].

3.4.2. Brown Macroalgae

Much less is known about the presence of prostaglandins in brown algae, and most studies have mainly focused on the brown algal kelp *Laminaria digitata*. Ritter et al. [19] showed that this brown alga uses the generation of oxylipins as a protective mechanism against stress conditions induced by an excess in copper (Table 2). Indeed, high concentrations of copper led to oxygen reactive species (ROS) accumulation in *L. digitata* cells, and consequently to a cascade of cellular responses. One of these responses was a significant release of PUFAs after 24 h of treatment, followed by the generation of oxylipins. Among complex oxylipins, also PGE$_1$ and PGD$_1$, deriving from ETrA and PGJ$_2$, PGA$_2$, 15-keto-PGE$_2$ and PGB$_2$, deriving from ARA were identified for the first time in brown algae [19]. Successively, the same authors showed that PGA$_2$ does not simply modulate but also triggers an oxidative response in *L. digitata* that, differently from the response induced by other molecules like methyljasmonate and lipopolysaccharides, occurs in seconds after treatment and in a dose-response-like manner. The authors hypothesized that PGA$_2$ can activate the generation of two different sources of ROS that can be used by the brown alga as defense molecules as in other marine organisms [68] (Figure 7).

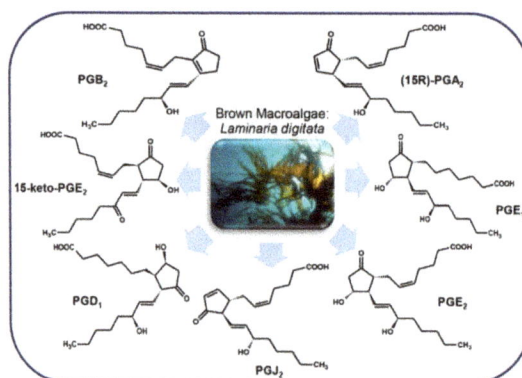

Figure 7. Brown algae prostaglandins: only *Laminaria digitata* has been studied for prostaglandins content. For details, refer to the text.

3.5. Microalgae

PGs were discovered for the first time in diatoms, phytoplanktonic marine microalgae, only in 2017 [23]. Diatoms are a rich source of polyunsaturated fatty acids (PUFA), that, in some species, are precursors of polyunsaturated aldehydes (PUAs), i.e., oxylipins with pro-apoptotic and anti-proliferative activity, with a defensive role against predator (copepods) grazing [87].

Di Dato et al. [23] explored the presence of PGs in some diatom species, i.e. *Skeletonema marinoi* Sarno & Zingone, 2005 (Figure 8a) (two different strains, FE7 and FE60) and *Thalassiosira rotula* Meunier, 1910 (Figure 8b) (Valeria Di Dato, Roberta Barbarinaldi, Alberto Amato, Federica Di Costanzo, Carolina Fontanarosa, Anna Perna, Angela Amoresano, Francesco Esposito, Adele Cutignano, Adrianna Ianora, Giovanna Romano. Variation in prostaglandin metabolism during growth of the diatom *Thalassiosira rotula*. *Sci Rep*, under review), identifying in their transcriptome genes involved in PGs biosynthesis, with some differences between the two species.

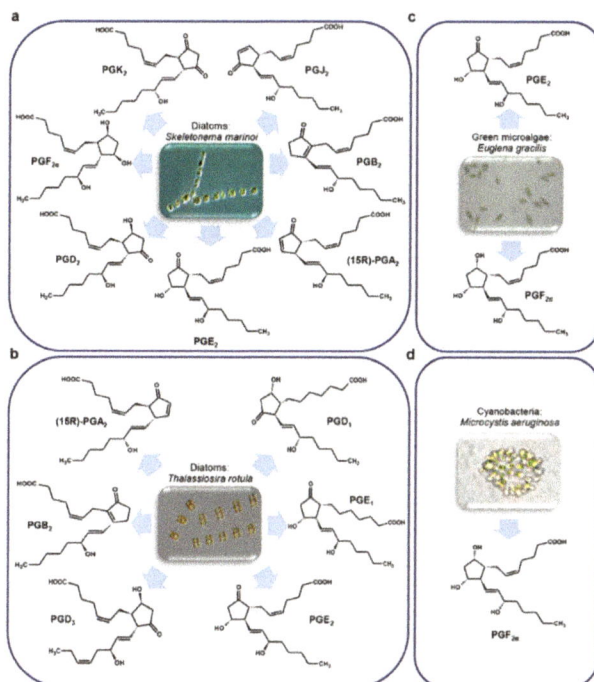

Figure 8. Microalgae prostaglandins. (**a**) *Skeletonema marinoi* (A. Ianora laboratory clones name FE7 and FE60); (**b**) *Thalassiosira rotula*; (**c**) *Euglena gracilis*; (**d**) *Microcystis aeruginosa*. For details, refer to the text.

More specifically, whereas cyclooxygenase-1 (COX-1) and microsomal prostaglandin E synthase 1 (mPTGES) were found in both species; prostaglandin H_2 D-isomerase (PTGDS) was found only in *S. marinoi*, while prostaglandin F synthase (PTGFS) was only detectable in *T. rotula*. The authors demonstrated the functioning of the pathway by measuring enzyme expression and molecule production by quantitative real time PCR (qPCR) and liquid chromatography/mass spectrometry (LC/MS) analysis, respectively. Interestingly, a wide set of PGs was revealed with representative molecules of each of the three series. In addition, a differential expression and concentration of molecules was reported among different species and strains of the same species, during different phases of growth and nutrient conditions [23]. However, the absence of PTGDS in *T. rotula* and of PTGFS in *S. marinoi* could be considered as a "potential absence." Indeed, the lack of a transcript in a transcriptome annotation can be due to a technical shortcoming and a limitation of the sequencing technology used, as in the case of very low expression levels of a target gene, that may fall under the detection limit.

It is interesting to note that, although the PGs pathway has been experimentally confirmed only in two diatom species, in silico analysis of transcriptomes from different species in different growth conditions, suggests the presence of PGs in many other diatom species [23].

Prostaglandins were identified also in the unicellular green alga *Euglena gracilis* G. A. Klebs, 1883 (Figure 8c), in which PGE$_2$ and PGF$_{2\alpha}$ were found at levels three times higher in cells grown in the dark than those grown in the light [88].

The presence of PGA, PGE, and PGF series and their esters have also been documented in the cyanobacteria of the taxa *Oscillatoria* and *Microcystidaceae* [89]. Indeed, PGF$_{2\alpha}$ was identified in *Microcystis aeruginosa* (Kützing) Kützing, 1846 [90] (Figure 8d).

Currently, to the best of our knowledge, no other marine microalga has been explored for the presence of PGs, and their role in diatoms is still under investigation. Di Dato and co-authors hypothesized that they can be used by diatoms for intercellular signaling and communication [23], in agreement with the role of these molecules in other organisms.

Microorganisms, and in particular microalgae such as diatoms, could represent a potential source of bioactive PGs, as alternative to their chemical synthesis to produce adequate amounts for pharmacological purposes as anti-inflammatory compounds. The biotechnological production of PGs from microalgae may also be convenient due to the natural presence of the full PGs pathway and the possibility to easily grow microalgae on a large scale in bioreactors under controlled culture conditions.

4. Marine Cyclopentenone Prostaglandins

Cyclopentenone prostaglandins are a sub-group of PGs characterized by the presence of a cyclopentenone moiety (CP) with a α,β-unsaturated ketone group in their cyclopentane ring. Their chemical reactivity is responsible for their anti-inflammatory, anti-tumoral and anti-viral activities [91], and the presence of the CP fragment in molecules with anticancer activity, can add more potency to these molecules. For instance, methyl-jasmonate increases its strength of action as an anti-tumor agent when a CP group is inserted in the molecule [92].

The group of cyclopentenone prostaglandins (CPPGs) includes canonical PGs of the A and J series, clavulones, and punaglandins.

Differently from the conventional PGs, that require receptor interaction to trigger their signal, cyclopentenone prostaglandins are actively transported inside the cells [91], where the CP group can interact with a wide variety of target molecules [92] including nuclear factors such as the heat shock protein 70 (HSP70) transcription factor, cyclin-dependent protein kinase (CDK), and NF-kB [35] and still not well defined mitochondrial factors [92].

4.1. Clavulones and Related Molecules

Clavulones (Figure 9) are acetoxy derivatives of PGA [91] characterized by a cyclopentenone fragment, a 12-S acetoxy function and two chains of different length: the α- and the ω-chain with respectively seven and eight carbon atoms [93]. These are anti-tumor marine prostanoids isolated from the soft coral *Clavularia viridis* Quoy & Gaimard, 1833, a single *Clavularia* genus that inhabits Okinawa bay in Japan [44,94,95].

Clavulones exists in three isoforms, I, II, and III and two stereoisomers at the C-4 and C-12 positions. These molecules possess a significant anti-inflammatory effect at a concentration of 30 μg/mL in a fertilized chicken egg assay (Table 1) [44,95]. The effects of clavulones on the growth of human cancer cells were first studied using clavulone I, the form that is more abundant in *C. viridis*. At concentration of 4.0 μM there was an impairment of DNA synthesis in human HL-60 leukemic cells after 1 h incubation, causing irreversible cytotoxic changes after 3 h of exposition [45]. In a more recent study, the anti-cancer activity of clavulone II on HL-60 cells has been deeply studied [46] revealing that low concentrations of clavulone II induce anti-proliferative effects by inducing the down-regulation of cyclin D1 with consequent arrest of the cell cycle in G1. On the contrary, higher concentrations of clavulone II induces apoptosis through the disruption of mitochondrial membrane potential and the activation of caspase-9, -8, and -3 and of B-cell lymphoma 2 (Bcl2)-family proteins (Table 1) [46]. It was suggested that corals might use clavulones as repellent and toxic substances against other marine organisms (Table 2) [45].

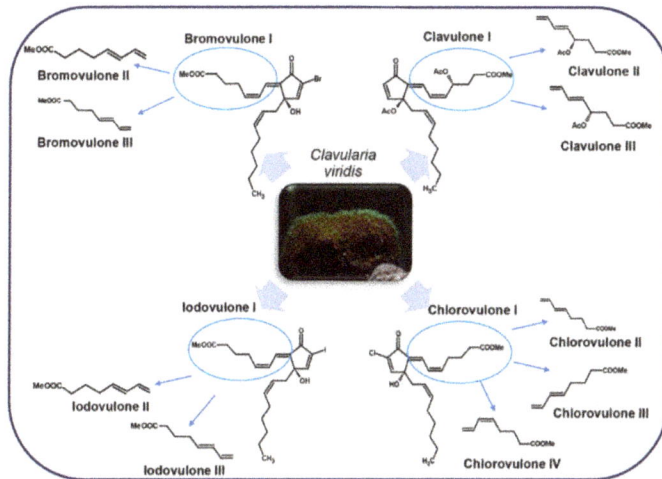

Figure 9. Clavulones and related molecules in *Clavularia viridis* (Cnidaria, soft corals). For details, refer to the text.

Clavulones, similarly to PGAs, also possess antiviral activity. In particular, clavulone II inhibits replication of the vesicular stomatitis virus (VSV) in infected mouse L929 fibroblasts, by blocking the transcription of viral RNA, and consequently the viral protein (Table 1) [47].

Interestingly, both the anti-proliferative and antiviral activities of clavulones are stronger than those of PGAs [47].

Other than clavulone I, II, and III, from the same stolonifer coral, 20-acetoxi-claviridenone b and 20-acetoxi-claviridenone c were discovered [96]. In addition to these, also four halogenated analogues, called chlorovulones I-IV were identified and, among these, chlorovulone I was shown to have anti-proliferative and cytotoxic activities (Table 1) [48]. The structure of an epoxy prostanoid with anti-proliferative activity was also identified in the same soft coral [49] together with bromovulone I and iodovulone I. Both had anti-proliferative and cytotoxic activities even though slightly lower than those of chlorovulone I [50]. All these molecules showed a stronger anti-tumor activity against HL-60 cells in vitro with respect to clavulone I (Table 1) [48–50].

More recently, seven new prostanoids were identified from the same soft coral: 4-deacetoxyl-12-O-deacetylclavulone I, 4-deacetoxyl-12-O-deacetylclavulone II, bromovulone II, iodovulone II, 4-deacetoxyl-12-O-deacetylclavulone III, bromovulone III, and iodovulone III. These molecules showed in vitro cytotoxic activity against human prostate carcinoma (PC-3) and colon adenocarcinoma (HT-29) cells and, among these, bromovulone III showed the highest anti-tumor activity, together with chlorovulone II and III, used as standard, that exhibited a slightly lower activity (Table 1) [51].

Through an assay-guided fractionation of a dichloromethane (CH$_2$Cl$_2$) extract of *C. viridis*, three new cytotoxic molecules were isolated: claviridenone E, claviridenone F, and claviridenone G. In particular, claviridenone F showed a significant cytotoxicity against human lung adenocarcinoma (A549), HT-29, and mouse lymphocytic leukemia cells (P-388), while claviridenone G exhibited a high cytotoxic activity only against A549 (Table 1) [52]. In addition to these molecules, there are clavulone-related oxylipins from *C. viridis*, named clavirins I and II, for which it was proposed a derivation from clavulone III and I, respectively, having growth-inhibitory activity against human cervix carcinoma cell line (HeLa S3) (Table 1) [53].

Other clavulone-related molecules that have been discovered are tricycloclavulone and clavubicyclone that may be derived from cycloaddition and electrocyclization of clavulone III, respectively. The latter molecule showed a moderate growth-inhibition activity against breast carcinoma (MCF-7) and ovarian carcinoma cells (OVCAR-3) in vitro (Table 1) [54]. Preclavulone lactone I and II and two minor chemical congeners, 17,18-dehydroclavulone I and clavulolactone I, were also isolated and characterized from *C. viridis*. Among these, 17,18-dehydroclavulone I has a (14Z,17Z)-double bond in the ω side chain, and this suggests that, differently from the other clavulones, it can derive from EPA instead of ARA [97].

Although there are structural similarities between prostaglandins and clavulones, the latter are not generated by a variant of the endoperoxide pathway, but from the lipoxygenase pathway by which arachidonic acid is converted into 8-(R)HPETE and then to preclavulone A [98]. Preclavulone A was identified also in an unrelated Caribbean coral, *Pseudoplexaura porosa* Houttuyn, 1772, suggesting that this molecule is widespread in corals [99]. In another study, the same authors isolated and defined the structures of 15 new halogenated iodo-, bromo-, and chlorovulones in *C. viridis* as minor constituents [100], but overall about 50 congeners of clavulones were identified in this soft coral [101].

4.2. Punaglandins

These molecules (Figure 10), structurally related to clavulones, were isolated in the Hawaiian octocoral *Telesto riisei* Duchassaing & Michelotti, 1860 [102].

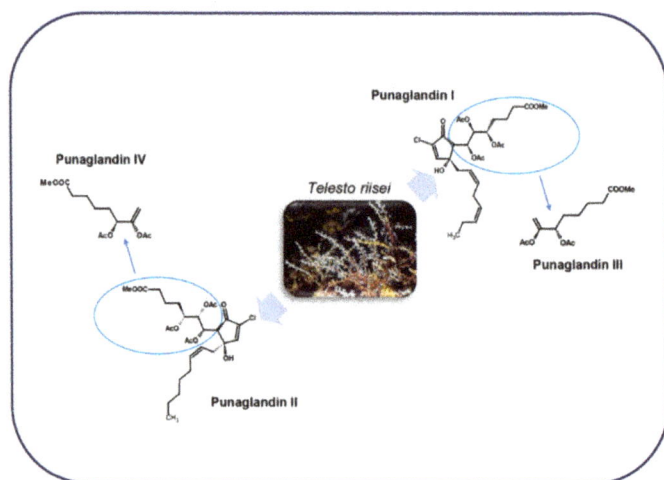

Figure 10. Punaglandins in *Telesto riisei* (Cnidaria, octocoral). For details, refer to the text.

The lack of symbiotic algae suggests that *T. riisei* is the source of these prostaglandins [103]. A total of 19 punaglandins were obtained from this octocoral, which also included acetate and epoxide versions of the four canonical punaglandins [104]. Punaglandins 3 and 4 formally results from elimination of acetic acid from punaglandins 1 and 2 respectively, and possess a cross-conjugated dienone structure [105]. They are halogenated derivatives of PGA [91] characterized by various oxygenations at C -5, -6, -7, and -12 and a 10-chloro-9-cyclopentenone function with a 5S, 6S, 12R stereochemistry [102].

At the moment of their discovery, there was great interest in the study of punaglandins, because of their anti-inflammatory and potent antitumor activities [104]. Indeed, these molecules, and in particular punaglandin 3, was shown to inhibit L1210 leukemia cell proliferation (IC$_{50}$ = 0.04 µM)

(Table 1) [102] with an activity 15-fold higher compared to the corresponding clavulone [55]. This cytotoxic activity is approximately equal to the one of vincristine and doxorubicin that are among the most effective anticancer molecules used today [103].

5. Marine Thromboxane

Thromboxanes (TXs) are closely relate to PGs that bind specific receptors, called thromboxane receptors (TP) and act as strong promoters of platelet aggregation and vaso- and broncho-constriction in mammals [106]. They are labile and biologically active molecules deriving from arachidonic acid in the cyclooxygenase pathway in human platelets. Thromboxane A_2 (TXA$_2$) has a short half-life (30 s in human blood) being rapidly converted to a stable B form (TXB$_2$), which is used as a marker for the presence of TXA$_2$ [69].

Other than in mammals, the presence of TXs is documented also in marine organisms.

TXB$_2$, along with prostaglandins, has been reported in aqueous homogenates of the mollusc *A. californica* J. G. Cooper, 1863 (Figure 4a) [74] using radioimmunoassay. In the marine bivalve *M. edulis* Linnaeus, 1758 (Figure 4a), arachidonic acid metabolism, in addition to PGs, leads to the production of TXs in the gills, mantle, and adductor tissues [107]. In the polychaetae *Arenicola marina* Linnaeus, 1758 small amounts of TXB$_2$ are detectable in the digestive and reproductive tracts [107].

Different species of fish also produce TXs [69]. In the plasma of the elasmobranch *Dasyatis sabina* Lesueur, 1824 (Figure 5b), the presence of an immunoreactive TXB$_2$ (iTXB$_2$) has been detected at concentrations of 0.57 ± 0.03 ng/mL. The level of iTXB$_2$ increased to 3.0 ± 0.27 ng/mL when the plasma clots, but decreased to 1.5 ± 0.17 ng/mL in the presence of indomethacin, a cyclooxygenase inhibitor. These findings suggest that TXA$_2$, the active thromboxane form, may be involved in blood clotting and may be generated by a cyclooxygenase-like enzyme as in mammals (Table 2) [69]. The binding of agonist (radiolabeled [125I]-BOP) and antagonist (L-657925 and L-657926) ligands of mammalian TP receptors to those of *D. sabina*, also demonstrates the similarity between this elasmobranch and mammalian TP receptors [69]. Three different species of shark (Figure 5b) (*Chiloscyllium griseum* Müller & Henle, 1838, *Carcharhinus plumbeus* Nardo, 1827 and *Carcharhinus melanopterus* Quoy & Gaimard, 1824) were also shown to produce TXB$_2$ as a major product of arachidonic acid metabolism suggesting that TXB$_2$ may be a biologically active prostanoid in these species [70].

Rowley et al. [78] tested the ability of leucocytes extracted from the blood of the dogfish *Scyliorhinus canicula* (Figure 5b) to produce and release PGs and TXs during their degranulation induced by the calcium ionophore A23187. While PGF$_{2\alpha}$, PGE$_2$, and PGD$_2$ levels were always high after the stimulus, the levels of TXB$_2$ were low and detectable in the supernatant only 5 min after the start of the stimulus, with levels increasing after 10 and 15 min [78].

Another direct evidence of the generation of TXB$_2$ in fish was demonstrated by the ability of washed whole blood cells from a variety of fishes of the Arabian Gulf to produce prostanoids from exogenous 14C-arachidonic acid in vitro [70]. In addition, rainbow trout thrombocytes, clotting cells similar to mammalian platelets, were shown to convert arachidonic acid mainly to TXB$_2$ [108,109]. These findings again suggest a role also for TXB$_2$, in rainbow trout as a vasodilator (Table 2), while in mammals TXB$_2$ has no significant biological activity [70]. However, not all fish thrombocytes have the ability to produce thromboxane, possibly suggesting that these molecules are not essential for thrombocyte aggregation in certain species [110].

6. Conclusions

Prostaglandins and their derivatives, although first identified in terrestrial organisms, are also widespread in the marine environment testifying the great importance of these molecules. Nevertheless, the eco-physiological role of marine PGs remains mostly unclear because of contrasting and often old data available in the literature, although it has been suggested that they have a possible role as defensive molecules against predators.

Interestingly, many marine organisms have been shown to produce classical PGs along with new derivatives that are not found in terrestrial animals, e.g., corals that are able to produce punaglandins and clavulones, which are specific of the marine environment and have shown potent pharmacological activity against inflammation, tumors, and viruses. These findings, together with the discovery of PGs in unicellular eukaryotic microalgae, provides new stimuli to pursue the search for new marine PG-derived molecules with anti-inflammatory activity.

Author Contributions: Conceptualization, V.D.D., G.R. and F.D.C.; methodology, V.D.D., G.R. and F.D.C.; resources, V.D.D., G.R. and F.D.C.; writing—original draft preparation, F.D.C., G.R. and V.D.D.; writing—review and editing, F.D.C., V.D.D., G.R. and A.I.; visualization, G.R. and A.I.; supervision, V.D.D., G.R. and A.I.; project administration, G.R.; funding acquisition, G.R.

Funding: This research was funded by Ministero dell'ambiente e della tutela del territorio e del mare, Italia, project name: "Genomics for a Blue Economy," grant number PGR00765.

Acknowledgments: We thank Adele Cutignano (Institute of Biomolecular Chemistry-National Research Council of Italy) for her help in drawing the molecules.

Conflicts of Interest: The authors declare no conflict of interest. The funders had no role in the design of the study; in the collection, analyses, or interpretation of data; in the writing of the manuscript, or in the decision to publish the results.

References

1. Cheung, R.C.F.; Ng, T.B.; Wong, J.H.; Chen, Y.; Chan, W.Y. Marine natural products with anti-inflammatory activity. *Appl. Microbiol. Biotechnol.* **2016**, *100*, 1645–1666. [CrossRef] [PubMed]
2. Mora, C.; Tittensor, D.P.; Adl, S.; Simpson, A.G.B.; Worm, B. How many species are there on Earth and in the ocean? *PLoS Biol.* **2011**, *9*, e1001127. [CrossRef] [PubMed]
3. Buckley, C.D.; Gilroy, D.W.; Serhan, C.N.; Stockinger, B.; Tak, P.P. The resolution of inflammation. *Nat. Rev. Immunol.* **2013**, *13*, 59–66. [CrossRef] [PubMed]
4. Fullerton, J.N.; Gilroy, D.W. Resolution of inflammation: A new therapeutic frontier. *Nat. Rev. Drug Discov.* **2016**, *15*, 551–567. [CrossRef] [PubMed]
5. Gilroy, D.; De Maeyer, R. New insights into the resolution of inflammation. *Semin. Immunol.* **2015**, *27*, 161–168. [CrossRef] [PubMed]
6. Headland, S.E.; Norling, L.V. The resolution of inflammation: Principles and challenges. *Semin. Immunol.* **2015**, *27*, 149–160. [CrossRef] [PubMed]
7. Ortega-Gómez, A.; Perretti, M.; Soehnlein, O. Resolution of inflammation: An integrated view. *EMBO Mol. Med.* **2013**, *5*, 661–674. [CrossRef] [PubMed]
8. Serhan, C.N.; Chiang, N.; Dalli, J.; Levy, B.D. Lipid mediators in the resolution of inflammation. *Cold Spring Harb. Perspect. Biol.* **2014**, *7*, a016311. [CrossRef] [PubMed]
9. Rajakariar, R.; Yaqoob, M.M.; Gilroy, D.W. COX-2 in inflammation and resolution. *Mol. Interv.* **2006**, *6*, 199–207. [CrossRef] [PubMed]
10. Murata, T.; Maehara, T. Discovery of anti-inflammatory role of prostaglandin D2. *J. Vet. Med. Sci.* **2016**, *78*, 1643–1647. [CrossRef] [PubMed]
11. Euler, U.S.v. Zur Kenntnis der pharmakologischen Wirkungen von Nativsekreten und Extrakten männlicher accessorischer Geschlechtsdrüsen. *Arch. Exp. Pathol. Pharmakol.* **1934**, *175*, 78–84. [CrossRef]
12. Goldblatt, M.W. Properties of human seminal plasma. *J. Physiol.* **1935**, *84*, 208–218. [CrossRef] [PubMed]
13. Wolfe, L.S. Eicosanoids: Prostaglandins, thromboxanes, leukotrienes, and other derivatives of carbon-20 unsaturated fatty acids. *J. Neurochem.* **1982**, *38*, 1–14. [CrossRef] [PubMed]
14. Piper, P.J. Introduction to the biosynthesis and metabolism of prostaglandins. *Postgrad. Med. J.* **1977**, *53*, 643–646. [CrossRef] [PubMed]
15. Bhakuni, D.S.; Rawat, D.S. *Bioactive Marine Natural Products*; Springer: New York, NY, USA; Anamaya: New Delhi, India, 2005; ISBN 978-1-4020-3472-5.
16. Nomura, T.; Ogata, H. Distribution of prostaglandins in the animal kingdom. *Biochim. Biophys. Acta* **1976**, *431*, 127–131. [PubMed]
17. Rowley, A.F.; Vogan, C.L.; Taylor, G.W.; Clare, A.S. Prostaglandins in non-insectan invertebrates: Recent insights and unsolved problems. *J. Exp. Biol.* **2005**, *208*, 3–14. [CrossRef] [PubMed]

18. Sajiki, J.; Kakimi, H. Identification of eicosanoids in the red algae, *Gracilaria asiatica*, using high-performance liquid chromatography and electrospray ionization mass spectrometry. *J. Chromatogr. A* **1998**, *795*, 227–237. [CrossRef]

19. Ritter, A.; Goulitquer, S.; Salaün, J.-P.; Tonon, T.; Correa, J.A.; Potin, P. Copper stress induces biosynthesis of octadecanoid and eicosanoid oxygenated derivatives in the brown algal kelp *Laminaria digitata*. *New Phytol.* **2008**, *180*, 809–821. [CrossRef]

20. Groenewald, E.G.; van der Westhuizen, A.J. Prostaglandins and related substances in plants. *Bot. Rev.* **1997**, *63*, 199–220. [CrossRef]

21. Ruggeri, B.; Thoroughgood, C. Prostaglandins in aquatic fauna: A comprehensive review. *Mar. Ecol. Prog. Ser.* **1985**, *23*, 301–306. [CrossRef]

22. Carté, B.K. Biomedical potential of marine natural products. Marine organisms are yielding novel molecules for use in basic research and medical applications. *BioScience* **1996**, *46*, 271–286.

23. Di Dato, V.; Orefice, I.; Amato, A.; Fontanarosa, C.; Amoresano, A.; Cutignano, A.; Ianora, A.; Romano, G. Animal-like prostaglandins in marine microalgae. *ISME J.* **2017**, *11*, 1722–1726. [CrossRef] [PubMed]

24. Nakanishi, M.; Rosenberg, D.W. Multifaceted roles of PGE2 in inflammation and cancer. *Semin. Immunopathol.* **2013**, *35*, 123–137. [CrossRef] [PubMed]

25. Lands, W.E.M. The biosynthesis and metabolism of prostaglandins. *Annu. Rev. Physiol.* **1979**, *41*, 633–652. [CrossRef] [PubMed]

26. Bos, C.L.; Richel, D.J.; Ritsema, T.; Peppelenbosch, M.P.; Versteeg, H.H. Prostanoids and prostanoid receptors in signal transduction. *Int. J. Biochem. Cell Biol.* **2004**, *36*, 1187–1205. [CrossRef] [PubMed]

27. Funk, C.D. Prostaglandins and leukotrienes: Advances in eicosanoid biology. *Science* **2001**, *294*, 1871–1875. [CrossRef] [PubMed]

28. Hansen, H.S. 15-hydroxyprostaglandin dehydrogenase. A review. *Prostaglandins* **1976**, *12*, 647–679. [CrossRef]

29. Wang, D.; DuBois, R.N. Prostaglandins and cancer. *Gut* **2006**, *55*, 115–122. [CrossRef]

30. Jakobsson, P.J.; Thorén, S.; Morgenstern, R.; Samuelsson, B. Identification of human prostaglandin E synthase: A microsomal, glutathione-dependent, inducible enzyme, constituting a potential novel drug target. *Proc. Natl. Acad. Sci. USA* **1999**, *96*, 7220–7225. [CrossRef]

31. Sykes, L.; MacIntyre, D.A.; Teoh, T.G.; Bennett, P.R. Anti-inflammatory prostaglandins for the prevention of preterm labour. *Reproduction* **2014**, *148*, R29–R40. [CrossRef]

32. Basu, S. Novel cyclooxygenase-catalyzed bioactive prostaglandin F2α from physiology to new principles in inflammation. *Med. Res. Rev.* **2007**, *27*, 435–468. [CrossRef] [PubMed]

33. Ricciotti, E.; FitzGerald, G.A. Prostaglandins and inflammation. *Arterioscler. Thromb. Vasc. Biol.* **2011**, *31*, 986–1000. [CrossRef] [PubMed]

34. Watanabe, T.; Nakao, A.; Emerling, D.; Hashimoto, Y.; Tsukamoto, K.; Horie, Y.; Kinoshita, M.; Kurokawa, K. Prostaglandin F2 alpha enhances tyrosine phosphorylation and DNA synthesis through phospholipase C-coupled receptor via Ca(2+)-dependent intracellular pathway in NIH-3T3 cells. *J. Biol. Chem.* **1994**, *269*, 17619–17625. [PubMed]

35. Straus, D.S.; Glass, C.K. Cyclopentenone prostaglandins: New insights on biological activities and cellular targets. *Med. Res. Rev.* **2001**, *21*, 185–210. [CrossRef] [PubMed]

36. Brown, J.A.; Bucknall, R.M. Antidiuretic and cardiovascular actions of prostaglandin E2 in the rainbow trout *Salmo gairdneri*. *Gen. Comp. Endocrinol.* **1986**, *61*, 330–337. [CrossRef]

37. Di Marzo, V.; Cimino, G.; Crispino, A.; Minardi, C.; Sodano, G.; Spinella, A. A novel multifunctional metabolic pathway in a marine mollusc leads to unprecedented prostaglandin derivatives (prostaglandin 1,15-lactones). *Biochem. J.* **1991**, *273 (Pt 3)*, 593–600. [CrossRef]

38. Weinheimer, A.J.; Spraggins, R.L. The occurrence of two new prostaglandin derivatives (15-epi-PGA2 and its acetate, methyl ester) in the gorgonian *Plexaura homomalla* chemistry of coelenterates. XV. *Tetrahedron Lett.* **1969**, *59*, 5185–5188. [CrossRef]

39. Light, R.J.; Samuelsson, B. Identification of prostaglandins in the gorgonian, *Plexaura homomalla*. *Eur. J. Biochem.* **1972**, *28*, 232–240. [CrossRef]

40. Schneider, W.P.; Hamilton, R.D.; Rhuland, L.E. Occurrence of esters of (15S)-prostaglandin A 2 and E 2 in coral. *J. Am. Chem. Soc.* **1972**, *94*, 2122–2123. [CrossRef]

41. Bayer, F.; Weinheimer, A. *Prostaglandins from Plexaura homomalla: Ecology, Utilization and Conservation of a Major Medical Marine Resource. A Symposium*; Studies in Tropical Oceanography; University of Miami Press on Behalf of the Upjohn Co.: Coral Gables, FL, USA, 1974.

42. Gerhart, D.J. Prostaglandin A_2: An agent of chemical defense in the Caribbean gorgonian *Plexaura homomalla*. *Mar. Ecol. Prog. Ser.* **1984**, *19*, 181–187. [CrossRef]

43. Reina, E.; Ramos, F.A.; Castellanos, L.; Aragón, M.; Ospina, L.F. Anti-inflammatory R-prostaglandins from Caribbean Colombian Soft Coral *Plexaura homomalla*. *J. Pharm. Pharmacol.* **2013**, *65*, 1643–1652. [CrossRef] [PubMed]

44. Kikuchi, H.; Tsukitani, Y.; Iguchi, K.; Yamada, Y. Absolute stereochemistry of new prostanoids clavulone I, II and III, from *Clavularia viridis* Quoy and Gaimard. *Tetrahedron Lett.* **1983**, *24*, 1549–1552. [CrossRef]

45. Honda, A.; Yamamoto, Y.; Mori, Y.; Yamada, Y.; Kikuchi, H. Antileukemic effect of coral-prostanoids clavulones from the stolonifer *Clavularia viridis* on human myeloid leukemia (HL-60) cells. *Biochem. Biophys. Res. Commun.* **1985**, *130*, 515–523. [CrossRef]

46. Huang, Y.-C.; Guh, J.-H.; Shen, Y.-C.; Teng, C.-M. Investigation of anticancer mechanism of clavulone II, a coral cyclopentenone prostaglandin analog, in human acute promyelocytic leukemia. *J. Biomed. Sci.* **2005**, *12*, 335–345. [CrossRef] [PubMed]

47. Bader, T.; Yamada, Y.; Ankel, H. Antiviral activity of the prostanoid clavulone II against vesicular stomatitis virus. *Antivir. Res.* **1991**, *16*, 341–355. [CrossRef]

48. Iguchi, K.; Kaneta, S.; Mori, K.; Yamada, Y.; Honda, A.; Mori, Y. Chlorovulones, new halogenated marine prostanoids with an antitumor activity from the stolonifer *Clavularia viridis* Quoy and Gaimard. *Tetrahedron Lett.* **1985**, *26*, 5787–5790. [CrossRef]

49. Iguchi, K.; Kaneta, S.; Mori, K.; Yamada, Y. A new marine epoxy prostanoid with an antiproliferative activity from the stolonifer *Clavularia viridis* Quoy and Gaimard. *Chem. Pharm. Bull.* **1987**, *35*, 4375–4376. [CrossRef] [PubMed]

50. Iguchi, K.; Kaneta, S.; Mori, K.; Yamada, Y.; Honda, A.; Mori, Y. Bromovulone I and iodovulone I, unprecedented brominated and iodinated marine prostanoids with antitumour activity isolated from the Japanese stolonifer *Clavularia viridis* Quoy and Gaimard. *J. Chem. Soc. Chem. Commun.* **1986**, 981–982. [CrossRef]

51. Shen, Y.-C.; Cheng, Y.-B.; Lin, Y.-C.; Guh, J.-H.; Teng, C.-M.; Ko, C.-L. New prostanoids with cytotoxic activity from Taiwanese octocoral *Clavularia viridis*. *J. Nat. Prod.* **2004**, *67*, 542–546. [CrossRef]

52. Duh, C.-Y.; El-Gamal, A.A.H.; Chu, C.-J.; Wang, S.-K.; Dai, C.-F. New cytotoxic constituents from the Formosan Soft Corals *Clavularia viridis* and *Clavularia violacea*. *J. Nat. Prod.* **2002**, *65*, 1535–1539. [CrossRef]

53. Iwashima, M.; Okamoto, K.; Iguchi, K. Clavirins, a new type of marine oxylipins with growth-inhibitory activity from the Okinawan soft coral, *Clavularia viridis*. *Tetrahedron Lett.* **1999**, *40*, 6455–6459. [CrossRef]

54. Iwashima, M.; Terada, I.; Okamoto, K.; Iguchi, K. Tricycloclavulone and clavubicyclone, novel prostanoid-related marine oxylipins, isolated from the Okinawan Soft Coral *Clavularia viridis*. *J. Org. Chem.* **2002**, *67*, 2977–2981. [CrossRef] [PubMed]

55. Baker, B.J.; Okuda, R.K.; Yu, P.T.K.; Scheuer, P.J. Punaglandins: Halogenated antitumor eicosanoids from the octocoral *Telesto riisei*. *J. Am. Chem. Soc.* **1985**, *107*, 2976–2977. [CrossRef]

56. Komoda, Y.; Kanayasu, T.; Ishikawa, M. Prostaglandin F 2 alpha from the Japanese coastal gorgonian, *Euplexaura erecta*. *Chem. Pharm. Bull.* **1979**, *27*, 2491–2494. [CrossRef] [PubMed]

57. Carmely, S.; Kashman, Y.; Loya, Y.; Benayahu, Y. New prostaglandin (PGF) derivatives from the Soft Coral. *Tetrahedron Lett.* **1980**, *21*, 875–878. [CrossRef]

58. Varvas, K.; Järving, I.; Koljak, R.; Vahemets, A.; Pehk, T.; Müürisepp, A.-M.; Lille, Ü.; Samel, N. *In vitro* biosynthesis of prostaglandins in the White Sea Soft Coral *Gersemia fruticosa*: Formation of optically active PGD2, PGE2, PGF2α and 15-keto-PGF2α from arachidonic acid. *Tetrahedron Lett.* **1993**, *34*, 3643–3646. [CrossRef]

59. Järving, R.; Järving, I.; Kurg, R.; Brash, A.R.; Samel, N. On the evolutionary origin of cyclooxygenase (COX) isozymes: Characterization of marine invertebrate COX genes points to independent duplication events in vertebrate and invertebrate lineages. *J. Biol. Chem.* **2004**, *279*, 13624–13633. [CrossRef]

60. Christ, E.J.; Van Dorp, D.A. Comparative aspects of prostaglandin biosynthesis in animal tissues. *Biochim. Biophys. Acta (BBA)—Lipids Lipid Metab.* **1972**, *270*, 537–545. [CrossRef]

61. Ogata, H.; Nomura, T.; Hata, M. Prostaglandin biosynthesis in the tissue homogenates of marine animals. *NIPPON SUISAN GAKKAISHI* **1978**, *44*, 1367–1370. [CrossRef]

62. Levine, L.; Kobayashi, T. Detection of compounds immunologically related to arachidonic acid transformation products in extracts of invertebrates. *Prostaglandins Leukot. Med.* **1983**, *12*, 357–369. [CrossRef]

63. Stanley-Samuelson, D.W. Physiological roles of prostaglandins and other eicosanoids in invertebrates. *Biol. Bull.* **1987**, *173*, 92–109. [CrossRef] [PubMed]

64. Tahara, D.; Yano, I. Maturation-related variations in prostaglandin and fatty acid content of ovary in the kuruma prawn (*Marsupenaeus japonicus*). *Comp. Biochem. Physiol. Part A Mol. Integr. Physiol.* **2004**, *137*, 631–637. [CrossRef] [PubMed]

65. Nomura, T.; Ogata, H.; Masao, I.T.O. Occurrence of prostaglandins in fish testis. *Tohoku J. Agric. Res.* **1973**, *24*, 138–144.

66. Nylund, G.M.; Weinberger, F.; Rempt, M.; Pohnert, G. Metabolomic Assessment of induced and activated chemical defence in the invasive red alga *Gracilaria vermiculophylla*. *PLoS ONE* **2011**, *6*, e29359. [CrossRef] [PubMed]

67. Cimino, G.; Crispino, A.; Di Marzo, V.; Spinella, A.; Sodano, G. Prostaglandin 1,15-lactones of the F series from the nudibranch mollusk *Tethys fimbria*. *J. Organ. Chem.* **1991**, *56*, 2907–2911. [CrossRef]

68. Zambounis, A.; Gaquerel, E.; Strittmatter, M.; Salaün, J.P.; Potin, P.; Küpper, F.C. Prostaglandin A$_2$ triggers a strong oxidative burst in *Laminaria*: A novel defense inducer in brown algae? *ALGAE* **2012**, *27*, 21–32. [CrossRef]

69. Cabrera, D.M.; Janech, M.G.; Morinelli, T.A.; Miller, D.H. A thromboxane A(2) system in the Atlantic stingray, *Dasyatis sabina*. *Gen. Comp. Endocrinol.* **2003**, *130*, 157–164. [CrossRef]

70. Thomson, M.; al-Hassan, J.M.; al-Saleh, J.; Fayad, S.; Ali, M. Prostanoid synthesis in whole blood cells from fish of the Arabian Gulf. *Comp. Biochem. Physiol. B Biochem. Mol. Biol.* **1998**, *119*, 639–646. [CrossRef]

71. Freas, W.; Grollman, S. Uptake and binding of prostaglandins in a marine bivalve, *Modiolus demissus*. *J. Exp. Zool.* **1981**, *216*, 225–233. [CrossRef]

72. Hampson, A.J.; Rowley, A.F.; Barrow, S.E.; Steadman, R. Biosynthesis of eicosanoids by blood cells of the crab, *Carcinus maenas*. *Biochim. Biophys. Acta* **1992**, *1124*, 143–150. [CrossRef]

73. Korotchenko, O.D.; Mishchenko, T.Y.; Isay, S.V. Prostaglandins of Japan Sea invertebrates—I. The quantitation of group B prostaglandins in echinoderms. *Comp. Biochem. Physiol. Part C Comp. Pharmacol.* **1983**, *74*, 85–88. [CrossRef]

74. Gerwick, W.H.; Nagle, D.G.; Proteau, P.J. Oxylipins from marine invertebrates. In *Marine Natural Products—Diversity and Biosynthesis*; Scheuer, P.J., Ed.; Springer: Berlin/Heidelberg, Germany, 1993; Volume 167, pp. 117–180. ISBN 978-3-540-56513-0.

75. Ogata, H.; Nomura, T. Isolation and identification of prostaglandin E2 from gastrointestinal tract of shark *Triakis scyllia*. *Biochim. Biophys. Acta* **1975**, *388*, 84–91. [PubMed]

76. Goetz, F.W.; Duman, P.; Ranjan, M.; Herman, C.A. Prostaglandin F and E synthesis by specific tissue components of the brook trout (*Salvelinus fontinalis*) ovary. *J. Exp. Zool.* **1989**, *250*, 196–205. [CrossRef]

77. Anderson, A.A.; Fletcher, T.C.; Smith, G.M. Prostaglandin biosynthesis in the skin of the plaice *Pleuronectes platessa* L. *Comp. Biochem. Physiol. C Comp. Pharmacol.* **1981**, *70*, 195–199. [CrossRef]

78. Rowley, A.F.; Barrow, S.E.; Hunt, T.C. Preliminary studies on eicosanoid production by fish leucocytes, using GC-mass spectrometry. *J. Fish Biol.* **1987**, *31*, 107–111. [CrossRef]

79. Cagen, L.M.; Qureshi, Z.; Nishimura, H. Synthesis of prostaglandin E2 and prostaglandin F2α by toadfish red blood cells. *Biochem. Biophys. Res. Commun.* **1983**, *110*, 250–255. [CrossRef]

80. Dang, T.H.; Lee, H.J.; Yoo, E.S.; Hong, J.; Choi, J.S.; Jung, J.H. The occurrence of 15-keto-prostaglandins in the red alga *Gracilaria verrucosa*. *Arch. Pharm. Res.* **2010**, *33*, 1325–1329. [CrossRef]

81. Hsu, B.-Y.; Tsao, C.-Y.; Chiou, T.-K.; Hwang, P.-A.; Hwang, D.-F. HPLC determination for prostaglandins from seaweed. *Food Control* **2007**, *18*, 639–645. [CrossRef]

82. Imbs, A.B.; Latyshev, N.A.; Svetashev, V.I.; Skriptsova, A.V.; Le, T.T.; Pham, M.Q.; Nguyen, V.S.; Pham, L.Q. Distribution of polyunsaturated fatty acids in red algae of the genus *Gracilaria*, a promising source of prostaglandins. *Russ. J. Mar. Biol.* **2012**, *38*, 339–345. [CrossRef]

83. De Almeida, C.L.F.; Falcão, H.d.S.; Lima, G.R.d.M.; Montenegro, C.d.A.; Lira, N.S.; de Athayde-Filho, P.F.; Rodrigues, L.C.; de Souza, M.d.F.V.; Barbosa-Filho, J.M.; Batista, L.M. Bioactivities from marine algae of the genus *Gracilaria*. *Int. J. Mol. Sci.* **2011**, *12*, 4550–4573. [CrossRef]

84. Kanamoto, H.; Takemura, M.; Ohyama, K. Identification of a cyclooxygenase gene from the red alga *Gracilaria vermiculophylla* and bioconversion of arachidonic acid to PGF(2α) in engineered *Escherichia coli*. *Appl. Microbiol. Biotechnol.* **2011**, *91*, 1121–1129. [CrossRef] [PubMed]

85. Bouarab, K.; Adas, F.; Gaquerel, E.; Kloareg, B.; Salaün, J.-P.; Potin, P. The innate immunity of a marine red alga involves oxylipins from both the eicosanoid and octadecanoid pathways. *Plant Physiol.* **2004**, *135*, 1838–1848. [CrossRef] [PubMed]

86. Andreou, A.; Brodhun, F.; Feussner, I. Biosynthesis of oxylipins in non-mammals. *Prog. Lipid Res.* **2009**, *48*, 148–170. [CrossRef] [PubMed]

87. Ianora, A.; Miralto, A. Toxigenic effects of diatoms on grazers, phytoplankton and other microbes: A review. *Ecotoxicology* **2010**, *19*, 493–511. [CrossRef] [PubMed]

88. Levine, L.; Sneiders, A.; Kobayashi, T.; Schiff, J.A. Serologic and immunochromatographic detection of oxygenated polyenoic acids in *Euglena gracilis* var. *bacillaris*. *Biochem. Biophys. Res. Commun.* **1984**, *120*, 278–285. [CrossRef]

89. Kafanova, T.V.; Busarova, N.G.; Isai, S.V.; Zvyagintseva, T.Y. Fatty acids and prostaglandins of thermal cyanobacteria. *Chem. Nat. Compd.* **1996**, *32*, 861–865. [CrossRef]

90. Krüger, G.H.J.; Groenewald, E.G.; de Wet, H.; Botes, P.J. The occurrence of prostaglandin F2α in procaryotic organisms. *S. Afr. J. Bot.* **1990**, *56*, 150–153. [CrossRef]

91. Narumiya, S.; Fukushima, M. Cyclopentenone prostaglandins: Anti-proliferative and anti-viral actions and their molecular mechanism. In *Eicosanoids and Other Bioactive Lipids in Cancer and Radiation Injury: Proceedings of the 1st International Conference 11–14 October 1989, Detroit, MI, USA*; Honn, K.V., Marnett, L.J., Nigam, S., Walden, T.L., Eds.; Developments in Oncology; Springer: Boston, MA, USA, 1991; pp. 439–448. ISBN 978-1-4615-3874-5.

92. Conti, M. Cyclopentenone: A special moiety for anticancer drug design. *Anticancer Drugs* **2006**, *17*, 1017–1022. [CrossRef]

93. Lis, L.G.; Zheldakova, T.A. New marine prostanoids, clavulones, halogenovulones, and punaglandins. *Chem. Nat. Compd.* **1993**, *29*, 259–274. [CrossRef]

94. Imbs, A.B. Prostaglandins and oxylipins of corals. *Russ. J. Mar. Biol.* **2011**, *37*, 325–334. [CrossRef]

95. Kikuchi, H.; Tsukitani, Y.; Iguchi, K.; Yamada, Y. Clavulones, new type of prostanoids from the stolonifer *Clavularia viridis* Quoy and Gaimard. *Tetrahedron Lett.* **1982**, *23*, 5171–5174. [CrossRef]

96. Kitagawa, I.; Kobayashi, M.; Yasuzawa, T.; Son, B.W.; Yoshihara, M.; Kyogoku, Y. New prostanoids from Soft Coral. *Tetrahedron* **1985**, *41*, 995–1005. [CrossRef]

97. Iwashima, M.; Okamoto, K.; Konno, F.; Iguchi, K. New marine prostanoids from the Okinawan Soft Coral, *Clavularia viridis*. *J. Nat. Prod.* **1999**, *62*, 352–354. [CrossRef] [PubMed]

98. Corey, E.J.; D'Alarcao, M.; Matsuda, S.P.T.; Lansbury, P.T.; Yamada, Y. Intermediacy of 8-(R)-HPETE in the conversion of arachidonic acid to pre-clavulone a by *Clavularia viridis*. Implications for the biosynthesis of marine prostanoids. *J. Am. Chem. Soc.* **1987**, *109*, 289–290. [CrossRef]

99. Corey, E.J.; Matsuda, S.P.T. Generality of marine prostanoid biosynthesis by the 2-oxidopentadienylcation pathway. *Tetrahedron Lett.* **1987**, *28*, 4247–4250. [CrossRef]

100. Watanabe, K.; Sekine, M.; Iguchi, K. Isolation and structures of new halogenated prostanoids from the Okinawan Soft Coral *Clavularia viridis*. *J. Nat. Prod.* **2003**, *66*, 1434–1440. [CrossRef] [PubMed]

101. Watanabe, K.; Sekine, M.; Iguchi, K. Isolation of three marine prostanoids, possible biosynthetic intermediates for clavulones, from the Okinawan Soft Coral *Clavularia viridis*. *Chem. Pharm. Bull.* **2003**, *51*, 909–913. [CrossRef]

102. Gerwick, W.H. Carbocyclic oxylipins of marine origin. *Chem. Rev.* **1993**, *93*, 1807–1823. [CrossRef]

103. Munro, M.H.G.; Luibrand, R.T.; Blunt, J.W. The search for antiviral and anticancer compounds from marine organisms. In *Bioorganic Marine Chemistry*; Scheuer, P.J., Ed.; Springer: Berlin/Heidelberg, Germany, 1987; pp. 93–176.

104. Baker, B.J.; Scheuer, P.J. The punaglandins: 10-chloroprostanoids from the octocoral *Telesto riisei*. *J. Nat. Prod.* **1994**, *57*, 1346–1353. [CrossRef]

105. Suzuki, M.; Morita, Y.; Yanagisawa, A.; Baker, B.J.; Scheuer, P.J.; Noyori, R. Prostaglandin synthesis 15. Synthesis and structural revision of (7E)- and (7Z)-punaglandin 4. *J. Org. Chem.* **1988**, *53*, 286–295. [CrossRef]

106. Armstrong, R.A.; Wilson, N.H. Aspects of the thromboxane receptor system. *Gen. Pharmacol.* **1995**, *26*, 463–472. [CrossRef]

107. Mustafa, T.; Srivastava, K.C. Prostaglandins (eicosanoids) and their role in ectothermic organisms. In *Advances in Comparative and Environmental Physiology*; Brouwer, M., Carr, W.E.S., Ellington, W.R., Engel, D.W., Gleeson, R.A., Korsgaard, B., Moerland, T.S., Mustafa, T., Prior, D.J., Sidell, B.D., et al., Eds.; Advances in Comparative and Environmental Physiology; Springer: Berlin/Heidelberg, Germany, 1989; pp. 157–207. ISBN 978-3-642-74510-2.

108. Kayama, M.; Sadō, T.; Iijima, N. The Prostaglandin synthesis in rainbow trout thrombocyte. *NIPPON SUISAN GAKKAISHI* **1986**, *52*, 925. [CrossRef]

109. Pettitt, T.R.; Barrow, S.E.; Rowley, A.F. Thromboxane, prostaglandin and leukotriene generation by rainbow trout blood. *Fish Shellfish Immunol.* **1991**, *1*, 71–73. [CrossRef]

110. Hill, D.J.; Hallett, M.B.; Rowley, A.F. Effect of prostanoids and their precursors on the aggregation of rainbow trout thrombocytes. *Am. J. Physiol.* **1999**, *276*, R659–R664. [CrossRef] [PubMed]

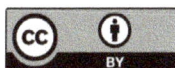

marine drugs

MDPI

Review

Intravenous Lipid Emulsions to Deliver Bioactive Omega-3 Fatty Acids for Improved Patient Outcomes

Philip C. Calder [1,2]

[1]   Human Development and Health, Faculty of Medicine, University of Southampton,
     Southampton SO16 6YD, UK; pcc@soton.ac.uk
[2]   NIHR Southampton Biomedical Research Centre, University Hospital Southampton NHS Foundation Trust
     and University of Southampton, Southampton SO16 6YD, UK

Received: 13 March 2019; Accepted: 6 May 2019; Published: 8 May 2019

Abstract: Lipids used in intravenous nutrition support (i.e., parenteral nutrition) provide energy, building blocks, and essential fatty acids. These lipids are included as emulsions since they need to be soluble in an aqueous environment. Fish oil is a source of bioactive omega-3 fatty acids (eicosapentaenoic acid and docosahexaenoic acid). Lipid emulsions, including fish oil, have been used for parenteral nutrition for adult patients post-surgery (mainly gastrointestinal). This has been associated with alterations in biomarkers of inflammation and immune defense, and in some studies, a reduction in length of intensive care unit and hospital stay. These benefits, along with a reduction in infections, are emphasized through recent meta-analyses. Perioperative administration of fish oil may be superior to postoperative administration, but this requires further exploration. Parenteral fish oil has been used in critically ill adult patients. Here, the influence on inflammatory processes, immune function, and clinical endpoints is less clear. However, some studies found reduced inflammation, improved gas exchange, and shorter length of hospital stay in critically ill patients if they received fish oil. Meta-analyses do not present a consistent picture but are limited by the small number and size of studies. More and better trials are needed in patient groups in which parenteral nutrition is used and where fish oil, as a source of bioactive omega-3 fatty acids, may offer benefits.

Keywords: fish oil; omega-3; eicosapentaenoic acid; docosahexaenoic acid; inflammation; eicosanoid; cytokine; surgery; critical illness; parenteral nutrition

1. Introduction

Eicosapentaenoic acid (EPA, 20:5n-3) and docosahexaenoic acid (DHA, 22:6n-3) are biologically active long-chain omega-3 (n-3) polyunsaturated fatty acids [1,2]. EPA and DHA are produced from simpler n-3 fatty acids in a metabolic pathway involving sequential desaturation and elongation of the precursor fatty acids (Figure 1). For a variety of reasons, endogenous synthesis of EPA and DHA through this pathway is considered to be relatively poor in humans [3], placing a focus on intake of preformed EPA and DHA. Naturally rich sources of EPA and DHA include many marine organisms particularly fatty fish like salmon, trout, mackerel, herring, and sardines [4]. The body oils of fatty fish (and the liver oils of nonfatty (lean) fish like cod) can be isolated; these oils are rich in EPA and DHA although the content and relative amounts of EPA and DHA present are dependent upon the fish source [4]. These oils are generically termed "fish oils" and "fish liver oils" and are commonly used as dietary supplements. Other sources of EPA and DHA include krill oil and algal oils. For most people on a Western style diet, intake of EPA and DHA is low, but this can be increased markedly by eating fatty fish regularly or by using supplements which contain EPA and DHA [4]. When intake of EPA and DHA is increased, the amounts of those fatty acids in blood, blood cells, and tissues is increased [5–7].

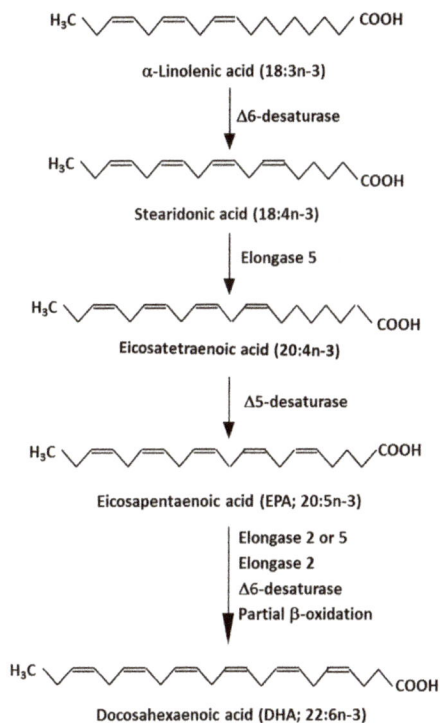

Figure 1. Pathway of biosynthesis of eicosapentaenoic acid (EPA) and docosahexaenoic acid (DHA) from precursor omega-3 (n-3) fatty acids.

EPA and DHA are readily incorporated into the phospholipids of cell membranes and this is central to their biological activity (Figure 2), including their effects on inflammation and immune responses [8,9]. For example, they have been shown to modulate the physical characteristics of the membrane (termed membrane order or membrane fluidity) and the formation of signalling platforms called lipid rafts in many cell types, including in cells involved in inflammatory and immune responses [8,9]. These alterations in membrane structure and function have been shown to modify the signals generated at the membrane level that go on to influence cytosolic and nuclear events. For example, the ability of DHA to suppress phosphorylation of the inhibitory subunit of the proinflammatory transcription factor nuclear factor kappa B (NFκB) and to inhibit proinflammatory protein production in cultured macrophages in response to bacterial lipopolysaccharide (LPS) [10] was identified to be due to disruption of the formation of lipid rafts that occurs when the cells are exposed to LPS [11]. This observation creates a direct link between the incorporation of n-3 fatty acids into membranes, altered membrane responses to external stimuli, initiation of signalling cascades, gene expression, and protein production in inflammatory cells.

EPA and DHA released from cell membrane phospholipids can be converted to bioactive lipid mediators through the action of cyclooxygenase, lipoxygenase, and cytochrome P450 enzymes (Figure 3). In this way, EPA and DHA are rather like the long-chain omega-6 (n-6) polyunsaturated fatty acid arachidonic acid (ARA, 20:4n-6), although the mediators produced from these three fatty acid substrates often have different biological activities or potencies [12,13].

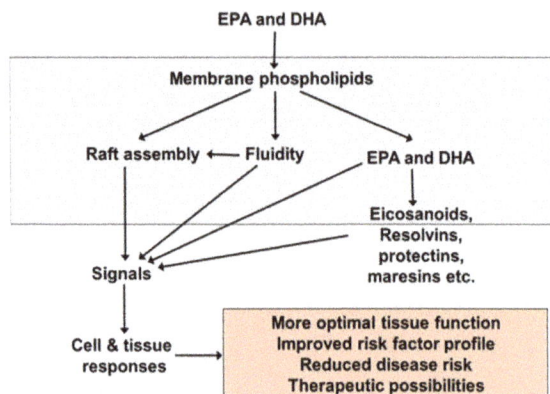

Figure 2. Generalized scheme of the mechanisms of action of eicosapentaenoic acid (EPA) and docosahexaenoic acid (DHA).

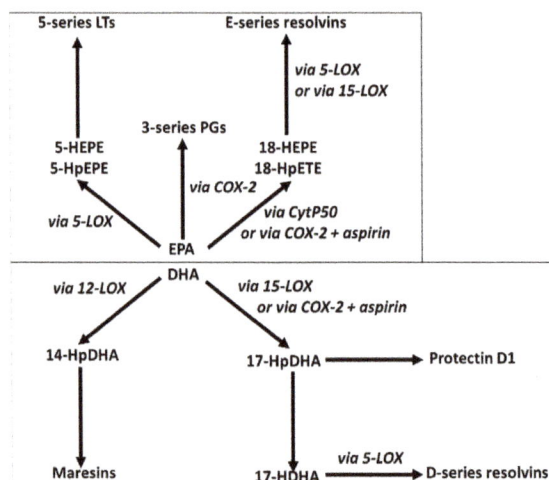

Figure 3. Overview of the pathways of conversion of eicosapentaenoic acid (EPA) and docosahexaenoic acid (DHA) to bioactive lipid mediators. EPA is metabolized via cyclooxygenase-2 (COX-2) to yield 3-series prostaglandins (PGs) and via 5-lipoxygenase (5-LOX) to yield 5-hydroperoxyeicosapenataenoic acid (HpEPE) which is converted to 5-hydroxyeicosapentaenoic acid (5-HEPE), the precursor of 5-series leukotrienes (LTs). EPA can also be metabolized to 18-HpETE by cytochrome P450 (CytP450) or by COX-2. In turn 18-HpEPE is converted to 18-HEPE which is metabolized by 5-LOX to resolvins E1 and E2 or by 15-lipoxygenase (15-LOX) to resolvin E3. DHA is metabolized via 12-lipoxygenase (12-LOX) to 14-hydroperoxydocosahexaenoic acid (14-HpDHA) which is converted to maresins. DHA can also be metabolized to 17-HpDHA by 15-LOX or by COX-2. 17-HpDHA is the precursor of protectin D1 and of 17-hydroxydocosahexaenoicacid (17-HDHA). 17-HDH is metabolized by 5-LOX to D-series resolvins. Different enantiomers of resolvins and protectins are produced in the absence or presence of aspirin.

EPA and DHA are incorporated into cell membranes at the expense of ARA, resulting in a shift in the pattern of the lipid mediators being produced. EPA, DHA, and their lipid mediator products also influence various transcription factors resulting in an altered expression of genes involved in many biological processes which include metabolism, immune function, and inflammation [9,12]. Consequently, through these actions from the membrane to the nucleus, EPA and DHA modify cell and tissue behavior and responses, and in general, these modifications are associated with more optimal function, an improved risk factor profile, a reduction in disease risk, and in some cases, therapeutic possibilities (Figure 2). EPA and DHA have long been recognized to have anti-inflammatory properties, including decreasing production of proinflammatory lipid mediators from ARA, decreasing production of key proinflammatory cytokines like tumor necrosis factor (TNF), interleukin (IL)-1β and IL-6, and reducing leukocyte-endothelium adhesion interactions [12,14]. More recently, EPA and DHA have been shown to be the precursors for potent inflammation resolving mediators termed resolvins, protectins, and maresins [15,16], which are produced through the pathways outlined in Figure 3. These molecules, collectively termed specialized pro-resolving mediators, have a range of potent actions including upregulating phagocytosis promoting clearance of damaged tissue and cellular debris and reducing production of classic inflammatory cytokines like TNF and IL-1β [15,16]. The combined actions of EPA and DHA suggest that they could be important in preventing, reducing the severity, and even treating chronic inflammatory conditions like rheumatoid arthritis [17–19]. Accumulation of EPA and DHA in cells and tissues from the diet or from oral supplements occurs over a time frame of days to weeks to months, depending upon the tissue involved [5–7]. In acute settings, more rapid delivery of EPA and DHA may be required. Lipid emulsions (LEs) that include fish oil as a source of EPA and DHA are commercially available for intravenous infusion as part of nutrition support for patients [20,21]. Intravenous administration of these LEs can quickly provide relatively high amounts of EPA and DHA if it is desired. This article will describe the rationale for the development of fish oil containing LEs and their application in surgical and critically ill patients.

2. Fish Oil Containing LEs for Intravenous Use

2.1. The Role of LEs in Intravenous Nutrition Support

It is not possible for some patients to consume food either transiently or in the longer term. If food intake beyond a few days is not possible, patients require what is termed "nutrition support" in order to maintain or restore optimal nutritional status and health. Nutrition support for patients should use the gastrointestinal tract whenever it is possible. However, there are instances where use of the gastrointestinal tract is not possible. These include patients with:

- a non-functional gastrointestinal tract due to:

  - surgical removal because of disease
  - intestinal blockage or leakage
  - impaired absorptive capacity

- severe gastrointestinal disease
- severe malnutrition
- trauma or critical illness

In such patients, the intravenous route should be used to provide nutrition support. This is referred to as parenteral nutrition. Parenteral nutrition should include a mix of macronutrients, as energy sources and substrates for biosynthesis, and micronutrients. It is important to include lipids as a component of parenteral nutrition. This is because the fatty acids within lipids are good sources of energy and reduce the need to provide large amounts of carbohydrates and they are building blocks for cell membranes required for tissue repair and host defenses. In addition, the provision of essential fatty acids is necessary to avoid a deficiency, which has been described in infants receiving long-term parenteral nutrition that was lipid free [22]. Finally, the fatty acids and the complex lipids that carry them may have bioactivities that affect the outcome for the patient [1,20,21]. In parenteral nutrition, lipids are provided as aqueous emulsions of oils that are mainly triglycerides, with a phospholipid monolayer which is usually phosphatidylcholine (lecithin) of soybean origin. A range of

LEs are commercially available comprising various mixtures of soybean oil, oil rich in medium chain triglycerides (MCTs), olive oil, and fish oil. The composition of these LEs is summarized in Table 1.

Table 1. Oil sources and major fatty acids (% of total) of commercially available lipid emulsions for use in parenteral nutrition.

	Pure Soybean Oil	Soybean Oil MCT Oil Blend	Restructured Soybean Oil MCT Oil Blend	Pure Fish Oil	Olive Oil Based	Fish Oil Blend 1	Fish Oil Blend 2
Oil source (%):							
Soybean	100	50	64	-	20	40	30
MCT	-	50	36	-	-	50	30
Olive	-	-	-	-	80	-	25
Fish	-	-	-	100	-	10	15
Fatty acids (%)							
Saturated	15	58	46	21	14	49	37
Monounsaturated *	24	11	14	23	64	14	33
Polyunsaturated	61	31	40	56	22	37	30
Omega-3	8	4	5	48	3	10	7
ALA	8	4	5	1	3	4	2
EPA	-	-	-	20	-	3.5	3
DHA	-	-	-	19	-	2.5	2
Omega-6 **	53	27	35	5	19	27	23

ALA, α-linolenic acid; EPA, eicosapentaenoic acid; DHA, docosahexaenoic acid. * mainly oleic acid (18:1n-9). ** Mainly linoleic acid (18:2n-6). Note that the fatty acid composition of fish oil is more variable than that of vegetable oils so that the precise contribution of different fatty acids may differ in different batches.

2.2. Rationale for Fish Oil Containing LEs

As outlined above, EPA and DHA have a number of bioactivities [1,2,9,12,20,21]. Through these bioactivities EPA and DHA can affect metabolism, inflammation, immune responses, oxidative stress, blood coagulation, organ function (e.g., liver, lung, muscle, brain), and wound healing amongst others [1]. These effects are likely to be of relevance to patients receiving parenteral nutrition support [20,21]. In this regard there has been significant attention on the ability of EPA and DHA to modulate inflammation and the immune response. This is because of the increasing recognition that uncontrolled inflammation and a period of immune paralysis can occur in certain groups or subgroups of patients, sometimes concurrently, and that these are linked with poor patient outcomes such as increased risk of infections, longer stay in hospital, and in more seriously ill patients increased mortality. For example, patients undergoing gastrointestinal surgery showed elevated plasma concentrations of the inflammatory cytokine interleukin (IL)-6 in the hours to days following surgery, with higher concentrations observed in the more severely stressed patients [23]. At the same time, there was a decline in T lymphocyte function in those patients [23]. Patients in the early stages of sepsis showed higher concentrations of TNF, IL-1β, and IL-6 than healthy controls and they had an elevated activation of the proinflammatory transcription factor NFκB in blood leukocytes [24]. Both the inflammatory cytokines and the activation of NFkB were higher in the patients who did not survive than in survivors [24], suggesting an association between hyperinflammation and mortality. Bozza et al. [25] identified that the concentrations of some plasma cytokines measured at entry to the intensive care unit (ICU) predicted 48-hour and 28-day mortality in patients with sepsis. Andaluz-Ojeda et al. [26] studied 29 mainly elderly male patients with infections of whom 17 survived and 12 did not. They found that the blood concentrations of IL-6, IL-8, IL-10, and monocyte chemoattractant protein-1 were higher on the first day of admission to the ICU in non-survivors than in survivors, and that these cytokines were associated with mortality at days three and 28 after adjusting for disease severity at ICU entry. These authors reported that 28-day survival was over 90% in those patients with IL-6, IL-8, and IL-10 concentrations all < 75th percentile on day one, while survival was around 30% in those patients with IL-6, IL-8, and IL-10 concentrations all > 75th percentile on day one [26]. These observations suggest an important association between a strong inflammatory response and a poor outcome, perhaps mediated through organ damage and failure (Figure 4). Likewise, immune paralysis could lead to a poor outcome related to an increased susceptibility to infections (Figure 4).

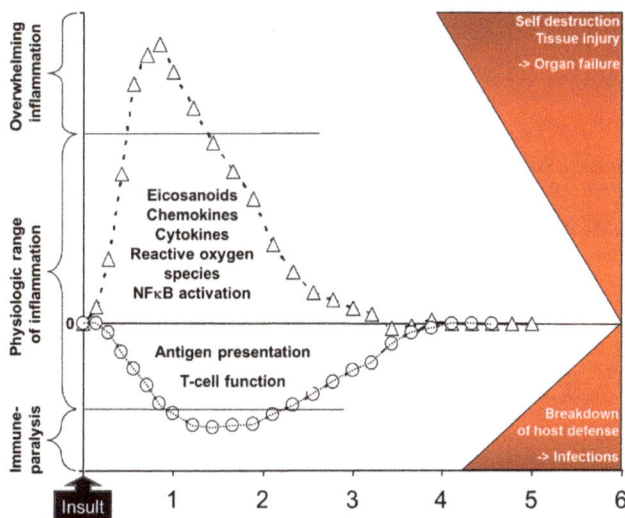

Figure 4. Schematic depiction of the response to insult with activation of inflammation and impairment of acquired immunity. It is considered that overwhelming inflammation and immune paralysis directly lead to adverse patient outcomes as depicted in the red area on the right. Examples of the "insult" include major surgery, wound or tissue injury, and the presence of infection. Modified from [27] with permission from Karger Publishers, Basel, Switzerland. Original figure Copyright © 2014, 2015 Karger Publishers, Basel, Switzerland.

Using cell culture and animal models, the effects of EPA and DHA have been demonstrated on the following: eicosanoids like prostaglandin E_2 and leukotriene B_4; chemokines like monocyte chemoattractant protein 1; cytokines like TNF, IL-1β, IL-6, and IL-10; reactive oxygen species production; and NFκB activation as reviewed elsewhere [12,14]. Although less well explored, effects of EPA and DHA on the function of antigen presenting cells [28] and T cells [29] are also described in the literature. These effects provide a rationale for inclusion of fish oil in LEs used for nutrition support in patients undergoing major surgery or with critical illness (Figure 5). Preclinical models strongly support this approach. For example, fish oil decreases vasoconstriction, hypertension, and vascular permeability and leakage in an animal model of lung injury [30]; decreases the metabolic and inflammatory response to endotoxin, improving heart and lung function and survival [30–32]; and enhances survival in some models of infection [29]. The pro-resolving effects of EPA- and DHA-derived lipid mediators may also be relevant in this regard. For example, Spite et al. [33] reported that DHA-derived resolvin D2 reduced bacterial load in blood and peritoneum and improved survival in a caecal ligation and a puncture model of sepsis in mice. This was associated with much reduced plasma levels of several inflammatory cytokines (TNF, IL-1β, IL-6, IL-10, IL-17) and chemokines, reduced leukocyte infiltration into the peritoneum, and reduced peritoneal concentrations of prostaglandin E_2 and leukotriene B_4. In a murine model of sepsis induced by caecal ligation and puncture, DHA-derived resolvin D1 decreased the bacterial load in the blood and peritoneum, decreased lung injury, decreased plasma concentrations of TNF, IL-6, IL-10, and interferon-γ, and improved survival [34]. In parallel with these effects on inflammation, resolvin D1 decreased the proportion of T lymphocytes undergoing apoptosis [34].

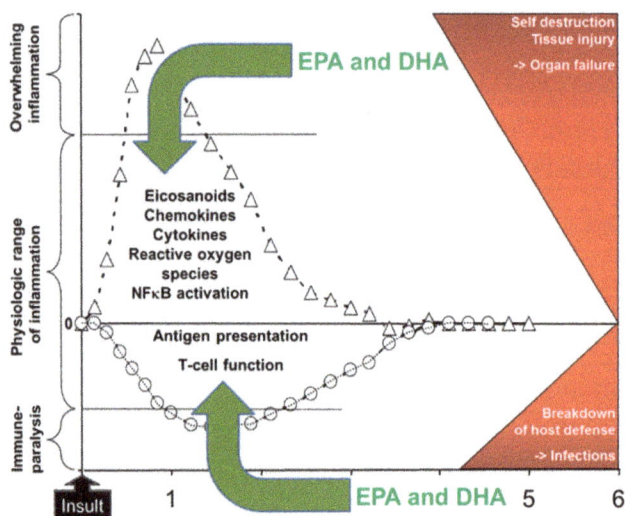

Figure 5. Rationale for inclusion of omega-3 fatty acids (eicosapentaenoic acid (EPA) and docosahexaenoic acid (DHA)) in intravenous nutrition support in patients at risk of or already displaying overwhelming inflammation and immune paralysis. Modified from [27] with permission from Karger Publishers, Basel, Switzerland. Original figure Copyright © 2014, 2015 Karger Publishers, Basel, Switzerland.

2.3. Anti-Inflammatory and Immune Enhancing Effects of Fish Oil Containing LEs in Patients

LEs that include fish oil are an effective way of delivering EPA and DHA directly into the circulation [35–37]. Infusion of a blend of soybean oil, MCTs, and fish oil (50:40:10 vol/vol/vol) daily for five days in septic patients in the ICU who were intolerant of enteral feeding resulted in an elevation in the content of EPA, though not DHA, in plasma phosphatidylcholine at the end of the infusion period [35]. Patients with hepatic colorectal metastases requiring resection received continuous infusion of a blend of soybean oil, MCTs, and fish oil (50:40:10 vol/vol/vol) for 72 h prior to surgery [36]. EPA in plasma phosphatidylcholine was higher than at study entry, and higher than in the control group at 20, 44, 68 and 72 h (Figure 6) [36]. Barros et al. [37] infused a pure fish oil LE into ICU patients receiving enteral nutrition for 6 h on each of 3 consecutive days; blood samples were collected prior to the first infusion, and 24 and 72 h after the third infusion. There was a significant increased appearance of EPA and DHA in plasma phosphatidylcholine at the latter two time points as compared with both the study entry and the control group [37].

It has been estimated that a daily oral dose of 2–2.5 g of EPA plus DHA is required to elicit an anti-inflammatory effect in humans [38]. LEs are typically infused at a rate of up to 1 g lipid/kg body weight per day, and therefore a 70 kg patient could receive 70 g of LE if the emulsion was infused continuously over an entire day. Depending upon the exact LE used (Table 1) this would provide 70, 7 or 10.5 g fish oil daily for pure fish oil, fish oil blend 1, and fish oil blend 2, respectively. This amount of fish oil would supply about 27, 4 or 3.5 g EPA plus DHA daily from these three LEs. Clearly these amounts would differ according to a patient's body weight, the LE infusion rate, and the infusion duration. Nevertheless, these figures indicate that anti-inflammatory doses of EPA and DHA can be delivered with LEs that are currently available. This is supported by the observations that using these fish oil containing LEs can decrease the blood concentrations or ex vivo production of proinflammatory eicosanoids [39,40] and cytokines [35,37,41] in surgical [39–41] and critically ill [35,37] patients. Randomized controlled trials (RCTs) of the effect of fish oil containing LEs on markers of inflammation and immune function in patients who had undergone surgery for gastrointestinal cancers were subject to a very recent meta-analysis [42]. Depending upon the biomarker, the analysis included between four and 13 RCTs and between 209 and 756 patients. It was determined that fish oil LEs resulted in significant decreases in the inflammatory markers TNF, IL-6, and C-reactive protein (all $P < 0.00001$) and significant increases in markers of acquired immunity including the numbers of lymphocytes ($P < 0.0001$), CD3 and CD4 cells and the CD4 to CD8 ratio (all $P < 0.00001$), and the concentrations of immunoglobulins A, M, and G (all $P < 0.00001$) [42]. These observations support the proposal shown in Figure 5 that fish oil containing LEs can be used to control inflammation and support immune function in patients receiving parenteral nutrition.

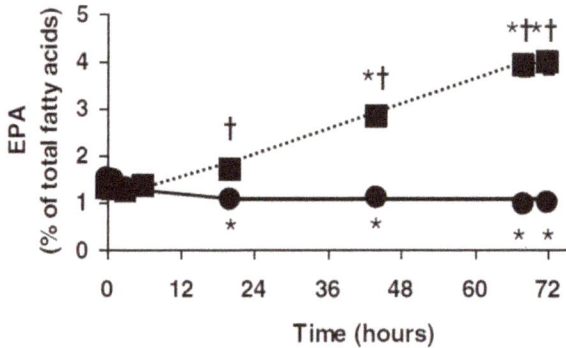

Figure 6. Plasma phosphatidylcholine eicosapentaenoic acid (EPA) in patients with hepatic colorectal metastases and receiving intravenous infusion of a blend of soybean oil, MCTs, and fish oil (closed squares) or soybean oil and MCTs (closed circles) daily for 72 h. * Indicates significantly different from study entry within the same group. † Indicates significant difference between groups at a given time point. Figure taken from Al Taan et al. [36].

3. Clinical Studies in Patients Undergoing Surgery

According to Figure 5, better control of inflammation and better support of immune defenses would be linked with improved patient outcomes. Section 2.3 describes that the use of fish oil containing LEs significantly decreases markers of inflammation and significantly increases markers of acquired immune defenses, especially in surgical patients. Therefore, it would be expected that fish oil LEs would improve patient outcomes in surgical patients. Whether this is the case has been mainly explored in patients undergoing gastrointestinal surgery usually for the removal of malignant tissue. LEs have mainly been used in the days immediately following surgery (usually days 1 to 5) although there are a small number of trials of longer duration or using perioperative administration. The clinical outcomes most often reported are infections and length of hospital stay, while length of ICU stay where patients went to the ICU post-surgery is also reported. Individual trials are discussed in detail elsewhere [20,21]. There have been a number of meta-analyses of the studies conducted with fish oil LEs in surgical patients [42–47]. These meta-analyses are summarized in Table 2. The findings of these meta-analyses are consistent and it is evident that compared with other LEs, usually based on pure soybean oil or a 50:50 (vol/vol) blend of soybean oil and MCT oil, fish oil containing LEs can decrease infections, the length of ICU stay, and the length of hospital stay in surgical patients. As indicated above, most of the studies have used LEs postoperatively but it would also seem advantageous to use fish oil containing LEs preoperatively for several days in cases of elective surgery in order to get the bioactive omega-3 fatty acids into the body in advance of the surgical insult.

Table 2. Summary of meta-analyses of randomized controlled trials of fish oil containing lipid emulsions (LEs) in surgical patients.

Meta-Analysis and Year	Effect of Fish Oil LE On		
	Infections	Length of ICU Stay	Length of Hospital Stay
Chen et al. (2010) [43]	Odds ratio 0.56 (0.32, 0.98) $P = 0.04$ $n = 7$ studies	−1.80 days (−3.04, −0.56) $P = 0.004$ $n = 5$ studies	−2.98 days (−4.65, −1.31) $P = 0.0005$ $n = 7$ studies
Wei et al. (2010) [44]	Risk ratio 0.49 (0.26, 0.93) $P = 0.03$ $n = 4$ studies	−2.07 days (−3.47, −0.47) $P = 0.004$ $n = 3$ studies	
Pradelli et al. (2012) [45] (non-ICU patients)	Risk ratio 0.53 (0.34, 0.82) $P = 0.004$ $n = 6$ studies		−1.86 days (−3.13, −0.59) $P = 0.0004$ $n = 6$ studies
Li et al. (2014) [46]	Odds ratio 0.53 (0.35, 0.81) $P = 0.003$ $n = 9$ studies		−2.14 days (−3.02, −1.27) $P < 0.00001$ $n = 11$ studies
Bae et al. (2017) [47]	Odds ratio 0.44 (0.30, 0.65) $P < 0.0001$ $n = 15$ studies		−2.70 days (−3.60, −1.79) $P < 0.00001$ $n = 10$ studies
Zhao and Wang (2018) [42]	Odds ratio 0.36 (0.20, 0.66) $P = 0.0008$ $n = 8$ studies		

4. Clinical Studies in Patients Requiring Critical Care

There are fewer studies that compare different intravenous LEs in critically ill patients to in surgical patients, yet critically ill patients are more likely to suffer the adverse effects of hyperinflammation and immune paralysis, are more likely to have poor outcomes like organ failure and death, are more likely to have a prolonged hospital stay, and are more likely to require nutrition support including parenteral support. The trials that have been performed most often report infections, respiratory function and need for ventilator support, length of ICU and hospital stay, and death. Individual trials of fish oil containing LEs in critically ill patients are reviewed in detail elsewhere [20,21,27,48,49]. There have been several meta-analyses of the studies conducted with fish oil LEs in critically ill patients [45,50–52]. These meta-analyses are summarized in Table 3. The outcomes of these meta-analyses reflect the mixed picture that emerges from the different trials, that is to say, different meta-analyses produce different findings for some outcomes. This may reflect the relatively small number of studies performed, the use of different fish oil containing LEs, and the heterogeneity of this patient population. Thus, at this stage it is difficult to make a conclusive statement about the role of fish oil containing LEs in critically ill patients, although the rationale, as depicted in Figure 5, remains highly relevant.

Table 3. Summary of meta-analyses of randomized controlled trials of fish oil containing lipid emulsions (LEs) in critically ill patients.

Meta-Analysis and Year	Effect of Fish Oil LE On				
	Infections	Length of ICU Stay	Length of Hospital Stay	Ventilation Requirement	Mortality
Pradelli et al. (2012) [45] (ICU patients)	Odds ratio 0.71 (0.45, 1.12) $P = 0.14$ $n = 5$ studies	−1.92 days (−3.27, −0.58) $P = 0.005$ $n = 8$ studies	−5.17 days (−8.35, −1.99) $P = 0.001$ $n = 8$ studies		
Palmer et al. (2013) [50]	Risk ratio 0.78 (0.43, 1.41) $P = 0.41$ $n = 5$ studies	−0.57 days (−5.05, 3.90) $P = 0.80$ $n = 6$ studies	−9.49 days (−16.51, −2.47) $P = 0.008$ $n = 3$ studies		Risk ratio 0.83 (0.57, 1.20) $P = 0.32$ $n = 8$ studies
Manzanares et al. (2014) [51]	Risk ratio 0.76 (0.42, 1.36) $P = 0.35$ $n = 3$ studies	−1.13 days (−8.96, 6.69) $P = 0.78$ $n = 3$ studies		−1.81 days (−3.98, 0.36) $P = 0.10$ $n = 3$ studies	Risk ratio 0.71 (0.49, 1.04) $P = 0.08$ $n = 5$ studies
Manzanares et al. (2015) [52]	Risk ratio 0.64 (0.44, 0.92) $P = 0.02$ $n = 5$ studies	−1.42 days (−4.53, 1.69) $P = 0.37$ $n = 7$ studies	−3.71 days (−9.31, 1.88) $P = 0.19$ $n = 7$ studies	−1.14 days (−2.67, 0.38) $P = 0.14$ $n = 6$ studies	Risk ratio 0.90 (0.67, 1.20) $P = 0.46$ $n = 9$ studies

Moving away from RCTs and closer to the real patient setting, Edmunds et al. [53] published an interesting secondary analysis of data from a prospective multicenter international study. The study included adults admitted to the ICU for more than 72 h and who were ventilated within 48 h. To be included in the secondary analysis, patients had to have received parenteral nutrition exclusively for more than 5 days and to have received a single type of LE during that time. Of the available 12,585 patients only 451 (3.5%) met these criteria, most (84.2%) having received enteral nutrition. Among the 451 patients included, 223 (49.4%) received pure soybean oil LE while only 19 (4.2%) received a LE that included fish oil. The findings of the study are summarized in Table 4. As compared with using pure soybean oil LE or a 50:50 blend of soybean oil and MCTs, use of fish oil was associated with fewer patient deaths by day 60, shorter lengths of ICU stay, and shorter lengths of hospital stay. Figure 7 shows that the use of fish oil containing LEs increased the likelihood of a patient being discharged alive from the ICU. These findings from a prospective study rather than from an RCT are indicative of a significant clinical benefit from fish oil LEs in critically ill patients. However, it needs to be recognized that the number of patients receiving intravenous fish oil was very small (4.2% of those receiving exclusive parenteral nutrition with one LE and only 0.15% of the entire patient cohort). Thus, the findings must be considered cautiously. Furthermore, it is possible that those centers that use fish oil LEs may use other innovative approaches that benefit their patients. Nevertheless, these findings are encouraging and support the design of improved trials for the future.

Table 4. Summary of findings of Edmunds et al. [53].

Outcome	Soybean Oil	Soybean Oil MCT Oil Blend	Fish Oil Blend
Patient died within 60 days (%)	28.3	30.8	10.5
Duration of mechanical ventilation (median days)	4.9	5.3	5.0
Length of ICU stay (median days)	10.9	9.6	7.05
Length of hospital stay (median days)	28.1	31.9	14.1

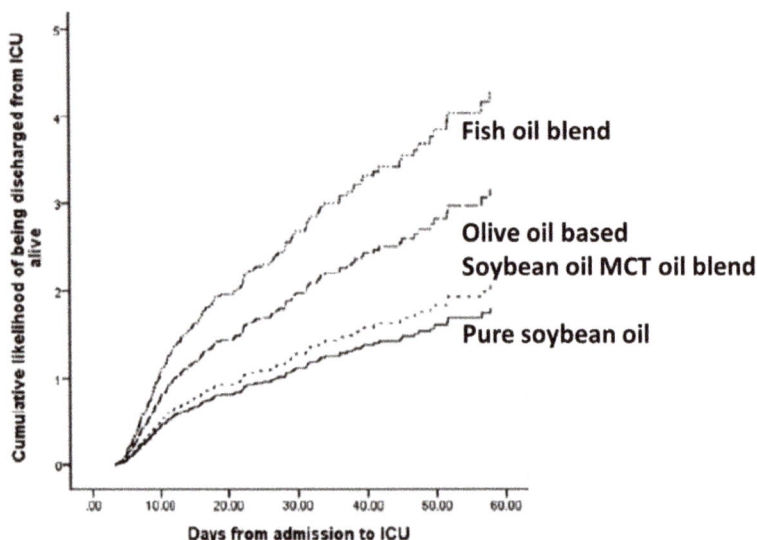

Figure 7. Cumulative likelihood of critically ill patients being discharged from the ICU alive according to the LE received. Modified with permission from C.E. Edmunds, R.A. Brody, J.S. Parrott, S.M. Stankorb, D.K. Heyland (2014) The effects of different IV fat emulsions on clinical outcomes in critically ill patients. Critical Care Medicine 42, 1168–1177 [53].

5. Summary and Conclusions

Lipids used in intravenous nutrition support (i.e., parenteral nutrition) provide energy, building blocks, and essential fatty acids. These lipids are included as emulsions since they need to be soluble in an aqueous environment. Fish oil is a source of bioactive omega-3 fatty acids (EPA and DHA) in contrast to the more traditional soybean oil which is rich in the omega-6 fatty acid linoleic acid. Preclinical research suggests that including fish oil in parenteral nutrition support may control adverse inflammatory responses and may support acquired immunity, thereby offering advantages to patients that would be seen through improved clinical outcomes. LEs, including fish oil, have been used for parenteral nutrition for adult patients post-surgery (mainly gastrointestinal). This has been associated with alterations in patterns of inflammatory mediators and in immune function, and in some studies, a reduction in length of ICU and hospital stay. These benefits, as well as a reduction in infections, are brought out by recent meta-analyses. Perioperative administration of fish oil may be superior to postoperative, but this requires greater exploration. Parenteral fish oil has been used in critically ill adults. Here, the influence on inflammatory processes, immune function, and clinical endpoints is not clear, because there are too few studies and those that are available report inconsistent findings. However, some studies found reduced inflammation, improved gas exchange, and shorter length of hospital stay in critically ill patients if they received fish oil. Meta-analyses do not provide a clear picture of the impact of fish oil containing LEs in critically ill patients, but these are limited by the small number and size of studies performed so far. A prospective study suggests a benefit from fish oil LEs in critically ill patients but in that study very few patients received fish oil. More and better trials are needed in patient groups in which parenteral nutrition is used and where fish oil may offer benefits.

Author Contributions: P.C.C. was solely responsible for all aspects of this publication.

Funding: This publication received no external funding.

Acknowledgments: P.C.C. is supported by the National Institute for Health Research through the Southampton Biomedical Research Centre.

Conflicts of Interest: P.C.C. has received advisory and/or speaking honoraria from Fresenius-Kabi, B. Braun, Baxter Healthcare, Abbott Nutrition, and Danone/Nutricia, sellers of parenteral and enteral feeds, and from Pronova BioPharma/BASF AS and Smartfish, sellers of products containing omega-3 fatty acids.

References

1. Calder, P.C. Functional roles of fatty acids and their effects on human health. *J. Parent. Ent. Nutr.* **2015**, *39* (Suppl. 1), 18S–32S. [CrossRef] [PubMed]

2. Calder, P.C. Very long-chain n-3 fatty acids and human health: Fact, fiction and the future. *Proc. Nutr. Soc.* **2018**, *77*, 52–72. [CrossRef] [PubMed]

3. Baker, E.J.; Miles, E.A.; Burdge, G.C.; Yaqoob, P.; Calder, P.C. Metabolism and functional effects of plant-derived omega-3 fatty acids in humans. *Prog. Lipid Res.* **2016**, *64*, 30–56. [CrossRef]

4. Calder, P.C. Omega-3: The good oil. *Nutr. Bull.* **2017**, *42*, 132–140. [CrossRef]

5. Katan, M.B.; Deslypere, J.P.; van Birgelen, A.P.J.M.; Penders, M.; Zegwaars, M. Kinetics of the incorporation of dietary fatty acids into serum cholesteryl esters, erythrocyte membranes and adipose tissue: An 18 month controlled study. *J. Lipid Res.* **1997**, *38*, 2012–2022.

6. Rees, D.; Miles, E.A.; Banerjee, T.; Wells, S.J.; Roynette, C.E.; Wahle, K.W.J.W.; Calder, P.C. Dose-related effects of eicosapentaenoic acid on innate immune function in healthy humans: A comparison of young and older men. *Am. J. Clin. Nutr.* **2006**, *83*, 331–342. [CrossRef] [PubMed]

7. Browning, L.M.; Walker, C.G.; Mander, A.P.; West, A.L.; Madden, J.; Gambell, J.M.; Young, S.; Wang, L.; Jebb, S.A.; Calder, P.C. Incorporation of eicosapentaenoic and docosahexaenoic acids into lipid pools when given as supplements providing doses equivalent to typical intakes of oily fish. *Am. J. Clin. Nutr.* **2012**, *96*, 748–758. [CrossRef]

8. Calder, P.C. The relationship between the fatty acid composition of immune cells and their function. *Prostagl. Leukotr. Essent. Fatty Acids* **2008**, *79*, 101–108. [CrossRef] [PubMed]

9. Calder, P.C. Mechanisms of action of (n-3) fatty acids. *J. Nutr.* **2012**, *142*, 592S–599S. [CrossRef]

10. Lee, J.Y.; Sohn, K.H.; Rhee, S.H.; Hwang, D. Saturated fatty acids, but not unsaturated fatty acids, induce the expression of cyclooxygenase-2 through Toll-like receptor. *J. Biol. Chem.* **2001**, *276*, 16683–16689. [CrossRef]

11. Wong, S.W.; Kwon, W.J.; Choi, A.M.; Kim, H.P.; Nakahira, K.; Hwang, D. Fatty acids modulate Toll-like receptor 4 activation through regulation of receptor dimerization and recruitment into lipid rafts in a reactive oxygen species-dependent manner. *J. Biol. Chem.* **2009**, *284*, 27384–27392. [CrossRef]

12. Calder, P.C. Marine omega-3 fatty acids and inflammatory processes: Effects, mechanisms and clinical relevance. *Biochim. Biophys. Acta Mol. Cell Biol. Lipids* **2015**, *1851*, 469–484. [CrossRef] [PubMed]

13. Wada, M.; DeLong, C.J.; Hong, Y.H.; Rieke, C.J.; Song, I.; Sidhu, R.S.; Yuan, C.; Warnock, M.; Schmaier, A.H.; Yokoyama, C.; et al. Enzymes and receptors of prostaglandin pathways with arachidonic acid-derived versus eicosapentaenoic acid-derived substrates and products. *J. Biol. Chem.* **2007**, *282*, 22254–22266. [CrossRef] [PubMed]

14. Calder, P.C. Omega-3 fatty acids and inflammatory processes: From molecules to man. *Biochem. Soc. Trans.* **2017**, *45*, 1105–1115. [CrossRef] [PubMed]

15. Bannenberg, G.; Serhan, C.N. Specialized pro-resolving lipid mediators in the inflammatory response: An update. *Biochim. Biophys. Acta Mol. Cell Biol. Lipids* **2010**, *1801*, 1260–1273. [CrossRef]

16. Serhan, C.N.; Chiang, N. Resolution phase lipid mediators of inflammation: Agonists of resolution. *Curr. Opin Pharmacol.* **2013**, *13*, 632–640. [CrossRef]

17. Miles, E.A.; Calder, P.C. Influence of marine n-3 polyunsaturated fatty acids on immune function and a systematic review of their effects on clinical outcomes in rheumatoid arthritis. *Brit. J. Nutr.* **2012**, *107*, S171–S184. [CrossRef]

18. Abdulrazaq, M.; Innes, J.K.; Calder, P.C. Effect of ω-3 polyunsaturated fatty acids on arthritic pain: A systematic review. *Nutrition* **2017**, *39-40*, 57–66. [CrossRef]

19. Senftleber, N.K.; Nielsen, S.M.; Andersen, J.R.; Bliddal, H.; Tarp, S.; Lauritzen, L.; Furst, D.E.; Suarez-Almazor, M.E.; Lyddiatt, A.; Christensen, R. Marine oil supplements for arthritis pain: A systematic review and meta-analysis of randomized trials. *Nutrients* **2017**, *9*, 42. [CrossRef] [PubMed]

20. Calder, P.C. Lipids for intravenous nutrition in hospitalised adult patients: A multiple choice of options. *Proc. Nutr. Soc.* **2013**, *72*, 263–276. [CrossRef]

21. Calder, P.C.; Adolph, M.; Deutz, N.E.; Grau, T.; Innes, J.K.; Klek, S.; Lev, S.; Mayer, K.; Michael-Titus, A.T.; Pradelli, L.; et al. Lipids in the intensive care unit: Recommendations from the ESPEN Expert Group. *Clin. Nutr.* **2018**, *37*, 1–18. [CrossRef] [PubMed]

22. Paulsrud, J.R.; Pensler, L.; Whitten, C.F.; Stewart, S.; Holman, R.T. Essential fatty acid deficiency in infants induced by fat-free intravenous feeding. *Am. J. Clin. Nutr.* **1972**, *25*, 897–904. [CrossRef] [PubMed]

23. Furukawa, K.; Yamamori, H.; Takagi, K.; Hayashi, N.; Suzuki, R.; Nakajima, N.; Tashiro, T. Influences of soybean oil emulsion on stress response and cell-mediated immune function in moderately or severely stressed patients. *Nutrition* **2002**, *18*, 235–240. [CrossRef]

24. Arnalich, F.; Garcia-Palomero, E.; López, J.; Jiménez, M.; Madero, R.; Renart, J.; Vázquez, J.J.; Montiel, C. Predictive value of nuclear factor kappaB activity and plasma cytokine levels in patients with sepsis. *Infect. Immun.* **2000**, *68*, 1942–1945. [CrossRef] [PubMed]

25. Bozza, F.A.; Salluh, J.I.; Japiassu, A.M.; Soares, M.; Assis, E.F.; Gomes, R.N.; Bozza, M.T.; Castro-Faria-Neto, H.C.; Bozza, P.T. Cytokine profiles as markers of disease severity in sepsis: A multiplex analysis. *Crit. Care* **2007**, *11*, R49. [CrossRef]

26. Andaluz-Ojeda, D.; Bobillo, F.; Iglesias, V.; Almansa, R.; Rico, L.; Gandía, F.; Resino, S.; Tamayo, E.; de Lejarazu, R.O.; Bermejo-Martin, J.F. A combined score of pro- and anti-inflammatory interleukins improves mortality prediction in severe sepsis. *Cytokine* **2012**, *57*, 332–336. [CrossRef]

27. Heller, A.R. Intravenous fish oil in adult intensive care unit patients. *World Rev. Nutr. Dietet.* **2015**, *112*, 127–140. [CrossRef]

28. Shaikh, S.R.; Edidin, M. Polyunsaturated fatty acids, membrane organization, T cells, and antigen presentation. *Am. J. Clin. Nutr.* **2006**, *84*, 1277–1289. [CrossRef]

29. Calder, P.C.; Yaqoob, P.; Thies, F.; Wallace, F.A.; Miles, E.A. Fatty acids and lymphocyte functions. *Brit. J. Nutr.* **2002**, *87*, S31–S48. [CrossRef]

30. Calder, P.C. N-3 fatty acids, inflammation and immunity—relevance to postsurgical and critically ill patients. *Lipids* **2004**, *39*, 1147–1161. [CrossRef]

31. Mascioli, E.; Leader, L.; Flores, E.; Trimbo, S.; Bistrian, B.; Blackburn, G. Enhanced survival to endotoxin in guinea pigs fed IV fish oil emulsion. *Lipids* **1988**, *23*, 623–625. [CrossRef]

32. Sadeghi, S.; Wallace, F.A.; Calder, P.C. Dietary lipids modify the cytokine response to bacterial lipopolysaccharide in mice. *Immunology* **1999**, *96*, 404–410. [CrossRef]

33. Spite, M.; Norling, L.V.; Summers, L.; Yang, R.; Cooper, D.; Petasis, N.A.; Flower, R.J.; Perretti, M.; Serhan, C.N. Resolvin D2 is a potent regulator of leukocytes and controls microbial sepsis. *Nature* **2009**, *461*, 1287–1291. [CrossRef]

34. Chen, F.; Fan, X.H.; Wu, Y.P.; Zhu, J.L.; Wang, F.; Bo, L.L.; Li, J.B.; Bao, R.; Deng, X.M. Resolvin D1 improves survival in experimental sepsis through reducing bacterial load and preventing excessive activation of inflammatory response. *Eur. J. Clin. Microbiol. Infect. Dis.* **2014**, *33*, 457–464. [CrossRef]

35. Barbosa, V.M.; Miles, E.A.; Calhau, C.; Lafuente, E.; Calder, P.C. Effects of a fish oil containing lipid emulsion on plasma phospholipid fatty acids, inflammatory markers, and clinical outcomes in septic patients: A randomized, controlled clinical trial. *Crit. Care* **2010**, *14*, R5. [CrossRef]

36. Al-Taan, O.; Stephenson, J.A.; Spencer, L.; Pollard, C.; West, A.L.; Calder, P.C.; Metcalfe, M.; Dennison, A.R. Changes in plasma and erythrocyte omega-6 and omega-3 fatty acids in response to intravenous supply of omega-3 fatty acids in patients with hepatic colorectal metastases. *Lipids Health Dis.* **2013**, *12*, 64. [CrossRef]

37. Barros, K.V.; Cassulino, A.P.; Schalch, L.; Della Valle Munhoz, E.; Manetta, J.A.; Noakes, P.S.; Miles, E.A.; Calder, P.C.; Flor Silveira, V.L. Supplemental intravenous n-3 fatty acids and n-3 fatty acid status and outcome in critically ill elderly patients in the ICU receiving enteral nutrition. *Clin. Nutr.* **2013**, *32*, 599–605. [CrossRef]

38. Calder, P.C. Omega-3 polyunsaturated fatty acids and inflammatory processes: Nutrition or pharmacology? *Brit. J. Clin. Pharmacol.* **2013**, *75*, 645–662. [CrossRef]

39. Wachtler, P.; König, W.; Senkal, M.; Kemen, M.; Köller, M. Influence of a total parenteral nutrition enriched with omega-3 fatty acids on leukotriene synthesis of peripheral leukocytes and systemic cytokine levels in patients with major surgery. *J. Trauma.* **1997**, *42*, 191–198. [CrossRef]

40. Grimm, H.; Mertes, N.; Goeters, C.; Schlotzer, E.; Mayer, K.; Grimminger, F.; Fürst, P. Improved fatty acid and leukotriene pattern with a novel lipid emulsion in surgical patients. *Eur. J. Nutr.* **2006**, *45*, 55–60. [CrossRef]

41. Weiss, G.; Meyer, F.; Matthies, B.; Pross, M.; Koenig, W.; Lippert, H. Immunomodulation by perioperative administration of n-3 fatty acids. *Brit. J. Nutr.* **2002**, *87* (Suppl. 1), S89–S94. [CrossRef]

42. Zhao, Y.; Wang, C. Effect of ω-3 polyunsaturated fatty acid-supplemented parenteral nutrition on inflammatory and immune function in postoperative patients with gastrointestinal malignancy: A meta-analysis of randomized control trials in China. *Medicine (Baltimore)* **2018**, *97*, e0472. [CrossRef]

43. Chen, B.; Zhou, Y.; Yang, P.; Wan, H.W.; Wu, X.T. Safety and efficacy of fish oil-enriched parenteral nutrition regimen on postoperative patients undergoing major abdominal surgery: A meta-analysis of randomized controlled trials. *J. Parent Enteral. Nutr.* **2010**, *34*, 387–394. [CrossRef]

44. Wie, C.; Hua, J.; Bin, C.; Klassen, K. Impact of lipid emulsion containing fish oil on outcomes of surgical patients: Systematic review of randomized controlled trials from Europe and Asia. *Nutrition* **2010**, *26*, 474–481.

45. Pradelli, L.; Mayer, K.; Muscaritoli, M.; Heller, A.R. N-3 fatty acid-enriched parenteral nutrition regimens in elective surgical and ICU patients: A meta-analysis. *Crit. Care* **2012**, *16*, R184. [CrossRef]

46. Li, N.N.; Zhou, Y.; Qin, X.P.; Chen, Y.; He, D.; Feng, J.Y.; Wu, X.T. Does intravenous fish oil benefit patients post-surgery? A meta-analysis of randomised controlled trials. *Clin. Nutr.* **2014**, *33*, 226–239. [CrossRef]

47. Bae, H.J.; Lee, G.Y.; Seong, J.M.; Gwak, H.S. Outcomes with perioperative fat emulsions containing omega-3 fatty acid: A meta-analysis of randomized controlled trials. *Am. J. Health Syst. Pharm.* **2017**, *74*, 904–918. [CrossRef]

48. Mayer, K.; Schaefer, M.B.; Seeger, W. Fish oil in the critically ill: From experimental to clinical data. *Curr. Opin. Clin. Nutr. Metab. Care* **2006**, *9*, 140–148. [CrossRef]

49. Mayer, K.; Schaefer, M.B.; Hecker, M. Intravenous n-3 fatty acids in the critically ill. *Curr. Opin. Clin. Nutr. Metab. Care* **2019**, *22*, 124–128. [CrossRef]

50. Palmer, A.J.; Ho, C.K.; Ajibola, O.; Avenell, A. The role of ω-3 fatty acid supplemented parenteral nutrition in critical illness in adults: A systematic review and meta-analysis. *Crit. Care Med.* **2013**, *41*, 307–316. [CrossRef]

51. Manzanares, W.; Dhaliwal, R.; Jurewitsch, B.; Stapleton, R.D.; Jeejeebhoy, K.N.; Heyland, D.K. Parenteral fish oil lipid emulsions in the critically ill: A systematic review and meta-analysis. *J. Parenter Enteral. Nutr.* **2014**, *38*, 20–28. [CrossRef]

52. Manzanares, W.; Langlois, P.L.; Dhaliwal, R.; Lemieux, M.; Heyland, D.K. Intravenous fish oil lipid emulsions in critically ill patients: An updated systematic review and meta-analysis. *Crit. Care* **2015**, *19*, 167. [CrossRef] [PubMed]

53. Edmunds, C.E.; Brody, R.A.; Parrott, J.S.; Stankorb, S.M.; Heyland, D.K. The effects of different IV fat emulsions on clinical outcomes in critically ill patients. *Crit. Care Med.* **2014**, *42*, 1168–1177. [CrossRef] [PubMed]

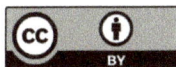

marine drugs

MDPI

Review

Chemically-Induced Production of Anti-Inflammatory Molecules in Microalgae

Zaida Montero-Lobato [1], María Vázquez [1], Francisco Navarro [2], Juan Luis Fuentes [1], Elisabeth Bermejo [1], Inés Garbayo [1], Carlos Vílchez [1,*] and María Cuaresma [1]

[1] Algal Biotechnology Group, CIDERTA, RENSMA and Faculty of Sciences, University of Huelva, 21007 Huelva, Spain; mariazaida.montero@alu.uhu.es (Z.M.-L.); maria.vazquez@ciecema.uhu.es (M.V.); jlfuentes@dqcm.uhu.es (J.L.F.); elisabeth.bermejo@dqcm.uhu.es (E.B.); garbayo@uhu.es (I.G.); maria.cuaresma@dqcm.uhu.es (M.C.)

[2] Department of Integrated Sciences, Cell Biology, Faculty of Experimental Sciences, University of Huelva, 21007 Huelva, Spain; fnavarro@dbasp.uhu.es

* Correspondence: cvilchez@uhu.es; Tel.: +34-959-217765

Received: 31 October 2018; Accepted: 28 November 2018; Published: 30 November 2018

Abstract: Microalgae have been widely recognized as a valuable source of natural, bioactive molecules that can benefit human health. Some molecules of commercial value synthesized by the microalgal metabolism have been proven to display anti-inflammatory activity, including the carotenoids lutein and astaxanthin, the fatty acids EPA (eicosapentaenoic acid) and DHA (docosahexaenoic acid), and sulphated polysaccharides. These molecules can accumulate to a certain extent in a diversity of microalgae species. A production process could become commercially feasible if the productivity is high and the overall production process costs are minimized. The productivity of anti-inflammatory molecules depends on each algal species and the cultivation conditions, the latter being mostly related to nutrient starvation and/or extremes of temperature and/or light intensity. Furthermore, novel bioprocess tools have been reported which might improve the biosynthesis yields and productivity of those target molecules and reduce production costs simultaneously. Such novel tools include the use of chemical triggers or enhancers to improve algal growth and/or accumulation of bioactive molecules, the algal growth in foam and the surfactant-mediated extraction of valuable compounds. Taken together, the recent findings suggest that the combined use of novel bioprocess strategies could improve the technical efficiency and commercial feasibility of valuable microalgal bioproducts production, particularly anti-inflammatory compounds, in large scale processes.

Keywords: anti-inflammatory; bioactive molecules; microalgae; polysaccharides; carotenoids; polyunsaturated fatty acids

1. Microalgae as Source of Anti-Inflammatory Compounds

In recent years, the pharmacy of the sea has become a new paradigm for the discovery and development of novel drugs and bioactive compounds. The increasing need for getting drugs with no or minimal toxic side effects is one of the main reasons that motivates the search for bioactive compounds from natural sources, including anti-inflammatory active molecules from microalgae.

Much has been written about the outstanding metabolic properties of microalgae that make them particularly attractive as a natural source for bioactive molecules production [1–3]. Regarding the topic of this review, a variety of microalgal metabolites which display anti-inflammatory activity can accumulate in the cells to a certain extent. The diversity in chemical nature, structures and biosynthesis pathways of the most abundant anti-inflammatory molecules synthesized by microalgae are well known and have been many times reported in several noticeable reviews [4–6]. Among them, some carotenoids, PUFA (polyunsaturated fatty acids) and carbohydrates displaying anti-inflammatory activity have been reported [7] which also comply with two requisites a target valuable product to be produced by microalgae or cyanobacteria should meet: (i) Being accumulated at relatively high concentrations in microalgal cells grown under standard cultivation conditions, and (ii) being over produced as an algal response to suboptimal cultivation conditions or when they are subjected to chemical and/or physical stress. These suboptimal or stress conditions can be related to changes in nutrient concentration, changes in physicochemical parameters, including pH, temperature, light quality and irradiance, or addition of chemicals triggering the overproduction of target molecules [3,8].

Table 1 summarizes some of the most marketed microalgae species used for accumulation of carotenoids, PUFA and carbohydrates, biochemical molecules groups that include the main anti-inflammatory microalgal compounds.

Table 1. Biochemical molecules groups of microalgae known to display anti-inflammatory activity.

Biochemical Group	Microalgae	References
Carotenoids	*Haematococcus pluvialis* *Dunaliella salina* *Chlorella sorokiniana* *Synechocystis* sp.	[9,10]
PUFA	*Phaeodactylum tricornutum* *Nannochloropsis gaditana*	[11]
Carbohydrates	*Chlorella vulgaris* *Phaeodactylum tricornutum* *Porphyridium* sp. *Tetraselmis suecica*	[12–14]

It is apparent that the proven anti-inflammatory activity of the biomolecules listed in Table 1 increases the value of the algal biomass as a source of functional components for the production of food supplements and novel foods or the production of natural ingredient-based health products. Before proven active against inflammation, some of the most valuable microalgal molecules, listed in Table 1, were reported to be commercially valuable due to their antioxidant properties which confer on the microalgal biomass high potential as a nutritional supplement. For instance, this is the case for the carotenoids astaxanthin (3,3′-dihydroxy-β,β-carotene-4,4′-dione), lutein (3R,3′R,6′R-β ε-carotene-3,3′-diol) and β-carotene (β,β-carotene), which are considered added-value molecules produced by microalgae traditionally demanded by the nutrition market for the production of food supplements [15,16]. The role of the aforementioned microalgal molecules in inflammation and chronic inflammation has been extensively described in a specific review [7], and other related papers [15,17]. Besides the anti-inflammatory activity, the antioxidant capacity displayed by many of these natural molecules increases their value as natural products with potential benefits to human health [18–20]. In addition to those molecules listed in Table 1, phycobiliproteins, phenolic compounds and several carotenoid-isomers are also among those microalgal compounds displaying anti-inflammatory activities and being potentially valuable for commercial applications related to human health care [7,21].

One of the main advantages of microalgae when used for the production of valuable compounds in large scale production systems is the high areal biomass productivities. The systematic production of microalgae biomass at large scale in addition to the high productivity of microalgal cultures under well established and controlled cultivation conditions [22] make them valuable as a natural source for the production of a range of bioactive compounds, including molecules displaying anti-inflammatory activity [3]. The low generation times of microalgal growth and the intensive control of cultivation parameters in photobioreactors make the production of bioactive compounds-enriched microalgal biomass technically and economically feasible at large scale throughout the year at suitable latitudes. Moreover, the algal metabolic plasticity and rapid response to changes in physicochemical conditions ease to address the accumulation of specific metabolic products in large-scale production processes.

In this review, the specific microalgae species and cultivation strategies that could be more suitable to enhance accumulation of anti-inflammatory microalgal molecules are discussed.

Only a few microalgae species are currently being produced with a commercial purpose in spite of the huge diversity existing in nature which according to literature accounts for about 300,000 species, out of which only 10% (30,000) have been documented [23]. Thus, most of the existing microalgae species are still to be discovered and tested for biotechnological exploitation. The worldwide microalgal market for food, feed or high-value ingredients production is mostly composed of a limited number of algal species belonging to the following genera: *Chlorella, Spirulina* (*Arthrospira*), *Dunaliella, Haematococcus, Nannochloropsis, Scenedesmus, Isochrysis, Porphyridium* and *Phaeodactylum* [16]. Until 2014, only a few high-value molecules produced with microalgae had reached the food and feed market: (i) Several pigments, such as the carotenoids β-carotene and astaxanthin, and the protein complex phycocyanin; and (ii) polyunsaturated fatty acids, such as EPA (eicosapentaenoic acid) and DHA (docosahexaenoic acid). All these compounds have been found to display anti-inflammatory activity, though most of them reached the market thanks to properties other than anti-inflammation. In addition, a peptide from *Phaeodactylum tricornutum* reached the market based on its anti-inflammatory properties only [16]. Thus, there is still a big room for discovering microalgae species with the capacity to accumulate anti-inflammatory compounds that could reach the market.

With no doubt genetic engineering techniques currently offer a large number of procedures to obtain modified strains which are designed to display specific functionalities. However, several factors still make the use of genetically modified microalgae difficult at commercial production scale; for instance, a still little positive consumer perception towards genetically modified organisms and the restrictive regulations on genetically modified organisms in many countries slow down development of industrial production of microalgae enriched in high-value compounds. However, the huge diversity of wild microalgae species that remain unexplored and unexploited should still for a long time allow addressing research on their natural potential for the production of target molecules by means of triggering key biosynthetic pathways through the use of specific chemicals and cultivation conditions [8,23]. This is one of the key messages of this review article, and the information and discussion below directly focus on this approach.

The biotechnological potential of most marketed microalgae species is actually very well known, and the expectations to unveil novel, abundant bioactive compounds from non-extremophilic microalgae are decreasing. In coming years, the production of novel microalgal compounds should expectedly be carried out from novel microalgal species isolated from locations where they could eventually be further produced at large scale. In this respect, extremophilic microalgae are microorganisms with unique metabolic capabilities yet unexploited, with a competitive advantage (as compared to non-extremophiles) to grow in open systems under restrictive cultivation conditions (for example, highly acid pH or very low temperature) which limit microbial contamination. For instance, *Dunaliella salina* is an outstanding example of extremophilic microalga commercially used for the production of a high value compound which displays anti-inflammatory activity, β-carotene [24].

2. Chemically-Induced Oxidative Stress to Improve Production of Anti-Inflammatory Compounds

2.1. Chemicals Triggering Accumulation of Anti-Inflammatory Compounds

Marketing of anti-inflammatory compounds obtained from microalgae is possible only if commercial feasibility of the product production process is achieved. A production process could become commercially feasible if the biosynthesis yields and productivity of target molecules are high and the overall production process costs are minimized. The productivity of anti-inflammatory molecules depends on each microalgal species and the specific cultivation conditions that boost the biosynthesis pathways involved. These conditions must be optimized for each microalgal species.

A number of anti-inflammatory molecules obtained from microalgae have also been shown to display high antioxidant capacity, thus they could in theory be produced under oxidative stress conditions. A list of the most abundant microalgal molecules with both anti-inflammatory and antioxidant activities should include the pigments β-carotene [25], astaxanthin [26], lutein [27], zeaxanthin [28] and phycobiliproteins [29]. The carotenoids exhibit high antioxidant activity which has been reported to positively impact human health, based on the chemical ability of carotenoids to scavenge reactive oxygen species (ROS) produced in the cell by the oxidative metabolism [7,15,30].

In addition to the aforementioned antioxidant pigments, LC-PUFAs (long chain polyunsaturated fatty acids, including EPA and DHA) have also been proven to exert antioxidant activity, which for instance was exemplified by studies in human vascular endothelial cells demonstrating reduced excretion of lipid peroxidation products after omega 3-intake and superoxide scavenging by LC-PUFAs [31]. The third group of anti-inflammatory molecules produced by microalgae, the polysaccharides, has also been proven to exert antioxidant activity, and their applications and benefits to human health can be found in several outstanding reviews published in recent years [7,32]. Polysaccharides isolated from *Porphyridium* [33] and *Rhodella* [34] are noticeable examples of antioxidant microalgae polysaccharides.

In addition to the above mentioned compounds, a number of other microalgal molecules have recently been reported which also have high antioxidant capacity besides anti-inflammatory activity: Phenolic compounds (flavonoids) [21], peptides [35], and the carotene isomers trans-β-carotene and 9-cis-β-carotene.

According to the aforementioned antioxidant capacity of a large number of microalgal molecules which also display anti-inflammatory activity, some of the main chemical strategies to enhance their biosynthesis and intracellular accumulation could be based on inducing oxidative stress in the cells which might result in increased production rates of antioxidant molecules. In this sense, ROS can act as chemical signals to specifically induce the biochemical production of antioxidant molecules, including the enzymes of the antioxidant cellular response to stress [36]. Therefore, the use of oxidative stress applied to microalgal cultures can be one of the strategies to achieve increased productivities of those specific target molecules.

In microalgal cultures, oxidative stress can be induced by a range of strategies which involve the use of chemicals. The knowledge of the chemical properties and reactivity of the main added-value molecules obtained from microalgae, as well as the principal metabolic steps of their biosynthesis have allowed to carry out novel research aimed at searching for chemical triggers that enhance accumulation of those molecules. The chemical triggers are different in nature and action mechanisms. According to the latter, these chemicals can be classified into several groups [8]: Oxidative stress inducers, metabolic regulators and metabolic precursors. Besides, chemicals can also be used to induce changes in the physicochemical conditions around the cell environment with the result of the intracellular accumulation of valuable molecules. For instance, surfactant addition to growing microalgal cultures results in foam production containing growing microalgal cells with shifted availability of carbon, oxygen and light [37]. This shifted environment induces physiological responses, including the shifted biochemical profile of valuable microalgal major biomolecules, as further discussed.

In a recent study, Franz et al. [38] described a screening of 42 chemicals for their roles on lipid metabolism in microalgae, and identified 12 chemicals that are capable of enhancing intracellular lipid levels by >100%. Three of these chemicals (epigallocatechin gallate, CDK2 inhibitor 2 and cycloheximide) enhanced intracellular lipids –PUFA included- by 200–400% based on Nile Red fluorescence intensity measurements. In addition, the researchers took a further step to verify these chemicals effectiveness in large-scale cultures and concluded that propyl gallate and butylated hydroxyanisole could be used in large-scale applications considering the low cost of the chemicals and the lipid content increases [38], demonstrating that the application of chemical enhancers could be a valuable, practical approach in addressing the enhanced productivity of microalgae-based products. The main algal molecules with both anti-inflammatory and antioxidant activity, the main chemicals triggering their accumulation and the induction mechanisms in the algal metabolism are summarized in Table 2.

Table 2. Chemical triggers for the production of anti-inflammatory molecules from microalgae.

Anti-Inflammatory Molecule	Chemical Trigger	Induction Mechanism	Microalgae	References
Astaxanthin	H_2O_2, SeO_3^2, Fe (II)	Oxidative stress	*Haematococcus pluvialis*	[39,40]
	MV	Oxidative stress	*Chlorococcum* sp.	[41]
	Fe (II)	Oxidative stress	*Cromochloris zofingiensis*	[42]
	Jasm., salic. acid	Oxidative stress	*Haematococcus pluvialis*	[43]
	N starvation, NaCl	Oxidative stress	*Haematococcus pluvialis*	[44–46]
Lutein	H_2O_2, NaClO	Oxidative stress	*Chlorella zoofingiensis*	[47,48]
	Fe (II), Cu (II)	Oxidative stress	*Coccomyxa onubensis*	[3,24,49]
	N starvation	Oxidative stress	*Coccomyxa onubensis*	[50]
	NaCl	Oxidative stress	*Botryococcus braunii*	[51]
EPA	Low oxygen	PUFA stimulation	*Pavlova lutheri*	[52]
	N, P repletion	PUFA stimulation	*Nannochloropsis oceanica*	[53]
DHA	Low oxygen	PUFA stimulation	*Schizochytrium* sp.	[54]
	N, P repletion	PUFA stimulation	*Pavlova lutheri*	[55]
Sulphated polysaccharides	N starvation	Oxidative stress	*Rhodella violacea*	[56]
	P starvation	Oxidative stress	*Phaeodactylum tricornutum*	[57]
	NaCl	Oxidative stress	*Dunaliella salina*	[58]
Phenolic compounds	Cu (II), Fe (II)	Oxidative stress	*Dunaliella tertiolecta*	[59]
	N repletion + Phe	Phenylpr. synth.	*Spirulina platensis*	[60]

Phe: Phenylalanine; Phenylpr. synth.: Phenylpropanoid synthesis stimulation; Jasm., salic. acid: Jasmonate, salicylic acid.

2.2. Induced-Oxidative Stress: A Key Strategy to Trigger Accumulation of Anti-Inflammatory Compounds

An increasing interest exists about how microalgae can cope with oxidative stress. Such interest is related to the microalgal potential for the large scale production of valuable molecules accumulated under oxidative stress, the so-called antioxidants. The primary microalgal antioxidant response to oxidative stress conditions imposed to their cultures consists of producing a range of enzymes, such as superoxide dismutase, ascorbate peroxidase, catalase, glutathione reductase and peroxidase, as well as other molecules, such as phytochelatins, pigments, polysaccharides, and polyphenols [61]. In addition, PUFA can also accumulate in response to oxidative stress as described below in this manuscript. As explained, polysaccharides, polyphenols, several pigments—particularly the oxygenated carotenoids called xantophylls—and some PUFA have been demonstrated to display anti-inflammatory activity. Thus, the production of such anti-inflammatory bioactive compounds could in theory be enhanced through chemically-induced oxidative stress of the microalgal cultures (Table 2). As well described by Cirulis et al. [61], chemically-induced production of antioxidant compounds from microalgae requires to research: (i) What chemicals induce oxidative stress in microalgae, (ii) which are the main microalgal metabolism responses to the imposed oxidative stress and what target molecules are produced most abundantly to dissipate the oxidative state, (iii) how to modulate the use of oxidative stress chemical triggers in order to simultaneously boost the accumulation of target molecules whilst obtaining high volumetric productivities, and (iv) how to integrate the acquired knowledge into production processes of target molecules both at laboratory and at large scale.

The simple fact that life occurs in an oxygenated atmosphere results in the continuous presence of oxygen in living cells. As a reactive molecule, oxygen takes part in many chemical and biochemical reactions by means of which ROS permanently arise. ROS are chemically reactive species containing oxygen. ROS include species with unpaired electrons and non-radical species, e.g., hydrogen peroxide, and form during oxygen metabolism through several well identified enzymatic pathways. DNA, proteins and membrane lipids, among other biomolecules, are direct targets of ROS which can alter the normal biological functions of those principal biomolecules: This is the so-called oxidative stress.

In photosynthetic cells like those of unicellular microalgae and cyanobacteria, ROS are produced in plastids, mitochondria and cytosol, among other organelles [62]. It is apparent that the light-dependent oxygen production largely contributes to an increase in ROS production in photosynthetic membranes: The greater the photosynthetic activity, the greater the oxygen production in the chloroplasts and, consequently, the potential oxidative damage produced by the ROS generated. Therefore, the reaction centers of photosystem II (PSII) and photosystem I (PSI) play a key role in the production of ROS (Figure 1). In the 1950s Mehler [63] unveiled and described the light-dependent reduction of oxygen to hydrogen peroxide in PSI, therefore superoxide anion being identified as primary reactive oxygen species generated in the chloroplasts [64]. Figure 1 shows details of the chloroplastic ROS-generating reactions (upper frame, a). As indicated, part of the electron flow derived from the water splitting reactions in PSII is derived to the chloroplastic photoreduction of oxygen.

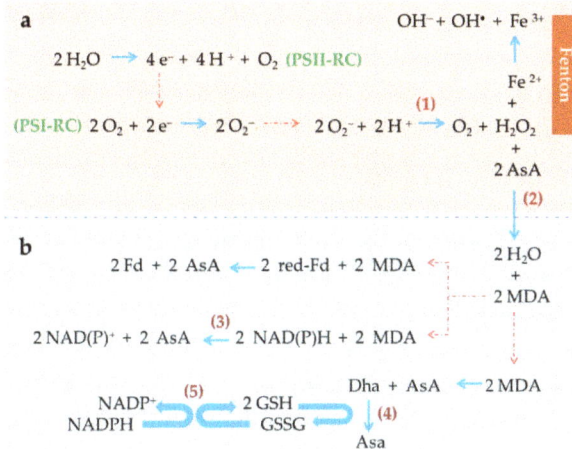

Figure 1. Reactive oxygen species (ROS) production and scavenging mechanisms in photosynthetic organisms. (**a**) Reactive oxygen species production mechanisms, and detoxification of hydrogen peroxide catalyzed by ascorbate peroxidase (2); (**b**) AsA recovery reactions: Enzyme-catalyzed (NAD(P)H-dependent) (3) and spontaneous (red-Fd dependent) biochemical mechanisms of monodehydroascorbate (MDA) reduction, spontaneous disproportion of MDA to Dha and AsA, and enzyme-catalyzed (4) biochemical mechanism of NADPH-GSSG dependent AsA recovery. PSII-RC, photosystem II reaction center; PSI-RC, photosystem I reaction center; AsA, reduced ascorbate; MDA, monodehydroascorbate; red-Fd, reduced ferredoxin; Dha, dehydroascorbate; GSSG, oxidized glutathione; GSH, reduced glutathione; (1) Superoxide dismutase; (2) Ascorbate peroxidase; (3) MDA reductase; (4) Dha reductase; (5) Glutathione reductase.

In order to minimize the ROS damage to key cellular processes and functionalities, the cells express diverse antioxidant biochemical mechanisms to neutralize, or at least minimize, the harmful effects of ROS (reviewed by Deawal et al. [18]). The primary antioxidant mechanisms in most organisms include molecules with antioxidant capacity, such as α-tocopherol (vitamin E), glutathione and ascorbic acid, and enzymes with antioxidant activity, such as superoxide dismutase, catalase, ascorbate peroxidase and glutathione peroxidase (Figure 1). In photosynthetic cells other molecules, such as carotenoids, PUFA and polysaccharides also contribute to cope with a harmful excess ROS. When ROS production exceeds the antioxidant capacity of the cells, harmful effects arise. The above referred antioxidant mechanisms contribute to keeping the intracellular physiological contents of ROS at low levels. In this sense, the enzyme superoxide dismutase catalyzes the subsequent disproportion of superoxide anion to oxygen and hydrogen peroxide [64], thus eliminating the oxidative risk associated with the superoxide anion but still generating a highly reactive, toxic compound, hydrogen peroxide. The main detoxification reaction for hydrogen peroxide is its enzyme-mediated reduction to water catalyzed by ascorbate peroxidase (APX). The subsequent group of reactions shown in Figure 1b expresses the reduced ascorbate (AsA) recovery reactions dependent of NAD(P)H or reduced ferredoxin (red-Fd).

The AsA-dependent enzyme-catalyzed reduction of hydrogen peroxide to water is a crucial step to produce an efficient detoxification of ROS. As shown in Figure 1 (frame a), the highly reactive hydrogen peroxide generated in the reduction of superoxide anion by the enzyme superoxide dismutase, can react with chemical species able to reduce it resulting in the production of additional, extremely active oxygen species. This is the case for Fe (II) which reduces hydrogen peroxide resulting in Fe (III), hydroxyl group and hydroxyl free radical production. This is the so-called Fenton reaction. Therefore, in presence of Fe (II), part of the hydrogen peroxide produced in photosynthetic cells can be diverted to ROS generation instead of being detoxified by the action of APX. Accordingly, Fe (II) can trigger oxidative stress in photosynthetic cells when added to a culture medium at optimized concentrations [36,39,44].

Some reports have been published which provide evidence of direct involvement of ROS in the enhanced biosynthesis of microalgal molecules with both antioxidant and anti-inflammatory properties, namely carotenoids and PUFAs. In 1994, Asada [36] described mechanisms of production and action of reactive oxygen species in photosynthetic cells, suggesting that such ROS might be acting as signal molecules to trigger the biosynthesis of a number of antioxidant molecules, carotenoids among them. Further studies have contributed to support the ROS function as signaling molecules and their action as signal transduction processes activators in response to stress. However, the knowledge on the chemical reactions involved in ROS production, their relative rates and the molecular mechanisms by which photosynthetic cells sense ROS is yet scarce. Particularly, for the activation of signaling cell events to happen, ROS with signaling functions (H_2O_2, $OH^{\cdot}$, O_2) must interact with specific molecular targets. The mechanisms of such interactions and whether each ROS is specifically recognized by a given mechanism or receptors remain unknown [62].

The role of antioxidants in inflammation has been recently reviewed by Arulselvan et al. [65]. In this respect, carotenoids, PUFA, polysaccharides and other natural molecules have been reported to exert antioxidant properties which may play a key role in the anti-inflammatory response [7,65]. Such antioxidant activity consists of scavenging ROS, and/or dissipating photons excess which cannot be photochemically quenched. The basic principle by which the anti-inflammatory microalgal unsaturated fatty acids and terpenoids (carotenoids, xantophylls) act as ROS scavengers is shown in Figure 2. Whether, and how, the biosynthesis of these antioxidant molecules is triggered by the action of ROS acting as signal transduction process activators remains unclear yet; however, many evidence have been published which prove enhanced biosynthesis and accumulation of those anti-inflammatory antioxidant molecules upon induced oxidative stress in microalgae. Consequently, the addition of certain chemicals which act as oxidative stress inducers should be expected to result in enhanced accumulation of carotenoids, PUFAs and/or polysaccharides and is indeed one of the strategies preferred in recent years [8].

The nature of chemicals that can induce oxidative stress in photosynthetic cells is diverse and the number of those can be enormous. Those being most commonly used in laboratory experiments currently are listed in Table 2 and include hydrogen peroxide, sodium hypochlorite, Fe (II and III), Cu (II), sodium chloride, selenite or selenate, herbicides, such as methyl viologen (MV), salicylic acid (SA), methyl jasmonate (MJ) and giberellic acid (GA), among other compounds. Some of them, for instance SA, MJ and GA, play roles in regulating expression of genes involved in the biosynthesis of anti-inflammatory xantophylls [8,66] and, more interestingly, they can play roles as oxidative stress inducers when used in concentrations that are relatively high in relation to the antioxidant capacity of the microalgal cells. Therefore, some of these compounds which are phytohormones and analogous molecules can trigger the accumulation of anti-inflammatory molecules by either playing regulatory roles in their biosynthetic pathways or directly acting as oxidative stress inducers when added in excess to the microalgal cultures [8]. Moreover, the cell response is mostly proportional to the concentration of the chemical trigger used which allows design production processes based on the modulate action of such a trigger compound on the algal metabolism. A productive process should be that one in which the target molecule accumulation is enhanced whilst growth rates remain sufficiently high as to keep overall productivity also high. From the practical point of view, the selection of an oxidative stress chemical inducer could be made according to at least the following criteria: (a) The chemical should induce modulate responses in algal growth and target molecules biosynthesis rates that are proportional to the inducer concentration, so that the productivity of target antioxidants can also be maximized accordingly; (b) the chemical should not be toxic to photosynthetic growth at low concentrations; (c) the chemical should be compatible with further biomass processing and with specific applications of the target molecules.

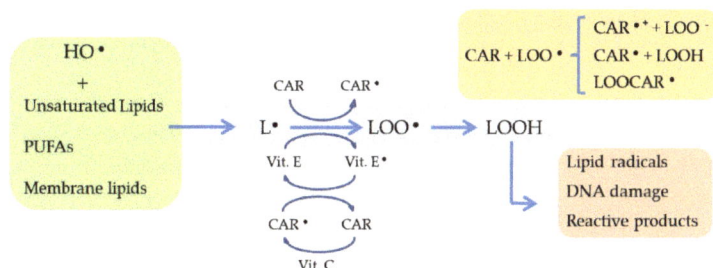

Figure 2. Joint action of ROS scavenging activity exerted by the microalgal anti-inflammatory molecules PUFA and carotenoids. PUFA (unsaturated lipids) and carotenoids are involved in scavenging reactive oxygen species (green frame, left; yellow frame, right); the resulting oxidized peroxidation products are chemically damaging for lipids and DNA, among other molecules (orange frame, right). CAR: Carotenoids; L: Lipid; LOO•: Peroxidized lipid; Vit C: Vitamin C; Vit E: Vitamin E.

In addition to the latter, other chemical strategies producing oxidative stress and addressing the accumulation of microalgal molecules with anti-inflammatory activity are commonly based on nutrient limitation or starvation. It should be noticed that nutrient starvation, particularly inorganic nitrogen, is an effective chemical tool to induce accumulation of lipids—including carotenes and xantophylls—and polysaccharides in microalgae. This subject has been widely reviewed [3,67]. In the following subsections, the most relevant strategies to address the chemically-induced accumulation of anti-inflammatory microalgal compounds are discussed.

2.3. Production of Pigments with Anti-Inflammatory Activity

Carotenoids have been found to positively impact the anti-inflammatory cellular response mechanisms and the immunoresponse modulation [7,68,69]. In addition, their antioxidant nature confers carotenoid-enriched diets properties to diminish the risk of suffering from degenerative diseases [70] and protect the eye macula from adverse photochemical reactions [71]. In people over the age of 65, visual sensitivity and vision loss directly has been found to be associated with lutein and zeaxanthin concentrations in the retina [15,72,73]. Astaxanthin, a powerful, natural antioxidant xanthophyll produced by the microalga *Haematococcus pluvialis*, has been proven effective as an anti-inflammatory [7,74–77]. In addition, astaxanthin was shown to be effective against benign prostatic hyperplasia and against prostatic cancer [70,78]. The protective action of astaxanthin involves an antioxidant mechanism based on the activation of its hydroxyl groups, which results in the formation of an ortho-dihydroxyconjugate polyene system. This polyene system acts as a chain-breaking antioxidant [79].

In photosynthetic organisms, carotenoids may act as accessory pigments in light harvesting functions during the light phase of photosynthesis and may also exert protection of the photosynthetic machinery from excess light and from other oxidative stress chemical factors (e.g., oxidative species, salt, and nutrient deficiency), by scavenging reactive oxygen species (ROS) [3,15,79]. In general, the level of carotenoids in microalgae increases with oxidative stress. Though chlorophyll is also a valuable antioxidant which has been described to display anti-inflammatory properties [80], its content in photosynthetic cells under oxidative stress usually decreases. Thus, the chlorophyll production is by far more efficient in microalgal cultures growing under non-limiting accumulation conditions, in highly dense cultures produced in controlled photobioreactors [81].

Only a limited number of microalgae genera are commonly used in research to test pigment accumulation under oxidative stress, such as *Haematococcus* for astaxanthin, *Chlorella*, *Scenedesmus* and *Botryococcus* for lutein, and *Dunaliella* for β-carotene [23]. A few reports demonstrate that direct addition of hydrogen peroxide triggered astaxanthin accumulation, for example in *Haematococcus pluvialis* [44], *Chlorococcum* [41] and *Chlorella zofingiensis* [47], showing maximal increased astaxanthin contents up to 30% higher than those of standard cultures. Astaxanthin accumulation can also be boosted indirectly, by intracellular production of hydrogen peroxide through oxidative stress induced by addition of selenite to the culture medium. Selenite-mediated oxidative stress induction was unveiled by significantly increased levels of the hydrogen peroxide antioxidant enzyme activity content of the microalgal cells upon selenite addition, which indirectly resulted in increased astaxanthin accumulation in *H. pluvialis* as part of the cellular antioxidant response [40]. Thus, the application of a suitable type and dosage of a given ROS can be potentially used as an efficient chemical tool for large-scale production of anti-inflammatory xanthophylls, such as astaxanthin.

The increased intracellular content of ROS that is required to boost astaxanthin accumulation can also be achieved by the addition of herbicides to microalgal cultures. Herbicides, such as methyl viologen, are commonly used in laboratory research and have been reported to enhance accumulation of astaxanthin in *Haematococcus* [44] and *Chlorococcum* [41] though it is a detriment to the microalgal growth and, obviously, to the quality of the microalgal products. Looking at the large-scale production process feasibility, the use of herbicides implies the associated problem of its toxicity and thus would not be suitable for industrial production. Interestingly, Ma and Chen [41] demonstrated that the hydroxyl (OH) radical might be a key ROS in the molecular signaling pathway that activates the astaxanthin biosynthesis, therefore suggesting a direct effect of a specific ROS on the astaxanthin production pathway induction. Indeed, an early study of Kobayashi et al. [39] demonstrated that several oxidant chemical species, including superoxide anion radical (O_2^-), hydrogen peroxide and 2,2'-azo-bis(2-amidinopropane)-dihydrochloride for peroxy radical (AO_2), and Fe (II), were capable of boosting astaxanthin accumulation in *H. pluvialis*. These chemical species might be playing a role as oxidizers in the oxidative enzyme reactions chain leading to astaxanthin biosynthesis [82].

The use of ferrous iron-Fe (II) as astaxanthin biosynthesis inducer is of particular interest. Fe (II) is an essential metal ion required for microalgal growth, therefore included in the culture medium composition. As described by Kobayashi et al. [39], Fe (II) catalyzes the so-called Fenton reaction by which OH radical generates. When added in excess, Fe (II) addresses the boosted generation of OH radical, thus largely increasing the oxidative state of the cells. As discussed above, OH radical triggers the molecular signaling pathway that activates astaxanthin biosynthesis. Thus, Fe (II) can be effectively used to enhance astaxanthin accumulation, as reported for example for *H. pluvialis* [83] and *Chromochloris zofingiensis* [42]. One of the advantages of Fe (II) as astaxanthin biosynthesis inducer is the dose-response of the microalgal growth II to this ion. This allows for the better control of chemical conditions (Fe (II) concentrations) that can simultaneously address astaxanthin accumulation and microalgal growth [84].

Nitrogen limitation or starvation and high salinity levels induce oxidative stress in microalgal cells and also the subsequent cellular antioxidant responses, including enhanced biosynthesis and accumulation of anti-inflammatory carotenes and xanthophylls [85]. Indeed, astaxanthin and other carotenoids displaying anti-inflammatory activity (e.g., lutein, β-carotene) can accumulate in microalgal cells in response to nitrogen limitation or starvation (astaxanthin, [45,46]; β-carotene, [67]; lutein [50]) and high salinity of the culture medium (astaxanthin, [39]; lutein [51]). Nitrogen starvation-based strategies come with the disadvantage of the time-limited cell viability of the microalgal cultures. Thus, the nitrogen starvation-based pigment production consists of a two-phase process, with the first phase of microalgal growth in nutrient replete medium followed by a second phase of incubation in a nitrogen-starved medium.

In spite of lutein being one of the most valuable carotenoids, chemically-induced accumulation of lutein has not been extensively studied in microalgae. Considering the valuable applications of lutein and the increasing market demand of natural sources of this pigment [16], this is with no doubt a challenging research field for algaers. In microalgae, lutein has been shown to accumulate in cultures subjected to oxidative stress. For instance, the lutein content of *Chlorella zoofingiensis* was shown to increase in response to ROS generated by low concentrations of H_2O_2 or NaClO [48]. The cultures were grown heterotrophically and the lutein increase accounted just for about 11% with respect to control cultures, which suggests there is still room for lutein production improvement under optimized process conditions. But not only the use of oxidants triggers lutein biosynthesis in microalgae; induction of oxidative stress based on nutrient starvation [50], or increased salinity (NaCl), have been found to induce increased accumulation of lutein in *C. onubensis*. Interestingly, lutein accumulates at a high intracellular concentration in Fe (II) or Cu (II)-added cultures of *C. onubensis*, an extremophilic microalgal species isolated from the highly acidic environment of Río Tinto (Southwestern Spain) [49]. The large lutein accumulation is probably one of the physiological microalgal responses to the oxidative conditions of acidic habitats which contain relatively high levels of solved metal ions, such as Fe (II), Mn (II), Al (III) and Zn (II) [24].

Almost no studies have been published dealing with ROS-mediated induction of β-carotene biosynthesis, probably due to the efficient chemical strategies applied for β-carotene mass production at industrial scale and the high intracellular β-carotene content and productivities achieved by the only β-carotene producing microalga *Dunaliella salina* which makes the search for novel chemical triggers unnecessary.

2.4. Production of Polyunsaturated Fatty Acids (PUFA) with Anti-Inflammatory Activity

The anti-inflammatory properties of PUFA from microalgae have been widely described and recently reviewed by several authors [7,32]. A large number of scientific papers described the effective therapeutic role of PUFA in a variety of inflammatory pathologies, such as Alzheimer, arthritis and lupus [7,86,87], with a demonstrated activity in chemopreventive functions when used as ω-3 PUFA-rich microalgal oil diet [88].

In photosynthetic cells, PUFA carry out a variety of cellular key functions. Besides the principal roles of PUFA as energy storage molecules, cell membrane components and in the physiology of photosynthetic cells, their antioxidant capacity is one of the cellular defense mechanisms against the harmful presence of ROS. In fact, PUFA show affinity towards ROS generated in algal cells subjected to oxidative stress conditions [89]. Indeed, PUFA have been described to react chemically with ROS (Figure 2), which results in the formation of lipid hydroperoxides [90,91] resulting in an altered profile of lipids. This is of course an inevitable consequence of oxygen-dependent life but is often ignored [33]. Particularly, PUFA autoxidation reaction is mediated by ROS, which results in the formation of lipid hydroperoxides as primary products. The lipid hydroperoxides can be further converted into more oxidized products, such as ketones and malonaldehyde. Other oxidation products are hydroxy alkenals which are formed by peroxidation of 4-hydroxy-2-nonenal (HNE), generated by peroxidation of ω-6 PUFAs.

Thus, together with carotenoids and polysaccharides, PUFA are included among the wide range of antioxidant compounds that are produced by microalgal cells to diminish the harmful consequences derived from oxidative stress [92]. However, such antioxidant role obviously causes the time course-dependent decreased proportion of PUFA with respect to saturated fatty acids, in microalgal cells. In spite of this fact, the production of microalgal PUFA can be improved under suitably controlled oxygen levels [33].

Besides the negative impact of ROS in the growth and high-value compounds accumulation of microalgae, ROS seem to play a relevant role in triggering lipid accumulation in microalgae [93,94] though experimental evidence of ROS-mediated lipid accumulation mechanisms is still lacking [33]. The aforementioned apparent contradiction suggests that lipid accumulation could be induced by suitable intracellular ROS levels which could be achieved by subjecting the microalgal cultures to controlled stress conditions, specifically through controlled oxygen levels. In this respect, bioprocess engineering can help to optimize the oxygen supply to the microalgal cultures. Sun et al. [33] suggest this can be done either by direct oxygen regulation strategies or through new bioreactor designs to improve oxygen supply. Overall, PUFA production can thus be enhanced by keeping oxygen concentration in the photobioreactor at relatively low levels, therefore favoring a ROS production low activity in the cells as a mean to stimulate PUFA accumulation whilst minimizing the excess ROS-dependent lipid peroxidation. As low oxygen concentrations are detrimental to the microalgal growth, the production of PUFA-enriched microalgae can be carried out in a two-step process: The first step of biomass production under normal aeration, followed by the second step of cultivation under low oxygen concentration for enhancing PUFA accumulation. This strategy was used by Qu et al. [54] to produce DHA-enriched biomass of *Schizochytrium* sp. Alternatively, simultaneous growth and PUFA production can be carried out at a constant, average oxygen concentration optimized in order to achieve maximal productivities, as described by Huang et al. [95] for growth and simultaneous accumulation of DHA.

As previously described above, chemical factors other than oxygen and ROS also generate oxidative stress. For example, nutrient limitation or deprivation (-N, -P) and high salinity cause increased intracellular ROS level in microalgae [96,97], thus triggering the expression of antioxidant defenses as carotenoids and lipids in the microalgal cells. If the intracellular ROS levels exceed the antioxidant cellular capacity, oxidative stress originates. Some of the consequences were aforementioned and include decreased PUFA proportion due to their reaction against ROS. For example, a reduced content of PUFA was observed in *Phaeodactylum tricornutum* cultures under nitrogen limitation [98], and a trend between increasing EPA yields and decreasing salinity was found in *Pavlova lutheri* [52], both results indirectly suggesting the intense oxidative state arose from nutrient limitation or increased salinity.

In spite of this negative correlation between accumulation of anti-inflammatory PUFA and nutrient limitation or salinity level, the accumulation of these compounds in microalgae can also be enhanced under nitrogen limitation or relatively high salinity but only if these conditions are optimized and applied to the right time of the stress phase, the accumulation being also species-dependent [99,100]. Although the connection between salinity or nutrient starvation and intracellular antioxidant capacity has been often reported [11,50,101], this does not necessarily imply systematic, continuous intracellular accumulation of antioxidants as they can also be involved in coping with intracellular ROS under intense oxidative stress, thus decreasing their concentration in the microalgal cells. Therefore, as the main conclusion, the oxidative stress-mediated accumulation of antioxidant, anti-inflammatory PUFA in microalgae should be carefully addressed by controlling the oxidative pressure and selecting the right experimental time to harvest the PUFA-enriched microalgal biomass.

Conversely, the reduced oxidative damage of microalgal cells growing in a replete culture medium can explain the highest EPA content displayed under nitrogen repletion conditions by *Nannochloropsis oceanica* (above 30% of total fatty acids cell content) [53], the highest DHA content observed in *Pavlova lutheri* (approximately 30% of total fatty acids cell content) [55] and the increased PUFA content in *Tetraselmis marina* [99]. Both nitrogen and phosphorus repletion conditions promote microalgal growth which implies the more active biosynthesis of cell membranes, and particularly tylakoid membranes in light limited high cell density cultures aimed at improving light capture [102].

2.5. Production of Sulphated Polysaccharides (sPS) with Anti-Inflammatory Activity

The anti-inflammatory properties of sPS from microalgae have been recently reviewed [32]. The anti-inflammatory properties of sPS-enriched microalgae have been proven in vivo and in vitro for diverse microalgae, such as species of *Chlorella* and *Phaeodactylum* [103,104]. According to the literature, probably the large majority of cyanobacterial polysaccharide structures contains sulfate groups [105] and thus can be considered to be sPS. However, the lack of knowledge on structural data of cyanobacterial polysaccharides limits the possibilities to establish relationships between their chemical structures and biological properties. In addition to it, the cyanobacterial polysaccharide structures can vary depending on species. Thus, further research on the structure of cyanobacterial polysaccharides is required before their real bioactive potential and applications to human health can be evaluated. The current knowledge on the production, extraction and characterization of cyanobacterial polysaccharides has been recently revised in an outstanding review by Delattre et al. [105].

In cyanobacteria, a large fraction of assimilated carbon can be diverted to the synthesis of polysaccharides [106]. Polysaccharides have the function of serving as carbon and energy reserves in microalgae. In addition, a fraction of the produced polysaccharides can be excreted to cover the cells with a mucilage layer to protect them from harsh environmental conditions and/or predators [105]. Some of these cyanobacterial polysaccharides have also been found to display antioxidant activity in addition to their reported anti-inflammatory activity. For example, antioxidant activity has been found in extracellular polysaccharides from *Rhodella reticulata* [34] and *Porphyridium* [107].

Cyanobacterial polysaccharides are also included among the antioxidant molecules produced by microalgae in response to oxidative stress. Cyanobacteria produce exopolysaccharides, which according to literature are sPS, up to more than 20 $g \cdot L^{-1}$ [108,109] in response to a range of physic-chemical conditions. Nutrient limitation and starvation, particularly lack of N, is the classical strategy to induce cyanobacterial polysaccharides accumulation [105], which most probably derives from the N/C ratio metabolic imbalance rather than from the antioxidant cellular response. N limitation, rather than N starvation, might be a more productive strategy. N limitation can be applied to one-phase production strategy in photobioreactors outdoors, by which N concentration is adjusted to limiting levels only when the cultivation conditions are suitable to boost sPS accumulation. Microalgal growth declines under N-limitation, but still a compromise between sPS intracellular accumulation and growth can be achieved in order to maximize sPS productivity. Limitation or starvation of main nutrients other than N, for instance P and S, can also result in polysaccharide accumulation [110], though their effectiveness depends much on the algal species and cultivation conditions, and it has to be specifically determined and optimized in each case [111,112]. As explained by Delattre et al. [105], almost no studies have been conducted to analyze what nutrient does really determine polysaccharides production and how to simplify the culture medium composition.

As explained above, salinity induces oxidative stress in microalgae. Accordingly, and considering the antioxidant character of microalgal polysaccharides, salinity could act as polysaccharide accumulation inducer in microalgae which could use the produced polysaccharides for protective roles. Indeed, the polysaccharide layer around the cells can limit the diffusion of ions through the cell cover [113]. Such this role might be played by polysaccharides produced by several species of cyanobacteria, for instance *Aphanocapsa*, *Anabaena* or *Synechocystis* [105,114,115], which should mostly be sulphated (sPS) and thus expected to display anti-inflammatory activity [32].

2.6. Production of Phenolic Compounds with Anti-Inflammatory Activity

Phenolic compounds are secondary metabolites produced by photosynthetic organisms and have awaked interest in recent years, particularly due to their antioxidant character. Based on such properties, the phenolic compounds are known for their benefits to human health. Specifically, the anti-inflammatory properties of microalgal phenolic compounds have been recently reported [116] and contribute to augment the industrial interest of microalgae as raw material for the generation of novel health products. The phenolic compounds found in microalgae and cyanobacteria and cited in the literature include phenolic acids and flavonoids, such as gallate, chlorogenate, cinnamate, gentisic acid, isoflavones, flavanones, flavonols, and dihydrochalcones [59,60].

The action mechanism of anti-inflammatory compounds is performed by a variety of inhibitory activities of pro-inflammatory mediators and/or gene expression [116]. In inflammation, pro-inflammatory cytokines induce the formation of nitric oxide (NO) by inducible nitric oxide synthase, and compounds that inhibit NO production have anti-inflammatory effects. Phenolic compounds, e.g., flavonoids, are among the molecules displaying inhibitory activities of pro-inflammatory mediators. In this regard, a study of Hämäläinen et al. [117] shows that the anti-inflammatory action of flavonoids is due to the inhibitory activity of lipopolysaccharide-induced NF-κB (nuclear factor kappa-light-chain-enhancer of activated B cells) activation. Anti-inflammatory effect of flavonoids consists of inhibiting NF-κB activation only, along with their inhibitory effect on nitric oxide synthase expression and nitric oxide production in activated macrophages.

Phenolic compounds accumulation in microalgae has been directly related to the antioxidant response mechanisms of the cells to increased intracellular oxidative states. Indeed, the anti-inflammatory activity of phenolic compounds is directly related to their antioxidant activity against ROS. Phenolic compounds have been described as radical scavengers based on their role as donors of hydrogen atoms or electrons, producing stable radical intermediates. They can also inhibit iron-mediated ROS formation to prevent the subsequent oxidative stress [92].

However, only a few studies have been reported so far which deal with the accumulation of phenolic compounds in microalgae as a specific cellular response to ROS generated under oxidative stress conditions, for instance, exposure to metal stress [61]. In this regard, a number of factors, such as nutrient level or presence of metal ions can trigger biosynthesis and accumulation of phenolic compounds in microalgae. As an example, El-Baky et al. [60] reported that intracellular accumulation of polyphenols in *Spirulina* was stimulated by nitrogen, both in inorganic ($NaNO_3$) or organic (L-phenylalanine) forms. Particularly, the authors reported the presence of phenolic acids and flavonoids predominantly with gallate, chlorogenate, cinnamate and *p*-OH-benzoates. Moreover, in relation to the microalgal antioxidant response, accumulation of phenolic compounds has been described in *Dunaliella tertiolecta* in response to stress produced by addition of Cu (II) or Fe (II). Cu-exposed (790 nmol·L^{-1}) *D. tertiolecta* cultures contained 1.4-fold higher intracellular levels of phenolic compounds than standard cultures [59], thus suggesting that the intracellular accumulation of phenolic compounds in microalgae can be triggered by a metal-induced enhanced oxidative state of the microalgal cells.

3. Surfactant-Facilitated Accumulation of Anti-Inflammatory Molecules

Microalgae cultivation in foam is a novel concept that consists of growing microalgal cells in surfactant-based foam [118]. A surfactant is a chemical compound that lowers the surface tension between two liquids, or a liquid and a solid, or a gas and a liquid. The chemical structure of a surfactant is composed of zones of different polarity, typically both a polar and a non-polar part. When mixed in culture medium at a given concentration (at least the so-called CMC, critical micelle concentration) and bubbled with air, foam arises. If the culture medium contains growing microalgal cells, microalgae-enriched foam with actively growing cells is produced. In doing so, microalgae can be continuously grown in foam for which specific foam-bed reactors should be designed [118].

The foam-bed photobioreactor is a novel bioengineering concept originally emerged at Wageningen University [119]. In a foam-bed photobioreactor the microalgal cells grow in liquid foams [118], and it has several advantages when compared to liquid cultures: Mass transfer increase, reduction in aeration and biomass harvesting costs, and minimization of water consumption. The successful performance of a foam-bead photobioreactor depends on several factors that have been recently studied [37,120]. Poloxamers, non-ionic surfactants, were demonstrated to be effective for microalgal growth in foam [37].

In the foam formed, the microalgal cells grow in the liquid layer that surrounds foam bubbles (Figure 3). The foam is formed by the air volume contained in micelles of surfactant molecules. The non-polar zone of a surfactant molecule is oriented towards the air inside the surfactant micelles whilst the polar zone points to the water layer around the bubble. The cell cover of microalgal cells usually presents electrical charge density which may change towards neutral values during growth. Accordingly, electrostatic interactions between either polar or non-polar zones of the microalgal cell cover and polar or non-polar zones of the surfactant molecules, respectively, may produce molecular disorders in the cell wall and thus influence their functions, including nutrient uptake. This can impact primary metabolism and growth of microalgal cells in foam [1,121], and can result in a modified biochemical composition of the cell. Consequently, cultivation in foam could be investigated as a tool to modify the major biochemical composition of the microalgal cells, i.e., total content of lipids and/or carbohydrates, which include molecules with anti-inflammatory activity as described above in this review.

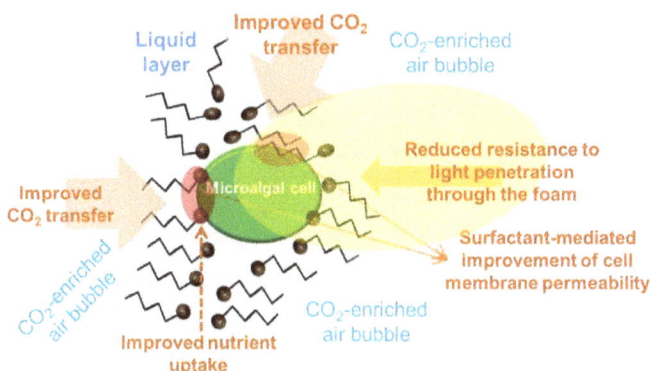

Figure 3. Scheme of physicochemical features that might contribute to enhanced growth and/or shifted biochemical composition of microalgae growing in liquid foams. Symbols: Black sphere with tail, surfactant molecules.

In a foam-bed photobioreactor, once foam reaches the top part of the cultivation vessel it has to be continuously broken to release the gas contained in the foam bubbles which can produce growth inhibition by oxygen, or lowered growth by carbon limitation. Foam can be broken at the top of the reactor by means of different procedures [118]. Thus, the gas is rapidly released to the atmosphere when foam breaks. This allows for a better control of the oxygen level in the reactor, which can be used to create conditions that stimulate accumulation of high-value compounds, for instance, anti-inflammatory PUFA. Indeed, oxygen concentration has been found to greatly influence the accumulation of value compounds in microalgae [122]. The accumulation of anti-inflammatory compounds in microalgae, such as specific PUFA and carotenoids, can be induced under low oxygen supply. Accordingly, bioprocess engineering strategies are required which lead to an oxygen supply adjusted to the specific demand, and efficient in the oxygen transfer from the gas phase to the culture broth particularly in heterotrophic production [123]. In this regard, novel cultivation strategies and reactor designs that improve mass transfer to the growing cells could help increase productivity of biomass and of the aforementioned target compounds. As described by Janoska et al. [118], the foam-bed photobioreactor has the advantage of high gas holdup which results in both increased mass transfer and lower pressure drop. The increased mass transfer results in higher both carbon and oxygen transfer rates from the gas bubbles to the microalgae cells that grow in the liquid layers between gas bubbles (Figure 3). The improved transfer rates in foam result in increased biomass productivity in well oxygenated microalgal cultures. The opposite, under low oxygen supply, the microalgal metabolism rapidly adapts to enhance PUFA biosynthesis, which can be due to the higher activity of the polyketide synthase (PKS) pathway as it does not require oxygen [124]. PKSs related to PUFA synthase are involved in the biosynthesis of long-chain polyhydroxy alcohols and contribute to the formation of the glycolipid envelope in cyanobacterial heterocysts [125].

The chemical interaction between the polar groups of surfactant molecules and the microalgal cell wall obviously results in a reduced charge density of the microalgal cell cover. In the case of positively charged groups in the surfactant structure, it has been speculated that their neutralization at the cell surface by negatively charged groups should be a reason for better surfactant adsorption to the algal cells [126]. Accordingly, the hydrophobic nature of the oxygen molecule should facilitate its diffusion to the theoretically less polar microalgal cell. Consequently, it could be suggested that the impact of either high or low oxygen concentrations in microalgal cells growing in foam should most probably be faster and more intense than in liquid cultures. This reasoning can partly explain results recently obtained which show that microalgae growing in foam are apparently more sensitive to stress than those growing in liquid cultures. This could be useful as a tool to address the faster accumulation of carbohydrate and lipids, the two major groups of biomolecules with anti-inflammatory activity, in microalgae growing in foam through suitable control of the oxygen and CO_2 levels in the gas supplied to the cultures, among other factors.

4. Conclusions

Besides being used as feed and food, microalgae are currently recognized as natural producers of highly valuable bioactive compounds. Several biomolecules produced by microalgae, namely carotenoids, polyunsaturated fatty acids, sulphated polysaccharides and phenolic compounds, have been found to display anti-inflammatory activity. This finding expands the range of applications of microalgal biomass from healthy diet ingredient in food to nutraceuticals that contribute to diminish the intensity of specific symptoms and/or to prevent specific pathologies related to inflammation processes. Many of those anti-inflammatory biomolecules have also high antioxidant capacity that has been reported to impact human health positively, in particular at advanced ages. Consequently, microalgae are considered to play a relevant role in the future map of novel strategies for the prevention and treatment of inflammatory diseases that includes the use of natural products obtained through well controlled biotechnological processes. The number of microalgae species still to be isolated from nature that could be promising for the accumulation of anti-inflammatory compounds is enormous. To achieve high productivities of target compounds, the isolation of fast-growth species and the enhancement of metabolic fluxes leading to increased biosynthesis of those target products are key aspects. In this sense, chemical tools such as specific triggers of target products and cell growth in foam, are being developed which will be very promising in the short term in order to exploit the production of microalgae enriched in molecules displaying anti-inflammatory activity.

Author Contributions: The authors' contributions were as follows: Z.M.-L. and C.V. studied and planned the topic of the review. Z.M.-L. and C.V. wrote Sections 1, 2.1 and 2.2. Z.M.-L., I.G. and E.B. wrote Section 2.3. F.N. wrote Section 2.4. Z.M.-L. and J.L.F. wrote Sections 2.5 and 2.6. M.V. and M.C. wrote Section 3. M.C. critically reviewed the manuscript. C.V., M.C. and I.G. took responsibility for the integrity of the work as a whole. All authors approved the final version of the manuscript for publication.

Funding: Z.M.-L. is beneficial of a predoctoral grant from "Plan Propio de Investigación" from the University of Huelva (Spain). Part of the scientific information reviewed in this paper (Section 3) was produced within the MIRACLES project which is supported by the European Commission Seventh Framework Programme under Grant Agreement No. 613588.

Conflicts of Interest: The authors declare no conflict of interest.

References

1. Singh, P.; Kumari, S.; Guldhe, A.; Misra, R.; Ismail, R.; Rawat, I.; Bux, F. Trends and novel strategies for enhancing lipid accumulation and quality in microalgae. *Renew. Sustain. Energy Rev.* **2016**, *55*, 1–16. [CrossRef]

2.   Thomas, N.V.; Kim, S.K. Beneficial effects of marine algal compounds in cosmeceuticals. *Mar. Drugs* **2013**, *11*, 146–164. [CrossRef] [PubMed]

3.   Forján, E.; Navarro, F.; Cuaresma, M.; Vaquero, I.; Ruíz-Domínguez, M.C.; Gojkovic, Ž.; Vázquez, M.; Márquez, M.; Mogedas, B.; Bermejo, E.; et al. Microalgae: Fast-growth sustainable green factories. *Crit. Rev. Environ. Sci. Technol.* **2015**, *45*, 1705–1755. [CrossRef]

4.   Gong, M.; Bassi, A. Carotenoids from microalgae: A review of recent developments. *Biotechnol. Adv.* **2016**, *34*, 1396–1412. [CrossRef] [PubMed]

5.   Khozin-Goldberg, I.; Iskandarov, U.; Cohen, Z. LC-PUFA from photosynthetic microalgae: occurrence, biosynthesis, and prospects in biotechnology. *Appl. Microbiol. Biotechnol.* **2011**, *91*, 905–915. [CrossRef] [PubMed]

6.   Uttaro, A.D. Biosynthesis of polyunsaturated fatty acids in lower eukaryotes. *Life* **2006**, *58*, 563–571. [CrossRef] [PubMed]

7.   Talero, E.; García-Mauriño, S.; Ávila-Román, J.; Rodríguez-Luna, A.; Alcaide, A.; Motilva, V. Bioactive compounds isolated from microalgae in chronic inflammation and cancer. *Mar. Drugs* **2015**, *13*, 6152–6209. [CrossRef] [PubMed]

8.   Yu, X.; Chen, L.; Zhang, W. Chemicals to enhance microalgal growth and accumulation of high-value bioproducts. *Front. Microbiol.* **2015**, *6*, 1–10. [CrossRef] [PubMed]

9.   Zhu, Y.H.; Jiang, J.G.; Chen, Q. Influence of daily collection and culture medium recycling on the growth and β-carotene yield of *Dunaliellasalina*. *J. Agric. Food Chem.* **2008**, *56*, 4027–4031. [CrossRef] [PubMed]

10. Panis, G.; Carreon, J.R. Commercial astaxanthin production derived by green alga *Haematococcuspluvialis*: A microalgae process model and a techno-economic assessment all through production line. *Algal Res.* **2016**, *18*, 175–190. [CrossRef]

11. Pérez, G.; Doldán, S.; Scavone, P.; Borsani, O.; Irisarri, P. Osmotic stress alters UV-based oxidative damage tolerance in a heterocyst forming cyanobacterium. *Plant Physiol. Biochem.* **2016**, *108*, 231–240. [CrossRef] [PubMed]

12. de Farias Silva, C.E.; Sforza, E. Carbohydrate productivity in continuous reactor under nitrogen limitation: Effect of light and residence time on nutrient uptake in *Chlorella vulgaris*. *Process Biochem.* **2016**, *51*, 2112–2118. [CrossRef]

13. Steinrücken, P.; Prestegard, S.K.; de Vree, J.H.; Storesund, J.E.; Pree, B.; Mjøs, S.A.; Erga, S.R. Comparing EPA production and fatty acid profiles of three *Phaeodactylum tricornutum* strains under western Norwegian climate conditions. *Algal Res.* **2018**, *30*, 11–12. [CrossRef] [PubMed]

14. Cesário, M.T.; da Fonseca, M.M.R.; Marques, M.M.; de Almeida, M.C.M.D. Marine algal carbohydrates as carbon sources for the production of biochemicals and biomaterials. *Biotechnol. Adv.* **2018**, *36*, 798–817. [CrossRef] [PubMed]

15. Vílchez, C.; Forján, E.; Cuaresma, M.; Bédmar, F.; Garbayo, I.; Vega, J.M. Marine carotenoids: biological functions and commercial applications. *Mar. Drugs* **2011**, *9*, 319–333. [CrossRef] [PubMed]

16. Enzing, C.; Ploeg, M.; Barbosa, M.; Sijtsma, L. Microalgae-based products for the food and feed sector: an outlook for Europe. In *JRC Scientific and Policy Reports*, 1st ed.; Vigani, M., Parisi, C., Rodriguez-Cerezo, E., Eds.; Publications Office of the European Union: Luxembourg, 2014; pp. 1–82. ISBN 978-92-79-34037-6.

17. Robertson, R.C.; Guihéneuf, F.; Bahar, B.; Schmid, M.; Stengel, D.B.; Fitzgerald, G.F.; Ross, R.P.; Stanton, C. The anti-inflammatory effect of algae-derived lipid extracts on lipopolysaccharide (LPS)-stimulated human THP-1 macrophages. *Mar. Drugs* **2015**, *13*, 5402–5424. [CrossRef] [PubMed]

18. Safafar, H.; van Wagenen, J.; Møller, P.; Jacobsen, C. Carotenoids, phenolic compounds and tocopherols contribute to the antioxidative properties of some microalgae species grown on industrial wastewater. *Mar. Drugs* **2015**, *13*, 7339–7356. [CrossRef] [PubMed]

19. Takaichi, S. Carotenoids in algae: distributions, biosyntheses and functions. *Mar. Drugs* **2011**, *9*, 1101–1118. [CrossRef] [PubMed]

20. Goiris, K.; Muylaert, K.; Fraeye, I.; Foubert, I.; de Brabanter, J.; de Cooman, L. Antioxidant potential of microalgae in relation to their phenolic and carotenoid content. *J. Appl. Phycol.* **2012**, *24*, 1477–1486. [CrossRef]

21. Blagojević, D.; Babić, O.; Rašeta, M.; Šibul, F.; Janjušević, L.; Simeunović, J. Antioxidant activity and phenolic profile in filamentous cyanobacteria: The impact of nitrogen. *J. Appl. Phycol.* **2018**, *30*, 2337. [CrossRef]

22. Norsker, N.; Barbosa, M.J.; Vermuë, M.H.; Wijffels, R.H. Microalgal production—A close look at the economics. *Biotechnol. Adv.* **2011**, *29*, 24–27. [CrossRef] [PubMed]

23. Richmond, A. *Handbook of Microalgae Culture: Biotechnology and Phycology*; Blackwell Science: Cambridge, UK, 2004.

24. Varshney, P.; Mikulic, P.; Vonshak, A.; Beardall, J.; Wangikar, P.P. Extremophilic micro-algae and their potential contribution in biotechnology. *Bioresour. Technol.* **2015**, *184*, 363–372. [CrossRef] [PubMed]

25. Ramos, A.A.; Polle, J.J.; Tran, D.; Cushman, J.C.; Jin, E.; Varela, J.C. The unicellular green alga *Dunaliella salina* Teod. as a model for abiotic stress tolerance: Genetic advances and future perspectives. *Algae* **2011**, *26*, 3–20. [CrossRef]

26. Yuan, J.P.; Peng, J.; Yin, K.; Wang, J.H. Potential health-promoting effects of astaxanthin: A high-value carotenoid mostly from microalgae. *Mol. Nutr. Food Res.* **2011**, *55*, 150–165. [CrossRef] [PubMed]

27. Shi, X.M.; Chen, F. High-yield production of lutein by the green microalga *Chlorella protothecoides* in heterotrophic fed-batch culture. *Biotechnol. Progr.* **2002**, *18*, 723–727. [CrossRef] [PubMed]

28. Lagarde, D.; Beuf, L.; Vermaas, W. Increased production of zeaxanthin and other pigments by application of genetic engineering techniques to *Synechocystis* sp. strain PCC 6803. *Appl. Environ. Microbiol.* **2000**, *66*, 64–72. [CrossRef] [PubMed]

29. Romay, Ch.; González, R.; Ledón, N.; Remirez, D.; Rimbau, V. C-phycocyanin: A biliprotein with antioxidant, anti-inflammatory and neuroprotective effects. *Curr. Protein Pept. Sci.* **2003**, *4*, 207–216. [CrossRef] [PubMed]

30. Fiedor, J.; Burda, K. Potential role of carotenoids as antioxidants in human health and disease. *Nutrients* **2014**, *6*, 466–488. [CrossRef] [PubMed]

31. Richard, D.; Kefi, K.; Barbe, U.; Bausero, P.; Visioli, F. Polyunsaturated fatty acids as antioxidants. *Pharmacol. Res.* **2008**, *57*, 451–455. [CrossRef] [PubMed]

32. De Jesus Raposo, M.F.; de Morais, R.M.S.C.; de Morais, A.M.M.B. Bioactivity and applications of sulphated polysaccharides from marine microalgae. *Mar. Drugs* **2015**, *11*, 233–252. [CrossRef] [PubMed]

33. Sun, L.; Wang, C.; Shi, Q.; Ma, C. Preparation of different molecular weight polysaccharides from *Porphyridium cruentum* and their antioxidant activities. *Int. J. Biol. Macromol.* **2009**, *45*, 42–47. [CrossRef] [PubMed]

34. Chen, B.; You, B.; Huang, J.; Yu, Y.; Chen, W. Isolation and antioxidant property of the extracellular polysaccharide from *Rhodella reticulata*. *World J. Microbiol. Biotechnol.* **2010**, *26*, 833–840. [CrossRef]

35. Wang, X.; Zhang, X. Separation, antitumor activities, and encapsulation of polypeptide from *Chlorella pyrenoidosa*. *Biotechnol. Progr.* **2013**, *29*, 681–687. [CrossRef] [PubMed]

36. Asada, K. Production and scavenging of reactive oxygen species in chloroplasts and their functions. *Plant Physiol.* **2006**, *141*, 391–396. [CrossRef] [PubMed]

37. Janoska, A.; Vázquez, M.; Janssen, M.; Wijffels, R.H.; Cuaresma, M.; Vílchez, C. Surfactant selection for a liquid foam-bed photobioreactor. *Biotechnol. Progr.* **2018**. [CrossRef] [PubMed]

38. Franz, A.; Danielewicz, M.; Wong, D.; Anderson, L.; Boothe, J. Phenotypic screening with oleaginous microalgae reveals modulators of lipid productivity. *ACS Chem. Biol.* **2013**, *8*, 1053–1062. [CrossRef] [PubMed]

39. Kobayashi, M.; Kakizono, T.; Nagai, S. Enhanced carotenoid biosynthesis by oxidative stress in acetate-induced cyst cells of a green unicellular alga, *Haematococcus pluvialis*. *Appl. Environ. Microbiol.* **1993**, *59*, 867–873. [PubMed]

40. Zheng, Y.; Li, Z.; Tao, M.; Li, J.; Hu, Z. Effects of selenite on green microalga *Haematococcus pluvialis*: Bioaccumulation of selenium and enhancement of astaxanthin production. *Aquat. Toxicol.* **2017**, *183*, 21–27. [CrossRef] [PubMed]

41. Ma, R.; Chen, F. Induction of astaxanthin formation by reactive oxygen species in mixotrophic culture of *Chlorococcum* sp. *Biotechnol. Lett.* **2001**, *23*, 519–523. [CrossRef]

42. Wang, Y.; Liu, Z.; Qin, S. Effects of iron on fatty acid and astaxanthin accumulation in mixotrophic *Chromochloris zofingiensis*. *Biotechnol. Lett.* **2013**, *35*, 351–357. [CrossRef] [PubMed]

43. Raman, V.; Ravi, S. Effect of salicylic acid and methyl jasmonate on antioxidant systems of *Haematococcus pluvialis*. *Acta Physiol. Plant* **2010**, *33*, 1043–1049. [CrossRef]

44. Kobayashi, M. In vivo antioxidant role of astaxanthin under oxidative stress in the green alga *Haematococcus pluvialis*. *Appl. Microbiol. Biotechnol.* **2000**, *54*, 550–555. [CrossRef] [PubMed]

45. Pirastru, L.; Darwish, M.; Chu, F.L.; Perreault, F.; Sirois, L.; Sleno, L.; Popovic, R. Carotenoid production and change of photosynthetic functions in *Scenedesmus* sp. exposed to nitrogen limitation and acetate treatment. *J. Appl. Phycol.* **2012**, *24*, 117–124. [CrossRef]

46. Boussiba, S.; Fan, L.; Vonshak, A. Enhancement and determination of astaxanthin accumulation in green alga *Haematococcus pluvialis*. *Methods Enzymol.* **1992**, *213*, 386–391. [CrossRef]

47. Ip, P.F.; Chen, F. Employment of reactive oxygen species to enhance astaxanthin formation in *Chlorella zofingiensis* in heterotrophic culture. *Process Biochem.* **2005**, *40*, 3491–3496. [CrossRef]

48. Wei, D.; Chen, F.; Chen, G.; Zhang, X.; Liu, L.; Zhang, H. Enhanced production of lutein in heterotrophic *Chlorella protothecoides* by oxidative stress. *Sci. China C Life Sci.* **2008**, *51*, 1088–1093. [CrossRef] [PubMed]

49. Vaquero, I.; Ruiz-Domínguez, M.C.; Márquez, M.; Vílchez, C. Cu-mediated biomass productivity enhancement and lutein enrichment of the novel microalga *Coccomyxa onubensis*. *Process Biochem.* **2012**, *47*, 694–700. [CrossRef]

50. Ruiz-Domínguez, M.C.; Vaquero, I.; Obregón, V.; de la Morena, B.; Vílchez, C.; Vega, J.M. Lipid accumulation and antioxidant activity in the eukaryotic acidophilic microalga *Coccomyxa* sp. (strain *onubensis*) under nutrient starvation. *J. Appl. Phycol.* **2015**, *27*, 1099–1108. [CrossRef]

51. Ambati, R.R.; Ravi, S.; Aswathanarayana, R.G. Enhancement of carotenoids in green alga *Botryococcus braunii* in various autotrophic media under stress conditions. *Int. J. Biomed. Pharm. Sci.* **2010**, *4*, 87–92.

52. Carvalho, A.P.; Malcata, F.X. Effect of culture media on production of polyunsaturated fatty acids by *Pavlova lutheri*. *Cryptogam. Algol.* **2000**, *21*, 59–71. [CrossRef]

53. Meng, Y.; Jiang, J.; Wang, H.; Cao, X.; Xue, S.; Yang, Q.; Wang, W. The characteristics of TAG and EPA accumulation in *Nannochloropsis oceanica* IMET1 under different nitrogen supply regimes. *Bioresour. Technol.* **2015**, *179*, 483–489. [CrossRef] [PubMed]

54. Qu, L.; Ji, X.J.; Ren, L.J.; Nie, Z.K.; Feng, Y.; Wu, W.J.; Ouyang, P.K.; Huang, H. Enhancement of docosahexaenoic acid production by *Schizochytrium* sp. using a two stage oxygen supply control strategy based on oxygen transfer coefficient. *Lett. Appl. Microbiol.* **2011**, *52*, 22–27. [CrossRef] [PubMed]

55. Tonon, T.; Harvey, D.; Larson, T.R.; Graham, I.A. Long chain polyunsaturated fatty acid production and partitioning to triacylglycerols in four microalgae. *Phytochemistry* **2002**, *61*, 15–24. [CrossRef]

56. Villay, A.; Laroche, C.; Roriz, D.; El Alaoui, H.; Delbac, F.; Michaud, P. Optimisation of culture parameters for exopolysaccharides production by the microalga *Rhodella violacea*. *Bioresour. Technol.* **2013**, *146*, 732–735. [CrossRef] [PubMed]

57. Abdullahi, A.S.; Underwood, G.J.C.; Gretz, M.R. Extracellular matrix assembly in diatoms (bacillariophyceae). V. Environmental effects on polysaccharide synthesis in the model diatom, *Phaeodactylum tricornutum*. *J. Phycol.* **2006**, *42*, 363–378. [CrossRef]

58. Mishra, A.; Jha, B. Isolation and characterization of extracellular polymeric substances from micro-algae *Dunaliella salina* under salt stress. *Bioresour. Technol.* **2009**, *100*, 3382–3386. [CrossRef] [PubMed]

59. López, A.; Rico, M.; Santana-Casiano, J.M.; González, A.G.; González-Dávila, M. Phenolic profile of *Dunaliella tertiolecta* growing under high levels of copper and iron. *Environ. Sci. Pollut. Res.* **2015**, *22*, 14820. [CrossRef] [PubMed]

60. El-Baky, H.H.A.; El Baz, F.K.; El-Baroty, G.S. Phenolics from *Spirulina maxima*: Over-production and in vitro protective effect of its phenolics on CCl₄ induced hepatotoxicity. *J. Med. Plants Res.* **2009**, *3*, 24–30. [CrossRef]

61. Cirulis, J.T.; Scott, J.A.; Ross, G.M. Management of oxidative stress by microalgae. *Can. J. Physiol. Pharmacol.* **2013**, *91*, 15–21. [CrossRef] [PubMed]

62. Tripathy, B.C.; Oelmüller, R. Reactive oxygen species generation and signaling in plants. *Plant Signal Behav.* **2012**, *7*, 1621–1633. [CrossRef] [PubMed]

63. Mehler, A.H. Studies on reactivities of illuminated chloroplasts. I. Mechanism of the reduction of oxygen and other Hill reagents. *Arch. Biochem. Biophys.* **1951**, *33*, 65–77. [CrossRef]

64. Asada, K.; Kiso, K.; Yoshikawa, K. Univalent reduction of molecular oxygen by spinach chloroplasts on illumination. *J. Biol. Chem.* **1974**, *249*, 2175–2181. [PubMed]

65. Arulselvan, P.; Fard, M.T.; Tan, W.S.; Gothai, S.; Fakurazi, S.; Norhaizan, M.E.; Kumar, S.S. Role of antioxidants and natural products in inflammation. *Oxid. Med. Cell Longev.* **2016**, *5276130*. [CrossRef] [PubMed]

66. Gao, Z.; Meng, C.; Zhang, X.; Xu, D.; Miao, X.; Wang, Y.; Yang, L.; Lv, H.; Chen, L.; Ye, N. Induction of salicylic acid (SA) on transcriptional expression of eight carotenoid genes and astaxanthin accumulation in *Haematococcus pluvialis*. *Enzyme Microb. Technol.* **2012**, *51*, 225–230. [CrossRef] [PubMed]

67. Lamers, P.P.; Janssen, M.; De Vos, R.C.H.; Bino, R.J.; Wijffels, R.H. Carotenoid and fatty acid metabolism in nitrogen-starved *Dunaliella salina*, a unicellular green microalga. *J. Biotechnol.* **2012**, *162*, 21–27. [CrossRef] [PubMed]
68. Le Marchand, L.; Hankin, J.H.; Kolonel, L.N.; Beecher, G.R.; Wilkens, L.R.; Zhao, L.P. Intake of specific carotenoids and lung cancer risk. *Cancer Epidemiol. Biomarkers Prev.* **1993**, *2*, 183–187. [PubMed]
69. Biesalski, H. Evidence from Intervention Studies. In *Functions of Vitamins beyond Recommended Dietary Allowances*; Walter, P., Hornig, D., Moser, U., Eds.; Woodhead Publishing Limited: Cambridge, UK, 2001; pp. 92–134.
70. Guerin, M.; Huntley, M.E.; Olaizola, M. *Haematococcus* astaxanthin: Applications for human health and nutrition. *Trends Biotechnol.* **2003**, *21*, 210–216. [CrossRef]
71. Landrum, J.T.; Bohne, R. Luteín, zeaxanthin and the macular pigment. *Arch. Biochem. Biophys.* **2001**, *385*, 28–40. [CrossRef] [PubMed]
72. Friedman, D.S.; O'Colmain, B.J.; Muñoz, B.; Tomany, S.C.; McCarty, C.; De Jong, P.T.; Nemesure, B.; Mitchell, P.; Kempen, J.; Congdon, N. Prevalence of age-related macular degeneration in the United States. *Arch. Ophthalmol.* **2004**, *122*, 564–572. [CrossRef] [PubMed]
73. Hammond, B.R.; Wooten, B.; Snodderly, D.M. Preservation of visual sensitivity of older individuals: Association with macular pigment density. *Invest. Ophthalmol. Vis. Sci.* **1998**, *39*, 397–406. [PubMed]
74. Lee, S.J.; Bai, S.K.; Lee, K.S.; Namkoong, S.; Na, H.J.; Ha, K.S.; Han, J.A.; Yim, S.V.; Chang, K.; Kwon, Y.G.; et al. Astaxanthin inhibits nitric oxide production and inflammatory gene expression by suppressing IκB kinase-dependent NF-κB activation. *Mol. Cells* **2003**, *16*, 97–105. [PubMed]
75. Akyön, Y. Effect of antioxidants on the immune response of *Helicobacter pylori*. *Clin. Microbiol. Infect.* **2002**, *8*, 438–441. [CrossRef] [PubMed]
76. Kim, S.H.; Jean, D.; Lim, Y.P.; Lim, C.; An, G. Weight gain limitation and liver protection by long-term feeding of astaxanthin in murines. *J. K. Soc. Appl. Biol. Chem.* **2009**, *52*, 180–185. [CrossRef]
77. Bolin, A.P.; Macedo, R.C.; Marin, D.P.; Barros, M.P.; Otton, R. Astaxanthin prevents in vitro auto-oxidative injury in human lymphocytes. *Cell Biol. Toxicol.* **2010**, *26*, 457–467. [CrossRef] [PubMed]
78. Anderson, M. Method of Inhibiting 5α-Reductase with Astaxanthin to Prevent and Treat Benign Prostate Hyperplasia (BPH) and Prostate Cancer in Human Males. U.S. Patent No. 6277417, 21 August 2001.
79. Zuluaga, M.; Gueguen, V.; Pavon-Djavid, G.; Letourneur, D. Carotenoids from microalgae to block oxidative stress. *BioImpacts* **2017**, *7*, 1–3. [CrossRef] [PubMed]
80. Olofsson, P.; Hultqvist, M.; Hellgren, L.I.; Holmdahl, R. Phytol: A chlorophyll component with anti-inflammatory and metabolic properties. In *Recent Advances in Redox Active Plant and Microbial Products*; Jacob, C., Kirsch, G., Slusarenko, A., Winyard, P., Burkholz, T., Eds.; Springer: Dordrecht, The Netherlands, 2014.
81. Cuaresma, M.; Janssen, M.; Vílchez, C.; Wijffels, R.H. Productivity of *Chlorella sorokiniana* in a short light-path (SLP) panel photobioreactor under high irradiance. *Biotechnol. Bioeng.* **2009**, *104*, 352–359. [CrossRef] [PubMed]
82. Beyer, P.; Kleinig, H. On the desaturation and cyclization reactions of carotenes. In *Chromoplast Membranes, Carotenoids*; Krinsky, N., Mathews-Roth, M., Taylor, R., Eds.; Springer: New York, NY, USA, 1989; pp. 195–206.
83. Harker, M.; Tsavalos, A.J.; Young, A.J. Factors responsible for astaxanthin formation in the chlorophyte *Haematococcus pluvialis*. *Bioresour. Technol.* **1996**, *55*, 207–214. [CrossRef]
84. Nahidian, B.; Ghanati, F.; Shahbazi, M.; Soltani, N. Effect of nutrients on the growth and physiological features of newly isolated *Haematococcus pluvialis* TMU. *Bioresour. Technol.* **2018**, *255*, 229–237. [CrossRef] [PubMed]
85. Minhas, A.K.; Hodgson, P.; Barrow, C.J.; Adholeya, A. A review on the assessment of stress conditions for simultaneous production of microalgal lipids and carotenoids. *Front. Microbiol.* **2016**, *7*, 1–19. [CrossRef] [PubMed]
86. Serini, S.; Bizzarro, A.; Piccioni, E.; Fasano, E.; Rossi, C.; Lauria, A.; Cittadini, A.; Masullo, C.; Calviello, G. EPA and DHA differentially affect in vitro inflammatory cytokine release by peripheral blood mononuclear cells from Alzheimer's patients. *Curr. Alzheimer Res.* **2012**, *9*, 913–923. [CrossRef] [PubMed]
87. Das, U.N. Can vagus nerve stimulation halt or ameliorate rheumatoid arthritis and lupus? *Lipids Health Dis.* **2011**, 10–19. [CrossRef] [PubMed]

88. Van Beelen, V.A.; Spenkelink, B.; Mooibroek, H.; Sijtsma, L.; Bosch, D.; Rietjens, I.M.C.M.; Alink, G.M. An n-3 PUFA-rich microalgal oil diet protects to a similar extent as a fish oil-rich diet against AOM-induced colonic aberrant crypt foci in F344 rats. *Food Chem. Toxicol.* **2009**, *47*, 316–320. [CrossRef] [PubMed]

89. Halliwell, B. Cellular stress and protection mechanisms. *Biochem. Soc. Trans.* **1996**, *24*, 1023–1027. [CrossRef] [PubMed]

90. Kiritsakis, A.K.; Dugan, L.R. Studies in photooxidation of olive oil. *J. Am. Oil Chem. Soc.* **1985**, *62*, 892–896. [CrossRef]

91. Li, M.; Hu, C.; Zhu, Q.; Chen, L.; Kong, Z.; Liu, Z. Copper and zinc induction of lipid peroxidation and effects on antioxidant enzyme activities in the microalga *Pavlova viridis* (Prymnesiophyceae). *Chemosphere* **2006**, *62*, 565–572. [CrossRef] [PubMed]

92. Li, H.B.; Cheng, K.W.; Wong, C.C.; Fan, K.W.; Chen, F.; Jiang, Y. Evaluation of antioxidant capacity and total phenolic content of different fractions of selected microalgae. *Food Chem.* **2007**, *102*, 771–776. [CrossRef]

93. Yilancioglu, K.; Cokol, M.; Pastirmaci, I.; Erman, B.; Cetiner, S. Oxidative stress is a mediator for increased lipid accumulation in a newly isolated *Dunaliella salina* strain. *PLoS ONE* **2014**. [CrossRef] [PubMed]

94. Yu, Y.; Li, T.; Wu, N.; Ren, L.; Jiang, L.; Ji, X.; Huang, H. Mechanism of arachidonic acid accumulation during aging in *Mortierella alpina*: A large-scale label-free comparative proteomics study. *J. Agric. Food Chem.* **2016**, *64*, 9124–9134. [CrossRef] [PubMed]

95. Huang, T.Y.; Lu, W.C.; Chu, I.M. A fermentation strategy for producing docosahexaenoic acid in *Aurantiochytrium limacinum* SR21 and increasing C22:6 proportions in total fatty acid. *Bioresour. Technol.* **2012**, *123*, 8–14. [CrossRef] [PubMed]

96. Ruenwai, R.; Neiss, A.; Laoteng, K.; Vongsangnak, W.; Dalfard, A.B.; Cheevadhanarak, S.; Petranovic, D.; Nielsen, J. Heterologous production of polyunsaturated fatty acids in *Saccharomyces cerevisiae* causes a global transcriptional response resulting in reduced proteasomal activity and increased oxidative stress. *Biotechnol. J.* **2011**, *6*, 343–356. [CrossRef] [PubMed]

97. Chokshi, K.; Pancha, I.; Ghosh, A.; Mishra, S. Salinity induced oxidative stress alters the physiological responses and improves the biofuel potential of green microalgae *Acutodesmus dimorphus*. *Bioresour. Technol.* **2017**, *244*, 1376–1383. [CrossRef] [PubMed]

98. Qiao, H.; Cong, C.; Sun, C.; Li, B.; Wang, J.; Zhang, L. Effect of culture conditions on growth, fatty acid composition and DHA/EPA ratio of *Phaeodactylum tricornutum*. *Aquaculture* **2016**, *452*, 311–317. [CrossRef]

99. Dahmen-Ben Moussa, I.; Chtourou, H.; Karray, F.; Sayadi, S.; Dhouib, A. Nitrogen or phosphorus repletion strategies for enhancing lipid or carotenoid production from *Tetraselmis marina*. *Bioresour. Technol.* **2017**, *238*, 325–332. [CrossRef] [PubMed]

100. Tsai, H.P.; Chuang, L.T.; Chen, C.N.N. Production of long chain omega-3 fatty acids and carotenoids in tropical areas by a new heat-tolerant microalga *Tetraselmis* sp. DS3. *Food Chem.* **2016**, *192*, 682–690. [CrossRef] [PubMed]

101. Burg, A.; Oshrat, L.O. Salt effect on the antioxidant activity of red microalgal sulfated polysaccharides in soy-bean formula. *Mar. Drugs* **2015**, *13*, 6425–6439. [CrossRef] [PubMed]

102. Fisher, T.; Berner, T.; Iluz, D.; Dubinsky, Z. The kinetics of the photoacclimation response of *Nannochloropsis* sp. (Eustigmatophyceae): A study of changes in ultrastructure and PSU density. *J. Phycol.* **1998**, *34*, 818–824. [CrossRef]

103. Guzmán, S.; Gato, A.; Lamela, M.; Freire-Garabal, M.; Calleja, J.M. Anti-inflammatory and immunomodulatory activities of polysaccharide from *Chlorella stigmatophora* and *Phaeodactylum tricornutum*. *Phytother. Res.* **2003**, *17*, 665–670. [CrossRef] [PubMed]

104. Matsui, M.S.; Muizzuddin, N.; Arad, S.; Marenus, K. Sulfated polysaccharides from red microalgae have antiinflammatory properties in vitro and in vivo. *Appl. Biochem. Biotechnol.* **2003**, *104*, 13–22. [CrossRef]

105. Delattre, C.; Pierre, G.; Laroche, C.; Michaud, P. Production, extraction and characterization of microalgal and cyanobacterial exopolysaccharides. *Biotechnol. Adv.* **2016**, *34*, 1159–1179. [CrossRef] [PubMed]

106. Passow, U. Transparent exopolymer particles (TEP) in aquatic environments. *Prog. Oceanogr.* **2002**, *55*, 287–333. [CrossRef]

107. Tannin-Spitz, T.; Bergman, M.; Van-Moppes, D.; Grossman, S.; Arad, S. Antioxidant activity of the polysaccharide of the red microalga *Porphyridium* sp. *J. Appl. Phycol.* **2005**, *17*, 215–222. [CrossRef]

108. Markou, G.; Nerantzis, E. Microalgae for high-value compounds and biofuels production: A new focus on cultivation under stress conditions. *Biotechnol. Adv.* **2013**, *31*, 1532–1542. [CrossRef] [PubMed]

109. Chi, Z.; Su, C.D.; Lu, W.D. A new exopolysaccharide produced by marine *Cyanothece* sp. 113. *Bioresour. Technol.* **2007**, *98*, 1329–1332. [CrossRef] [PubMed]

110. Underwood, G.J.C.; Boulcot, M.; Raines, C.A.; Waldron, K. Environmental effects on exopolymer production by marine benthic diatoms–dynamics, changes in composition and pathways of production. *J. Phycol.* **2004**, *40*, 293–304. [CrossRef]

111. Guerrini, F.; Cangini, M.; Boni, L.; Trost, P.; Pistocchi, R. Metabolic responses of the diatom *Achnanthes brevipes* (Bacillariophyceae) to nutrient limitation. *J. Phycol.* **2000**, *36*, 882–890. [CrossRef]

112. Alcoverro, T.; Conte, E.; Mazzella, L. The production of mucilage by the epipelic diatom *Cylindrotheca closterium* from the Adriatic Sea under nutrient limitation. *J. Phycol.* **2000**, *36*, 1087–1095. [CrossRef]

113. Kumar, A.S.; Mody, K.; Jha, B. Bacterial exopolysaccharides–a perception. *J. Basic Microbiol.* **2007**, *47*, 103–117. [CrossRef] [PubMed]

114. Su, C.; Zhenming, C.; Weidong, L. Optimization of medium and cultivation conditions for enhanced exopolysaccharide yield by marine *Cyanothece* sp. 113. *Chin. J. Oceanol. Limnol.* **2007**, *25*, 411–417. [CrossRef]

115. Ozturk, S.; Aslim, B. Modification of exopolysaccharide composition and production by three cyanobacterial isolates under salt stress. *Environ. Sci. Pollut. Res.* **2010**, *17*, 595–602. [CrossRef] [PubMed]

116. Sanjeewa, K.K.A.; Fernando, I.P.S.; Samarakoon, K.W.; Lakmal, H.H.C.; Kim, E.A.; Kwon, O.N.; Dilshara, M.G.; Lee, J.B.; Jeon, Y.J. Anti-inflammatory and anti-cancer activities of sterol rich fraction of cultured marine microalga *Nannochloropsis oculata*. *Algae* **2016**, *31*, 277–287. [CrossRef]

117. Hämäläinen, M.; Nieminen, R.; Vuorela, P.; Heinonen, M.; Moilanen, E. Anti-inflammatory effects of flavonoids: genistein, kaempferol, quercetin, and daidzein inhibit STAT-1 and NF-κB activations, whereas flavone, isorhamnetin, naringenin, and pelargonidin inhibit only NF-κB activation along with their inhibitory effect on iNOS expression and NO production in activated macrophages. *Mediat. Inflamm.* **2007**. [CrossRef]

118. Janoska, A.; Lamers, P.P.; Hamhuis, A.; van Eimeren, Y.; Wijffels, R.H.; Janssen, M. A liquid foam-bed photobioreactor for microalgae production. *Chem. Eng. J.* **2017**, *313*, 1206–1214. [CrossRef]

119. Janssen, M.; Lamers, P.P.; de Haan, M.; Wijffels, R.H. Growing Microalgae or Cyanobacteria in Liquid-Based Foam. International Patent WO 2014072294 A1, 15 May 2014.

120. Vázquez, M.; Fuentes, J.L.; Hincapié, A.; Garbayo, I.; Vílchez, C.; Cuaresma, M. Selection of microalgae with potential for cultivation in surfactant-stabilized foam. *Algal Res.* **2018**, *31*, 216–224. [CrossRef]

121. Taoka, Y.; Nagano, N.; Okita, Y.; Izumida, H.; Sugimoto, S.; Hayashi, M. Effect of Tween 80 on the growth, lipid accumulation and fatty acid composition of *Thraustochytrium aureum* ATCC 34304. *J. Biosci. Bioeng.* **2011**, *111*, 420–424. [CrossRef] [PubMed]

122. Sun, X.M.; Geng, L.J.; Ren, L.J.; Ji, X.J.; Hao, N.; Chen, K.Q.; Huang, H. Influence of oxygen on the biosynthesis of polyunsaturated fatty acids in microalgae. *Bioresour. Technol.* **2018**, *250*, 868–876. [CrossRef] [PubMed]

123. Bailey, R.B.; Dimasi, D.; Hansen, J.M.; Mirrasoul, P.J.; Ruecker, C.M.; Iii, G.T.; Kaneko, T.; Barclay, W.R. Enhanced Production of Lipids Containing Polyenoic Fatty Acid by Very High Density Cultures of Eukaryotic Microbes in Fermentors. US Patent 8206956, 29 May 2012.

124. Ren, L.J.; Ji, X.J.; Huang, H.; Qu, L.; Feng, Y.; Tong, Q.Q.; Ouyang, P.K. Development of a stepwise aeration control strategy for efficient docosahexaenoic acid production by *Schizochytrium* sp. *Appl. Microbiol. Biotechnol.* **2010**, *87*, 1649–1656. [CrossRef] [PubMed]

125. Shelest, E.; Heimerl, N.; Fichtner, M.; Sasso, S. Multimodular type I polyketide synthases in algae evolve by module duplications and displacement of AT domains *in trans*. *BMC Genomics* **2015**, *16*, 1015. [CrossRef] [PubMed]

126. Shen, Z.; Li, Y.; Wen, H.; Ren, X.; Liu, J.; Yang, L. Investigation on the role of surfactants in bubble-algae interaction in flotation harvesting of *Chlorella vulgaris*. *Sci. Rep.* **2018**, *8*, 3303. [CrossRef] [PubMed]

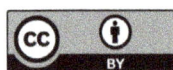

MDPI

St. Alban-Anlage 66

4052 Basel

Switzerland

Tel. +41 61 683 77 34

Fax +41 61 302 89 18

www.mdpi.com

Marine Drugs Editorial Office

E-mail: marinedrugs@mdpi.com

www.mdpi.com/journal/marinedrugs